THROMBOLYTIC AND ANTITHROMBOTIC THERAPY FOR STROKE

THROMBOLYTIC AND ANTITHROMBOTIC THERAPY FOR STROKE

Editors

Julien Bogousslavsky MD

Professor and Chairman
University Department of Neurology
Chief of Neurology Services
Centre Hospitalier Universitaire Vaudois
Lausanne
Switzerland

and

Werner Hacke MD PhD FAHA FESC

Professor and Head
Department of Neurology
University of Heidelberg
Heidelberg
Germany

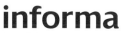

informa
healthcare

© 2006 Informa UK Ltd

First published in the United Kingdom in 2006
by Informa UK Ltd
4 Park Square, Milton Park,
Abingdon, Oxon OX14 4RN

Tel: +44 (0)20 7017 6000
Fax: +44 (0)20 7017 6699
Email: info.medicine@tandf.co.uk
Website: www.tandf.co.uk/medicine

Although every effort has been made to ensure that all owners of copyright material have been acknowledged in this publication, we would be glad to acknowledge in subsequent reprints or editions any omissions brought to our attention.

Although every effort has been made to ensure that drug doses and other information are presented accurately in this publication, the ultimate responsibility rests with the prescribing physician. Neither the publishers nor the authors can be held responsible for errors or for any consequences arising from the use of information contained herein. For detailed prescribing information or instructions on the use of any product or procedure discussed herein, please consult the prescribing information or instructional material issued by the manufacturer.

A CIP record for this book is available from the British Library.

Library of Congress Cataloging-in-Publication Data

Data available on application

ISBN10 1 84184 203 6
ISBN13 978 1 84184 203 5

Distributed in North and South America by

Taylor & Francis
6000 Broken Sound Parkway, NW, (Suite 300)
Boca Raton, FL 33487, USA

Within Continental USA
Tel: 1(800) 272 7737; Fax: 1(800) 374 3401
Outside Continental USA
Tel: (561) 994 0555; Fax: (561) 361 6018
Email: orders@crcpress.com

Distributed in the rest of the world by
Thomson Publishing Services
Cheriton House
North Way
Andover, Hampshire SP10 5BE, UK
Tel: +44 (0)1264 332424
Email: tps.tandfsalesorder@thomson.com

Composition by C&M Digitals (P) Ltd., Chennai, India
Printed and bound in Spain by Grafos SA

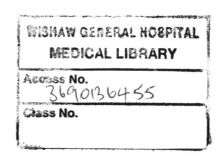

Contents

Contributors

Heinrich J Audebert, MD
Department of Neurology
Munich–Harlaching Hospital
Munich
Germany

Jürg-Hans Beer
Chefartz Innere Medicine
Kantonsspital Baden
Baden
Switzerland

Eivind Berge MD PhD
Department of Internal Medicine
Ullevaal University Hospital
Oslo
Norway

Julien Bogousslavsky MD
Professor and Chairman
University Department of Neurology
Chief of Neurology Service
Centre Hospitalier Universitaire Vaudois
Lausanne
Switzerland

Patrícia Canhão MD
Department of Neurosciences and
    Mental Health
Hospital de Santa Maria
University of Lisbon
Lisbon
Portugal

Louis R Caplan MD
Department of Neurology
Beth Israel Hospital
Boston, MA
USA

Ángel Chamorro MD
Stroke Unit Neurology Service
Hospital Clinic Universitari
Barcelona
Spain

Désiré Collen MD PhD
Center for Molecular and Vascular Biology
KU Leuven
Leuven
Belgium

Laszlo Csiba MD PhD
Department of Neurology
University of Debrecen
Debrecen
Hungary

Antoni Dávalos MD
Section of Neurology
Hospital Doctor Josep Trueta
Girona
Spain

Stephen M Davis MD FRACP
Professor and Director of Neurology
Royal Melbourne Hospital and
University of Melbourne
Melbourne
Australia

Geoffrey Donnan MD FRACP
National Stroke Research Institute
Department of Neurology
University of Melbourne
Austin
and
Repatriation Medical Centre
Heidelberg
Victoria
Australia

José M Ferro MD PhD
Department of Neurosciences and Mental Health
Hospital de Santa Maria
University of Lisbon
Lisbon
Portugal

Jochen B Fiebach MD
Department of Neuroradiology
University of Heidelberg
Heidelberg
Germany

Marc Fisher MD
Department of Neurology
Memorial Hospital
Worcester, MA
USA

Anthony J Furlan MD
Section Head, Stroke and Neurologic Intensive Care
The Cleveland Clinic Foundation
Cleveland, OH
USA

Werner Hacke MD
Professor and Head
Department of Neurology
University of Heidelberg
Heidelberg
Germany

Peter J Hand MD FRACP
Deputy Director of Neurology and
Co-Head, Stroke Care Unit
Royal Melbourne Hospital and
University of Melbourne
Melbourne
Australia

Gerhard F Hamann MD
Professor and Head
Department of Neurology
Dr Horst Schmidt Kliniken GmbH
Wiesbaden
Germany

Graeme J Hankey MD FRACP
Clinical Professor
School of Medicine and Pharmacology
Royal Perth Hospital
Perth
Western Australia

Michael Hennerici MD
Department of Neurology
University of Heidelberg
Mannheim
Germany

Guntram W Ickenstein, MD
Department of Neurology
University of Regensburg
Regensburg
Germany

Daniel Jenni MD
Department of Medicine
Kantonsspital Baden
Baden
Switzerland

Vincent Larrue MD
Department of Neurology
University of Toulouse
Toulouse
France

Jacques R Leclerc
Lilly Research Laboratories
Lilly Corporate Center
Indianapolis, IN
USA

Kennedy R Lees MD
Professor of Cerebrovascular Medicine/Honorary
Consultant Physician and
Clinical (Research) Director
Acute Stroke Unit
Western Infirmary
Glasgow
UK

Roger Lijnen PhD
Center for Molecular and Vascular Biology
KU Leuven
Leuven
Belgium

Svetlana Lorenzano MD
Stroke Unit
Department of Neurological Sciences
University 'La Sapienza'
Rome
Italy

Romesh Markus PhD FRACP
National Stroke Research Institute
Department of Neurology
University of Melbourne
Austin
and
Repatriation Medical Centre
Heidelberg
Victoria
Australia

Patrik Michel MD
Director, Acute Stroke Unit
Lausanne University Hospital
Lausanne
Switzerland

Nobuo Nagai
Center for Molecular and Vascular Biology
KU Leuven
Leuven
Belgium

György Németh MD PhD
Division of Medical Science
Gedeon Richter Limited
Budapest

Peter A Ringleb MD
Department of Neurology
University of Heidelberg
Heidelberg
Germany

Peter Sandercock DM FRCPE FMedSci
Professor of Medical Neurology
Clinical Neurosciences
Western General Hospital
Edinburgh
UK

Peter D Schellinger MD PhD
Associate Professor of Neurology
Department of Neurology
University of Heidelberg
Heidelberg
Germany

Magdy Selim MD PhD
Assistant Professor of Neurology
Department of Neurology –
    Stroke Division
Beth Israel Deaconess Medical Center
Boston, MA
USA

Danilo Toni MD PhD
Stroke Unit
Department of Neurological Sciences
University 'La Sapienza'
Rome
Italy

Simone Wagner MD
Department of Neurology
University of Heidelberg
Heidelberg
Germany

Nils Gunnar Wahlgren MD PhD
Professor of Neurology
Karolinska University Hospital
Stockholm
Sweden

Max Wintermark MD
Assistant Professor of Radiology
Department of Radiology,
    Neuroradiology Section
University of California, San Francisco
San Francisco, CA
USA

Herman Zeumer MD
Department of Neuroradiology
University Hospital Eppendorf
Hamburg
Germany

Preface

Stroke is one area of medicine that has greatly evolved over the last few years – this is particularly true for its treatment and prevention. Only 20 years ago acute stroke remained an untreated condition in most instances. It has now become one of the most critical emergency conditions for which sophisticated, new paradigms have been developed. Acute stroke units and teams can now provide the framework to which most modern management and treatment programs can be applied; this has led to a dramatic decrease in mortality, and delayed sequelae and disability. Thrombolytic and antithrombotic treatments constitute the mainstay of the pharmacological approach to acute ischemic stroke therapy and enable the modification of the course and fate of a large number of stroke victims when they have been referred to hospital in due time. Several antithrombotic agents also have a major place in the stroke prevention strategies, both in the acute and more chronic phases.

Despite these advances, no other book has focused on thrombolytic and antithrombotic therapy for stroke, which is the reason we have launched this monograph. We would like to thank our outstanding and expert colleagues from around the world for their invaluable help. We hope that this book will provide useful support for all individuals involved in stroke management and therapy.

Julien Bogousslavsky
Werner Hacke

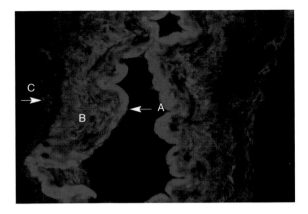

Figure 4.1
Immunofluorescence image of a cerebral artery from the rat stained with collagen type IV and detected by TRITC fluorescence. A, intima; B, media; C, adventitia. Magnification 50x.

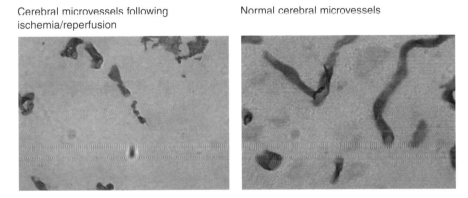

Figure 4.3
Loss in microvascular basal lamina staining following cerebral ischemia/reperfusion: basal ganglia of the rat, anti-collagen IV immunohistochemistry.[60] Magnification 400x.

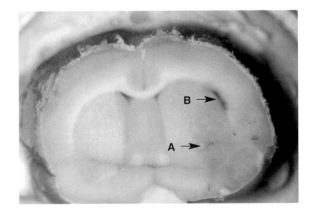

Figure 4.4
Coronal section of an ischemic rat brain: A, petechial bleeding in the infarcted basal ganglia; B, bleeding in the left ventricle.

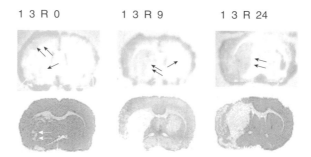

Figure 4.7
Brain section with an overlay containing plasminogen. The plasminogen activators from the underlying brain generate plasmin. Plasmin digests casein in the overlay, and clear lysis zones become visible at the sites of plasminogen activator activity. There is a steady increase in plasminogen activator activity over prolonged periods of ischemia/reperfusion.

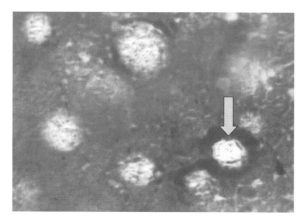

Figure 4.8
High magnification (400x) of a gelatin overlay on brain tissue with an acute infarct. Holes (see arrow) are produced from gelatinolytic activity from the underlying brain.[72]

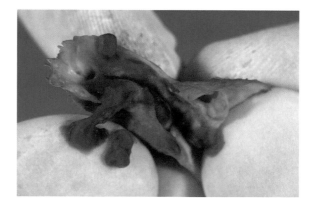

Figure 5.2
Endarterectomy specimen showing thrombus in the internal carotid artery.

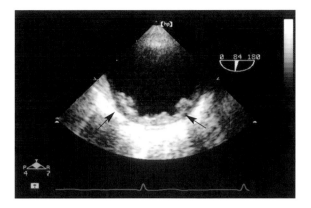

Figure 5.5
Transesophageal echocardiogram showing protruberent atheromatous plaques in the aortic arch (arrows).

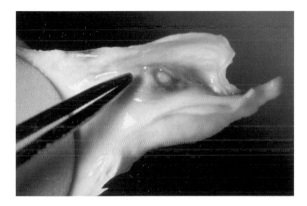

Figure 5.7
Endarterectomy specimen showing an ulcerated plaque.

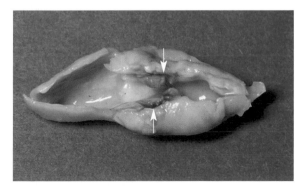

Figure 5.8
Endarterectomy specimen showing intraplaque hemorrhage (arrows).

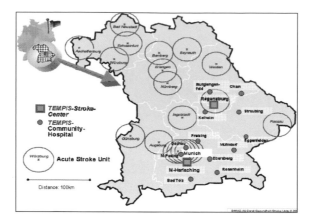

Figure 15.4
Institutions for specialized stroke care in Bavaria.

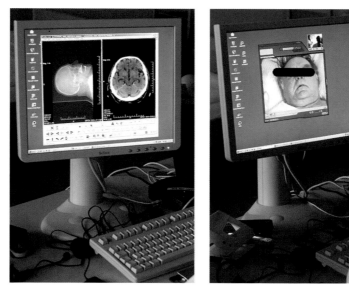

Figure 15.6
Screenshots of a telestroke conference in the TEMPIS project.

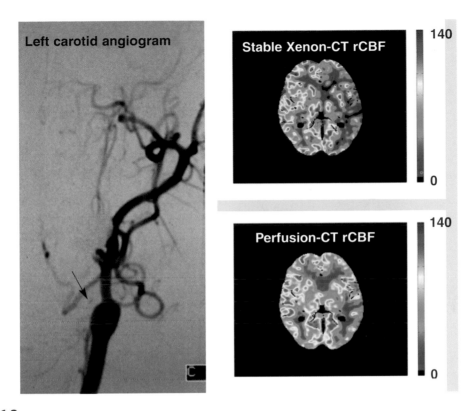

Figure 16.2

A 58-year-old male patient admitted for repeated transitory ischemic accidents. The postero-anterior angiographic view demonstrates a complete chronic occlusion of the left internal carotid artery (arrow), whereas both stable xenon-CT and perfusion-CT display a lowered regional cerebral blood flow (rCBF) in the left middle cerebral artery (MCA) territory. This area with lowered rCBF relates to an ischemic area, superimposed on a context of chronic arterial occlusion, and explains the patient's symptomatology. The perfusion-CT rCBF map (ml/100 g/min) relates closely to the corresponding reference stable xenon-CT map (ml/100 g/min), in both the gray and the white matter, as well as in the pathological ischemic area.

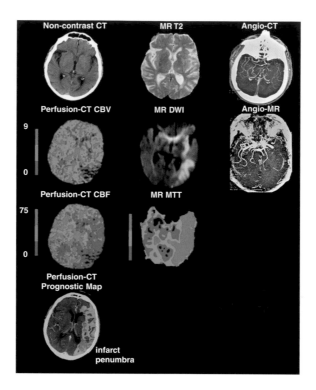

Figure 16.3

A 71-year-old male patient admitted for sudden onset of a right hemisyndrome, associated with nonfluent aphasia. Non-enhanced cerebral CT/perfusion-CT and DWI/PWI were performed 2 and 2.3 h after symptomatology onset, respectively. Non-enhanced cerebral CT demonstrates a left insula ribbon sign and left parietal hypodensity. The more sensitive perfusion-CT prognostic map clearly identifies a posterior and deep left MCA infarct (red), with penumbra (green) involving the remaining left MCA territory. Regional cerebral blood flow (rCBF) (ml/100 g/min) is lowered in both the infarct and the penumbra, whereas regional cerebral blood volume (rCBV) (ml × 100 g) is lowered in the infarct, and preserved or increased in the penumbra, because of the autoregulation processes. The cerebral infarct on perfusion-CT shows a similar size to the DWI abnormality, and the cerebral ischemic lesion (infarct plus penumbra) on perfusion-CT shows similar size to the MRI MTT abnormality. Stroke in this patient was related to an M1 occlusion, demonstrated on both CT angiography and MRA. The patient underwent unsuccessful thrombolysis.

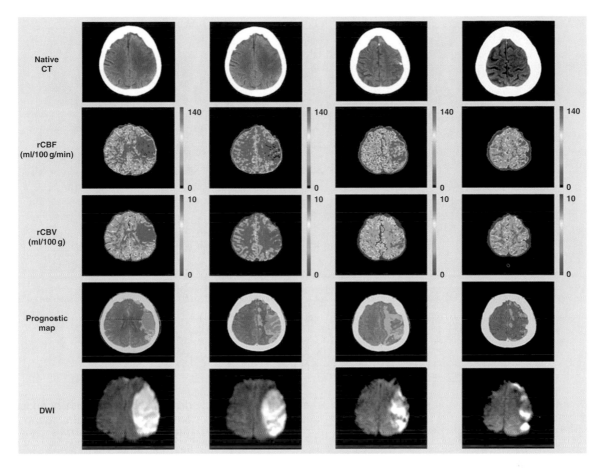

Figure 16.4

A hypertensive 43-year-old female patient was admitted at our institution 3.5h after sudden onset of a right hemisyndrome, associated with right homonymous hemianopsia and global aphasia. Since it was contra-indicated, thrombolysis was not performed. The non-enhanced cerebral CT scan obtained 30min after admission (top row) displays a subtle loss of the cortical ribbon in the left sylvian territory, whereas the more sensitive perfusion-CT prognostic map (fourth row) clearly identifies a posterior left MCA infarct (red), with a limited rim of penumbra (green). Due to the persistent occlusion of the left MCA (demonstrated by admission CT-angiography and delayed MRA obtained 2 days after admission), the penumbra described on the admission perfusion-CT evolved towards infarct and was completely replaced by it, as demonstrated by a close correlation of the whole ischemic area (penumbra plus infarct) as seen on the perfusion-CT with the infarct displayed on the delayed DWI (fifth row).

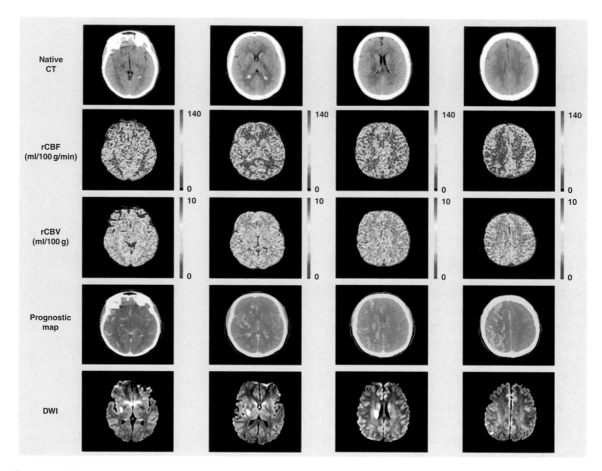

Figure 16.5

A 46-year-old female patient with suspected deep right sylvian artery stroke. The non-enhanced cerebral CT (top row) obtained on admission, 4 h after symptomatology onset, features a hypodensity and a gray matter–white matter dedifferentiation in the right internal capsule. The more sensitive perfusion-CT prognostic map (fourth row) identifies a more extensive deep left MCA penumbra (green), with a very limited infarct (red) located on the right internal capsule. No thrombolysis was performed due to time delay. six days after admission, DWI (fifth row) demonstrates the residual irretrievable infarct, which closely correlates with the one described on the perfusion-CT prognostic map. Recanalization of the right MCA, demonstrated by delayed MRA, afforded recovery of the penumbra described on the admission perfusion-CT.

1

Thrombosis and therapeutic antidotes: historical aspects

Louis R Caplan

Thrombosis takes center stage

Physicians now take for granted the concept that infarction is due to lack of blood supply and nutrition caused by obstruction of arteries that supply regions of ischemia. Early observers referred to focal necrotic regions using nonspecific descriptive terms such as softenings, ramollissements, and encephalomalacia. These softenings were not clearly attributed to ischemia until the middle of the 19th century.[1] Physicians had known for centuries that coagulation occurred within the vascular system. Vesalius, in the middle of the 16th century, described 'unnatural deposits' within the left atrium in patients with gangrene of the extremities.[2] Diseased vessels were also well described. Thomas Willis, writing in the middle years of the 17th century, noted instances in which 'both carotid arteries were choked up so that not the least drop of blood could pass through either of them'.[3] Others also found thrombi and coagula in the vascular system at necropsy, but debated whether or not these formed postmortem or during life. During the late 18th and early 19th centuries, two major figures, John Hunter in England and Cruveilhier in France, thought that coagula were caused by inflammation in the veins.[1] Hunter, writing at the end of the 18th century, noted the frequency of vein inflammation after surgery and after phlebotomies and postulated that venous thrombi formed as exudates from the walls of blood vessels.[4] Cruveilhier, in 1829, wrote that coagulation in veins was the earliest sign of phlebitis.[1] Thrombi within arteries and the heart were attributed at that time to similar inflammatory conditions.

Rudolph Virchow (1821–1902) deserves the major credit for describing in situ antemortem thrombosis with subsequent embolism. In a remarkable series of observations and experiments, he analyzed the relationship between thrombi and infarction, locally and at a distance. Among 76 necropsies performed in 1847, Virchow found thrombi in extremity veins in 18 patients and within the pulmonary arteries in 11,[1,5] and reasoned that the bloodstream emanating from these veins must have been the conduit for transportation of the thrombi to distant sites such as the arteries of the lung. Virchow then used animal experiments to study the fate of foreign materials placed in veins. He subsequently sought and found obstruction of brain, splenic, renal, and limb arteries at necropsy in patients who had cardiac valve disease and left atrial thrombi. Virchow showed systematically that in situ thrombosis and embolism were the cause of infarction and that the process was unrelated to inflammation. Virchow described his classic triad of vascular thrombosis: (1) stasis of blood in a vessel, (2) injury to the wall of the blood vessel, and (3) an abnormality in the balance between blood procoagulant and anticoagulant factors. Before Virchow's studies and reports, blood factors and thrombosis were given little attention.

Despite this demonstration by Virchow, physicians did not appreciate the clinical features of coronary thrombosis and myocardial infarction until the report of James Herrick in 1912,[6] and cardiologists did not clarify the relationship between angina pectoris, coronary artery occlusion, and myocardial infarction until the work of Blumgart and colleagues in the 1940s,[7] which showed the importance of thrombosis of coronary artery atherosclerotic lesions.

Interest in the causes of brain ischemia probably began with Wepfer, who recognized that, at necropsy, there was often an obstruction of blood flow caused by disease of arterial walls.[8] In 1896, Chiari described a single patient who had an intra-arterial embolism that had apparently arisen from a thrombus in the internal carotid artery in the neck.[9] During the 1920s, Charles Foix (1882–1927) and his French colleagues, analyzed the distribution of brain softenings (ramollissements) in various arterial territories and correlated the anatomy with clinical findings.[10] The early writings of Foix were concerned mostly with vascular anatomy, distribution of infarcts, and clinical–anatomical correlation. Only a few weeks before his premature death, Foix and his colleagues Hillemand and Ley presented a very preliminary report to the Medical Society of the Hospitals of Paris on the vascular pathology found in arteries supplying regions of brain softenings.[10,11] Among 56 cases, the artery supplying the infarct was completely occluded in only 12 patients and subtotally occluded in 14 – but in 30, the supply artery was widely patent. Foix and his colleagues proposed four possible explanations for the frequent lack of arterial occlusion at necropsy: (1) occlusion might *follow* brain softening and might have developed later; (2) embolism with passage of embolic material by the time of autopsy; (3) insufficiency ('l'insuffisance cardio-artérielle'), i.e. more proximally located circulatory failure; and (4) vasospasm ('spasme artérielle').[10,11] Miller Fisher's report on carotid artery occlusion published in 1951 emphasized the occurrence of intra-arterial embolism arising from proximal arterial atherosclerotic lesions with superimposed occlusive thrombosis as a very important cause of ischemic stroke.[12]

Only recently, during the last quarter of the 20th century, have studies documented the great importance and ubiquity of intracranial embolism, both cardiogenic and intra-arterial, as the major cause of transient brain ischemia and infarction. In the Harvard Stroke Registry, angiography performed within 48 h after onset of symptoms of ischemic stroke showed a high incidence of intracranial arterial occlusion, while studies after 48 hours were often normal.[13] Ringelstein and colleagues studied the pathogenesis of brain infarcts in 107 patients with internal carotid artery occlusions in the neck.[14]

Angiography in 15 of 21 patients (71%) showed an 'occlusio supra occlusionem', i.e. intra-arterial emboli blocking intracranial arteries.[14] Fieschi and colleagues performed angiography within 6 h of onset of symptoms of brain ischemia and showed complete arterial occlusions by thrombi in 76% of patients, the majority of which (66%) were intra-cranial.[15] In a study of patients screened for acute treatment with recombinant tissue-type plasminogen activator (rtPA), 112 of 139 (80%) had arterial occlusions on angiography performed within 8 h of symptom onset.[16]

Antithrombotic treatment

Hirudin

The first anticoagulant strategy used clinically employed leeches. For centuries, leeches had been used to promote healing, but in the late 19th century and early years of the 20th century, physicians noted that bleeding from leech bites was difficult to stop and the active anticoagulant in leeches was isolated and named hirudin.[17] Interest in hirudin as an anticoagulant has increased recently. Hirudin is the most potent naturally occurring inhibitor of thrombin and it has now been produced using recombinant DNA technology.

Heparin

Heparin, which occurs naturally in human and animal tissues, was the second substance to be used as an anticoagulant. McLean, then a medical student at Johns Hopkins, first investigated a substance then called cephalin.[17,18] He attempted to isolate it from the brain, but could not be certain of its purity and so turned, with more success, to isolating substances from the heart (cuorin) and liver (heparphosphatide). These proved identical and were named heparin by Howell and Holt in 1918.[19] Hedenius, with his colleague Wilander, experimented with self-injection of heparin and determined that an anticoagulant dose could be ascertained with precision.[17,20] Hedenius and colleagues, in 1941, collected and reported results among 85 patients treated with heparin; these patients included 10 instances of embolism (6 to the brain), 33 cases called cerebral or cerebellar thrombosis, and 38 instances of venous thrombosis in the limbs.[20] Nineteen of the patients did well, and Hedenius commented that 'this physiological anti-coagulation will in the future be useful as a reliable therapeutic medium in the treatment of thrombo-embolic disease'.[20] As early as 1950, trials were organized to study the effect of heparin (usually followed by dicumerol, which had by then also been discovered).

Heparin is a mixture of sulfated mucopolysaccharides. Most presently available heparin preparations are derived from either bovine lungs or porcine intestines. Heparin is composed of about 21 different compounds ranging in molecular weight from 3 to 37.5 kDa.[21,22] The anticoagulant properties of heparin are due to the ability of its components to bind to antithrombin III (ATIII). ATIII slowly binds to thrombin and the serine protease factors VIIa, IXa, Xa, XIa, and XIIa, and neutralizes these compounds. Heparin binds to ATIII and dramatically accelerates the formation of complexes of ATIII with thrombin and also with the coagulation factors Xa and XIa.[22,23] The anticoagulant functions of naturally occurring heparin were clarified during the 1960s and early 1970s.

Unfractionated heparin increases platelet aggregation in response to various stimuli and promotes the synthesis of thromboxane by activated platelets. Unfortunately, the anticoagulant activity of various commercially available heparin preparations varies among sources and even varies from batch to batch. Low-molecular-weight fractions of heparin (LMWH) contain most of the anticoagulant effects, are potent in inhibiting factor Xa, by doing so prevent the generation of large amounts of thrombin, and do not activate platelets.[24,25]

LMWH began to become popular in the 1980s. It is prepared by depolymerization of unfractionated heparin using chemical or enzymatic methods. LMWH in commercial use has an average molecular weight of 4–6 kDa. Reduced binding to plasma proteins results in a more predictable and reliable anticoagulant response. LMWH has a high bioavailability and longer half-life than unfractionated heparin. These pharmacological properties of LMWH make it possible to give the agent subcutaneously once or twice daily, even on an outpatient basis. LMWH causes less platelet activation and a lower frequency of thrombocytopenia compared with unfractionated heparins. Commercially available low-molecular-weight synthetic heparinoids have recently become available, and their utility has been examined in clinical randomized trials.

Heparin, LMWH and heparinoids have been studied most often in trials of patients with brain ischemia[26–30] on with dural sinus venous thrombosis.[31–33] Unfortunately, in most of these trials, the causative vascular lesions were not well defined by modern brain and vascular imaging. Controversy still surrounds the use of heparin in patients with brain ischemia.[34,35] Many clinicians have used and continue to use heparin compounds in patients with brain embolism, but the timing of their use and the necessity for preceding warfarin administration with heparins is still unsettled.

Warfarin compounds

During the 1920s in North America, a hemorrhagic disorder of cattle developed that had considerable economic significance. Cattle in North Dakota, USA and Alberta, Canada often died of internal bleeding or from blood seepage after minor injuries or surgery. Investigators eventually deduced that the cause of the hemorrhagic disorder was the ingestion of spoiled hay made from sweet clover.[17] Bleeding could be prevented by infusing blood from normal cows that had not eaten the spoiled hay. The odor of the new-mown hay was related to a compound called coumarin. Karl Link and colleagues found that the naturally ocurring coumarin in the hay was changed during spoilage to 4-hydroxycoumarin. Two molecules of 4-hydroxycoumarin were coupled together to form a compound dubbed dicoumarol, which became the first commercially available oral anticoagulant.[17,36] In the 1940s, warfarin and other anticoagulants derived from 4-hydroxycoumarin began to become available.

Warfarin is a water-soluble derivative of coumaric acid; it is absorbed by the small intestine and transported in the blood, loosely bound to albumin. The therapeutic effect is derived from the ability of the compound to inhibit the action of vitamin K, which is necessary for the biological synthesis of factors II (prothrombin), VII, IX, and X.[37] By depressing these procoagulant factors, warfarin affects both the so-called intrinsic cascade and the extrinsic coagulation pathway.[37]

Early observational studies showed the effectiveness of warfarin in patients with rheumatic mitral stenosis who had brain embolism.[38–40] Warfarin, often preceded by heparin, was also proven to be effective in patients with thrombophlebitis and pulmonary embolism, and in preventing brain embolism in patients with acute myocardial infarction. During the 1950s and 1960s, clinicians began to study the effect of 4-hydroxycoumarin derivatives in patients with brain ischemia.[41–45] These studies antedated computed tomography (CT) and other modern imaging techniques and had mixed, rather inconclusive, results. They used prothrombin times to monitor the intensity of anticoagulation. Prothrombin times (PTs) were maintained at generally higher levels than are now used, and the frequency of brain and major systemic bleeding was relatively high. In the early 1980s, Wessler and Gitel provided data that persuasively show that the dosage at which warfarin protects against thrombosis is probably far below that needed to cause bleeding.[37] In one study of 96 patients with venous thromboses treated with various intensities of oral anticoagulation, higher-intensity therapy (i.e. more prolonged PTs) caused more bleeding, and less intense therapy was equally effective in preventing recurrent thromboembolism.[46] Others later corroborated the safety and effectiveness of less intense warfarin anticoagulation.

Because of the wide variation in thromboplastin reagents used in testing anticoagulation, in 1977, the World Health Organization (WHO) designated a single batch of human brain thromboplastin as an international standard.[47] Manufacturers calibrate their reagent against the international standard and calculate an International Sensitivity Index (ISI), which relates their reagent to the international standard. Using the ISI and the PT, the International Normalized Ratio (INR) can be readily calculated.

Various expert groups have published recommendations for the intensity of anticoagulation based on the international system, but the intensity is still debated. A large Dutch trial (SPIRIT: Stroke Prevention in Reversible Ischemia Trial) that compared the effectiveness of aspirin versus oral anticoagulation (INR target range 3.0–4.5) was stopped prematurely after an interim analysis showed an unacceptable rate of hemorrhage in the anticoagulant-treated group.[48]

As a result of this trial, most clinicians now recommend less intense anticoagulation, aiming at INR range of 1.8–2.5. The Atrial Fibrillation Investigators analyzed the results of five trials of anticoagulation in patients with atrial fibrillation (INR target range 1.4–4.2), and recommended a target range of 2.0–3.0 as having the best benefit/risk results.[49,50] Unfortunately, until recently, the effectiveness of warfarin administration had not been tested in modern randomized trials in patients with known pathologies. During the last decade, trials of stroke prophylaxis in patients with atrial fibrillation who did not have valvular heart disease have documented a dramatic benefit of warfarin treatment.[51–56] Warfarin is about 50% more effective than aspirin in reducing the rate of stroke in patients with atrial fibrillation who do not have valvular disease.

Warfarin compounds continue to be studied in patients with cerebrovascular disease. A retrospective nonrandomized study suggested that warfarin might be superior to aspirin treatment in preventing strokes in patients with angiographically documented intracranial disease.[57] More recently, a multicenter randomized trial did not show any superiority of warfarin over aspirin in any diagnostic group.[58] Clinicians now agree that warfarin is indicated in patients with atrial fibrillation and high-risk cardiac embolic sources, but continue to debate and explore its utility in other stroke-related conditions.

The major limitation on the use of warfarin is the difficulty in maintaining therapeutic INR levels. In two major randomized trials, an important proportion of patients could not be maintained in the target INR ranges (2–2.5).[58–60] Even when directions for warfarin dosage are managed by anticoagulation clinics, the target INR ranges are difficult to maintain. This is mostly because warfarin works through an effect on prothrombin, and the action of prothrombin is affected by many variables, including diet, liver function, and the use of other medicines.

Direct thrombin inhibitors

Recently, agents that inhibit thrombin directly have been introduced into medical practice. These agents have the advantage of having fixed doses and not requiring monitoring of INR levels. Argabatran, a direct thrombin inhibitor that is given intravenously, was first tested in animals[61,62] and has now been introduced in humans.[63,64] It is now widely used in Asia in preference to heparin.

Oral direct thrombin inhibitors are under investigation. One such agent, ximelagatran was tested widely in trials of patients with phlebothrombosis[65,66] and atrial fibrillation.[66,67] Compared with warfarin, ximelagatran was equally effective, easier to control, and associated with less bleeding. Liver function abnormalities were an important adverse effect of this drug. Other oral thrombin inhibitors are being investigated. These agents work rapidly, so that their use would obviate the need for heparin. They could be used as single agents, eliminating the use of heparin and warfarin.

Substances that inhibit platelet functions

Since the discovery that platelets and white platelet–fibrin thrombi play an important role in promoting thrombosis in arteries, substances that modify platelet adhesion and aggregation have become of great clinical interest in thrombotic disorders, particularly ischemic stroke. The first clinical observations of aspirin as an anticoagulant were probably made by a dental practitioner, Craven, when noted that his patients bled more if they had used aspirin, and so urged friends and patients to take one or two aspirin tablets a day.[17] In the mid-1950s, Craven published details on the effectiveness of this strategy in preventing coronary and cerebral thrombosis among 8000 men in articles in the *Mississippi Valley Medical Journal* – not a periodical on every physician's bookshelf.[17,68,69] Some 20 years later, case reports from the USA and UK on the effectiveness of aspirin in preventing attacks of transient monocular blindness brought the subject to more general attention.[70,71] Trials of aspirin in the USA and Canada soon ensued in the late 1970s.[72,73]

Aspirin and other nonsteroidal anti-inflammatory drugs (NSAIDs) such as indomethacin, phenylbutazone, and ibuprofen inhibit platelet release reactions, secondary ADP-induced platelet aggregation, and platelet adhesion to collagen, when tested in vitro.[74] Aspirin probably inhibits platelet aggregation and secretion by preventing the synthesis of prostaglandins and thromboxane A_2(TxA_2). This action is achieved by inhibiting the cyclo-oxygenase enzyme that converts arachidonic acid to prostaglandin G_2 (PGG_2) the precursor of TxA_2.[74]

During the 1980s and 1990s, trials explored the optimal dosage of aspirin[75] and the utility of other newer agents that inhibited platelet function. These trials considered the effectiveness of dipyridamole in immediate release[76,77] and extended-release[78,79] forms when added to aspirin, ticlopidine,[80,81] and clopidogrel.[82] With the realization that, for the most part, these agents acted on only some platelet functions, clinicians then began to explore the use of more than one 'antiplatelet agent' (e.g. aspirin and clopidogrel and extended-release dipyridamole with aspirin). At the turn of the century, trials began to study the utility of glycoprotein (GP)IIb/IIIa inhibitors, which are active on the final bond between platelets and fibrinogen.[83,84]

Thrombolysis

During the late 1950s, clinicians began to give stroke patients thrombolytic agents in an attempt to open thrombosed arteries. Early attempts used bovine or human thrombolysins or streptokinase.[85] During the early 1960s, Meyer and colleagues randomized 73 patients with worsening strokes to receive streptokinase intravenously and/or concomitant anticoagulants within 3 days of stroke onset.[86,87] Clots were lysed in some patients, but 10 patients treated with streptokinase died, and some patients had brain hemorrhages. After these studies, streptokinase was thought to be too dangerous to use, and its use for systemic and cardiac thromboembolism was considered contraindicated in the presence of brain lesions or past strokes.

During the 1980s, stimulated by the successful use of thrombolytic agents for the treatment of pulmonary embolism[88,89] and coronary artery thrombosis,[90,91] clinicians turned again to these 'clot busters' to treat cerebrovascular thromboembolism.[85,92,93] Streptokinase and urokinase were the commonest early substances used. Following the success of an endogenous substance, tissue-type plasminogen activator (tPA), in recanalizing coronary arteries,[97] researchers turned to recombinant tPA (rtPA) in patients with arterial occlusive cerebrovascular lesions. Factor XII and the release of tPA and other substances promote the conversion of plasminogen to plasmin, the active fibrinolytic enzyme.[85,94] Plasmin activity is concentrated at the sites of fibrin deposition. Once rtPA promotes entry of plasmin into a thrombus, fibrinolysis can progress.

The first trials involved intra-arterial instillation of thrombolytic agents into patients with arteriographically confirmed occlusion of the intracranial anterior and posterior circulation arteries. Clinicians then began to investigate the intravenous administration of thrombolytic drugs to patients with angiographically confirmed intracranial thrombi. Most of these studies involved drug delivery within 8 h of symptom onset, and all analyzed the effectiveness of thrombolysis by estimating the degree of vascular recanalization, as well as the clinical outcome.[92,93,95,96] Recanalization depended heavily on the location of the thrombi and the timing of drug delivery. Intracranial hemorrhage was a serious complication, occurring in 5–10% of patients – rather more with intravenous delivery. These early trials were mostly uncontrolled and patients were not randomized.

The first reported randomized trial was ECASS (European Cooperative Acute Stroke Study).[95] In this study, 620 patients with acute hemispheral strokes were recruited in 75 hospitals in 14 European countries; angiography or other vascular imaging was not included. Treatment was given within 6 h of the onset of symptoms of brain ischemia, with 313 patients being randomized to receive rtPA (1.1 mg/kg) and 307 patients to receive placebo. CT findings of brain hemorrhage or major early infarct signs involving more than one-third of the middle cerebral artery territory were exclusion criteria, but the reading of CT scans at the study sites proved unreliable and more than 100 patients who should have been excluded received rtPA. In the target population who met predetermined inclusion and exclusion criteria, there was a significantly better outcome in the rtPA-treated patients as measured by combined Barthel Index and modified Rankin Scale scores at 90 days. Intracerebral hemorrhages and mortality were higher in the rtPA-treated patients, but these differences were not statistically significant. Large parenchymal hematomas were more often found in patients treated with rtPA. Patients treated within 3 h did better after rtPA

than controls and those treated with rtPA between 3 and 6 h.[97] ECASS showed that the treatment of patients with early infarct signs on CT scan was particularly dangerous. Initial analysis of the CT scans at local hospitals was often unreliable. Some hemorrhages and many early infarcts were missed by local physicians.

The next randomized trial reported was the NINDS (National Institute of Neurological Disorder and Stroke) study.[98] The major differences between this study and ECASS were a lower dose of rtPA, earlier treatment (302 patients were treated within 90 min and 322 between 90 and 180 min after ischemic symptom onset), and nonexclusion of patients because of brain ischemia found on entry CT scans. There was a statistically significant benefit for rtPA over placebo for all outcome measures at 3 months. Symptomatic intracerebral hemorrhages were more common in patients treated with rtPA (6.4% vs 0.6%) and in particular were more common in patients with more severe neurologic deficits at entry and in patients aged 75 years or older.

Publication of the results of the NINDS study in 1995[98] gave momentum to a movement to quickly introduce intravenous thrombolysis into the treatment of patients with acute ischemic stroke. During the summer of 1996, the US Food and Drug Administration (FDA) approved the use of rtPA for the treatment of stroke patients when the drug was given within the first 3 hours. Subsequent nearly identical published treatment protocols adopted by committees of the American Heart Association[99] and the American Academy of Neurology[100] recommend intravenous administration of rtPA (0.9 mg/kg, to maximum of 90 mg) given in a 10% bolus followed by an infusion lasting 60 min to patients within 3 hours of onset of ischemic stroke. The recommendations stipulate that a CT scan reformed before the infusion should not show major infarction, mass effect, edema, or hemorrhage. Neither the NINDS rtPA Study Group nor the American Heart Association nor the American Academy of Neurology committees require or suggest vascular tests before treatment, and all are silent regarding who can or should administer and supervise the treatment.

The next published randomized trial was the ECASS II study.[101] Investigators treated 800 patients from Europe, Australia, and New Zealand with rtPA or placebo within 6 h of stroke onset. Stroke patients were treated with the same dose as used in the NINDS trial rather than the higher dose used in ECASS I. Patients with major infarcts on CT scan were excluded, but vascular imaging was not required before treatment. Guidelines for the control of hypertension were more explicit than in ECASS I. In ECASS II, 36.6% of patients in the placebo-treated group had favorable outcomes – a much better result than in ECASS I and the NINDS trial. Among the rtPA-treated group, 40.3% had favorable outcomes; this was not statistically significantly different from the placebo-treated group.[101] During the interval between ECASS I and ECASS II, dedicated stroke units and stroke teams had become well developed in Europe. ECASS II showed that stroke unit care was important and could dramatically improve the morbidity and mortality of stroke. Treatment results and frequency of hemorrhages were similar in the 0–3 h and 3–6 h treatment groups.

There have been three therapeutic trials of intravenous streptokinase in patients without identification of the vascular lesions: ASK (Australian Streptokinase Trial), MAST-I (Multicenter Acute Stroke Trial – Italy) and MAST-E (Multicenter Acute Stroke Trial – Europe).[102–104] All were stopped prematurely because of the high rate of brain hemorrhages in patients treated with intravenous streptokinase.

In 1999, the results of a randomized trial of intra-arterial pro-urokinase (PRoAct II) were published.[105] This study showed unequivocally that patients with angiographically confirmed middle cerebral artery occlusions treated with intra-arterial drug within 6 hours of symptom onset had much more frequent and complete recanalization and improved clinically much more than those not so treated. Inexplicably, the FDA failed to approve intra-arterial therapy, although the use of this therapy gained considerable

ground and became widely prevalent in the USA after the trial report.

Since the planning of the NINDS trial and ECASS I, major advances were made in brain and vascular imaging and the newer technologies became more widely available in some countries. Unfortunately, none of the published randomized trials used modern noninvasive brain and vascular imaging techniques to select or evaluate patients. At the time of writing, the topic of stroke thrombolysis continues to be hotly debated. Although rtPA has been released and approved for use in stroke patients in the USA for more than 5 years, less than 10% of eligible patients receive the drug. Clinicians and regulators continue to discuss who should receive the treatment, using what technology, using what criteria, during what time intervals, at what sites, and given by whom.

The advent of modern magnetic resonance imaging (MRI), including magnetic resonance angiography (MRA) and diffusion and perfusion imaging as well as gradient-echo T2*-weighted imaging, and modern CT studies using CT angiography (CTA) and CT perfusion imaging, has changed the approach to thrombolysis in many centers.[106–109] The decision on whether or not to administer thrombolytics should be based on an analysis of the size and location of brain infarction, the location and severity of any occlusive thromboemboli, and the tissue still at risk for infarction – and not only on the clock. Mechanical clot retrieval devices are also being introduced. Their use will provide interventionists with a menu of different techniques – chemical thrombolyis, angioplasty/stenting, and mechanical clot retrievers – that could be used to reperfuse potentially ischemic tissues.[109]

References

1. Fisher CM. The history of cerebral embolism and hemorrhagic infarction. In: Furlan A (ed). The Heart and Stroke. Berlin: Springer-Verlag, 1987:3–16.

2. Vesalius A. De humani corporis fabrica. Basilae: J Oporini, 1543.

3. Willis T. Cerebri anatome: cui accessit nervorum descriptio et usus. London: J Flesher, 1664.

4. Hunter J. Observations on the inflammation of the internal coats of veins. Trans Soc Improv Med Cirurg Knowledge Lond 1793;1:18–29.

5. Virchow R. Ueber die akut entzundung der arterien. Virchows Arch Path Anat 1847;1:272–378.

6. Herrick JB. Clinical features of sudden obstruction of the coronary arteries. JAMA 1912;59:2015–20.

7. Blumgart HL, Schlesinger MJ, Davis D. Studies on the relation of the clinical manifestation of angina pectoris, coronary thrombosis, and myocardial infarction to the pathological findings. Am Heart J 1940; 19:1–9.

8. Wepfer JJ. Observationes anatomicae ex cadaveribus eorum, quos sustulit apoplexia, cum exercitatione de ejus loco affecto. Schaffhausen: J Caspari Suteri, 1658.

9. Chiari H. Über das verhalten des Teilungswinkels der carotis communis bei der endarteritis chronica deformans. Verhandl Deutsch path Gesellsch 1905; 9:326–30.

10. Caplan LR. Charles Foix, the first modern stroke neurologist. Stroke 1990;21:348–56.

11. Foix C, Hillemand P, Ley J. Relativement au ramollissement cerebral a sa frequence et a son siege et al'importance relative des obliterations arterielles, completes ou incompletes dans sa pathogenie. Rev Neurol 1927;43:217–18.

12. Fisher CM. Occlusion of the internal carotid artery. Arch Neurol Psychiatr 1951;65:346–77.

13. Mohr J, Caplan LR, Melski J, et al. The Harvard Cooperative Stroke Registry: a prospective registry. Neurology 1978;28:754–62.

14. Ringelstein EB, Zeumer H, Angelou D. The pathogenesis of strokes from internal carotid artery occlusion: diagnostic and therapeutical implications. Stroke 1983;14:867–75.

15. Fieschi C, Argentino C, Lenzi GL, et al. Clinical and instrumental evaluation of patients with ischemic stroke within the first six hours. J Neurol Sci 1989; 91:311–21.

16. Wolpert SM, Bruchman H, Greenlee R, et al. Neuroradiologic evaluation of patients with acute stroke treated with recombinant tissue plasminogen activator. AJNR Am J Neuroradial 1993;14:333–47.

17. Fields WS, Lemak NA. A History of Stroke: Its Recognition and Treatment. New York: Oxford University Press, 1989.

18. McLean J. The discovery of heparin. Circulation 1958;19:75–78.

19. Howell WH, Holt E. Two new factors in blood coagulation – heparin and pro-antithrombin. Am J Physiol 1918;47:328–41.

20. Hedenius P. Use of heparin in internal disease. Acta Med Scand 1941;107:170–7.

21. Wu K. New pharmacologic approaches to thromboembolic disorders. Hosp Prac 1985;20:101–20.

22. Caplan LR. Review: anticoagulation for cerebral ischemia. Clin Neuropharm 1986;9:399–414.

23. Damus P, Hicks M, Rosenberg R. Anticoagulant action of heparin. Nature 1973;246:355–7.

24. Rosenberg R, Lam L. Correlation between structure and function of heparin. Proc Natl Acad Sci USA 1979;76:3198–202.

25. Weitz JI. Low-molecular-weight heparins. N Engl J Med 1997;337:688–98.

26. Ramirez-Lassepas M, Quinones MR, Nino HH. Treatment of acute ischemic stroke: open trial with continuous intravenous heparinization. Arch Neurol 1986;42:386–90.

27. Duke RJ, Bloch RF, Alexander GG, et al. Intravenous heparin for the prevention of stroke progression in acute partial stable stroke: a randomized controlled trial. Ann Intern Med 1986;105:825–8.

28. Gordon DL, Linhardt R, Adams HP. Low-molecular-weight heparins and heparinoids and their use in acute or progressing ischemic stroke. Clin Neuropharm 1990;13:522–43.

29. Kay R, Wong KS, Yu YL, et al. Low-molecular-weight heparin for the treatment of acute ischemic stroke. N Engl J Med 1995;333:1588–93.

30. The Publications Committee for the Trial of ORG 10172 in Acute Stroke Treatment (TOAST) Investigators. Low molecular weight heparinoid, ORG 10172 (Danaparoid), and outcome after acute ischemic stroke. A randomized controlled trial. JAMA 1998; 279:1265–72.

31. Einhaupl KM, Villringer A, Meister W, et al. Heparin treatment in sinus venous thrombosis. Lancet 1991; 338:597–600.

32. Meister W, Einhaupl K, Villringer A, et al. Treatment of patients with cerebral sinus and vein thrombosis with heparin. In: Einhaupl K, Kempski O, Baethmann A (eds). Cerebral Sinus Thrombosis. Experimental and Clinical Aspects. New York: Plenum, 1990:225–30.

33. de Bruijn SFTM, Stam J, for the Cerebral Venous Sinus Thrombosis Study Group. Randomized, placebo-controlled trial of anticoagulant treatment with low-molecular-weight heparin for cerebral venous sinus thrombosis. Stroke 1999;30:484–8.

34. Simon RP, Powers WJ. Debate. Anticoagulation in acute ischemic stroke: not indicated. In: Choi D, Dacey RG, Hsu CY, Powers WJ (eds). Cerebrovascular Disease: Momentum at the End of the Second Millennium. New York: Futura, 2001.

35. Caplan LR, Debate. Heparin should be used to treat patients presenting with acute stroke or stroke-in-evolution: affirmative position. In: Choi D, Dacey RG, Hsu CY, Powers WJ (eds). Cerebrovascular Disease: Momentum at the End of the Second Millennium. New York: Futura, 2001.

36. Link KP. The discovery of dicoumarol and its sequels. Circulation 1959;19:97–107.

37. Wessler S, Gitel S. Warfarin: from bedside to bench. N Engl J Med 1984;311:645–52.

38. Fleming HA, Bailey SM. Mitral valve disease, systemic embolism and anticoagulants. Postgrad Med J 1971; 47:599–604.

39. Adams GF, Merrett JD, Hutchinson WM, Pollock AM. Cerebral embolism and mitral stenosis: survival with and without anticoagulants. J Neurol Neurosurg Psychiatry 1974;37:378–83.

40. Carter AB. Prognosis of cerebral embolism. Lancet 1965;ii:514–19.

41. Wright I, McDevitt E. Cerebral vascular disease: Significance, diagnosis, and present treatment, including selective use of anticoagulant substances. Ann Intern Med 1954;41:682–98.

42. Millikan C, Siekert RG, Whisnant JP. Anticoagulant therapy in cerebral vascular disease – current status. JAMA 1958;166:587–92.

43. Marshall J, Shaw DA. Anticoagulant therapy of cerebrovascular disease. Proc R Soc Med 1959;52:547–9.

44. Veterans Administration. An evaluation of anticoagulant therapy in the treatment of cerebrovascular disease. Neurology 1961;11:132–8.

45. Baker RN, Broward JA, Fang HC, et al. Anticoagulant therapy in cerebral infarction. *Neurology* 1962;12: 823–35.

46. Hull R, Hirsch J, Jay R, et al. Different intensities of oral anticoagulant therapy in the treatment of proximal-vein thrombosis. N Engl J Med 1982;307: 1676–81.

47. Hirsh J, Poller L, Deykin D, et al. Optimal therapeutic range for oral anticoagulants. Chest 1989;95(Suppl): 5S–11S.

48. The Stroke Prevention in Reversible Ischemia Trial (SPIRIT) Study Group. A randomized trial of anticoagulants versus aspirin after cerebral ischemia of presumed arterial origin. Ann Neurol 1997;42:857–65.

49. Atrial Fibrillation Investigators: Risk factors for stroke and efficacy of antithrombotic therapy in atrial fibrillation: analysis of pooled data from 5 randomized clinical trials. Arch Intern Med 1994;154:1949–57.

50. Hart RG. Oral anticoagulation for secondary prevention of stroke. Cerebrovasc Dis 1997;7(Suppl 6):24–29.

51. The Boston Area Anticoagulation Trial for Atrial Fibrillation Investigators. The effect of low-dose warfarin on the risk of stroke in patients with nonrheumatic atrial fibrillation. N Engl J Med 1990;323:1505–11.

52. Petersen P, Godtfredsen J, Boysen G, et al. Placebo-controlled, randomized trial of warfarin and aspirin for prevention of thromboembolic complications in chronic atrial fibrillation: The Copenhagen AFASAK Study. Lancet 1989;i:175–9.

53. The Stroke Prevention in Atrial Fibrillation Investigators. The Stroke Prevention in Atrial Fibrillation Study: final results. Circulation 1991;84: 527–39.

54. EAFT (European Atrial Fibrillation Trial) Study Group. Secondary prevention in non-rheumatic atrial fibrillation after transient ischaemic attack or minor stroke. Lancet 1993;342:1255–62.

55. Stroke Prevention in Atrial Fibrillation Investigators. Warfarin versus aspirin for prevention of thrombo-embolism in atrial fibrillation: Stroke Prevention in Atrial Fibrillation II Study. Lancet 1994;343:687–91.

56. Stroke Prevention in Atrial Fibrillation Investigators. Adjusted-dose warfarin versus low-intensity, fixed-dose warfarin plus aspirin for high-risk patients with atrial fibrillation: Stroke Prevention in Atrial Fibrillation III randomised clinical trial. Lancet 1996; 348:633–8.

57. Chimowitz MI, Kokkinos J, Strong J, et al. The Warfarin–Aspirin Symptomatic Intracranial Disease Study. Neurology 1995;45:1488–93.

58. Mohr JP, Thompson JLP, Lazar RM, et al. A comparison of warfarin and aspirin for the prevention of recurrent ischemic stroke. N Engl J Med 2001; 345:1444–51.

59. Chimowitz MI, Lynn MJ, Howlett-Smith H, et al. Comparison of warfarin and aspirin for symptomatic intracranial arterial stenosis. N Engl J Med 2005; 352:1305–16.

60. Koroshetz W. Warfarin, aspirin, and intracranial vascular disease. N Engl J Med 2005;352:1368–70.

61. Tamoa Y, Kikumoto R. Effect of argabatran, a selective thrombin inhibitor, on animal models of cerebral thrombosis. Semin Thromb Hemost 1997; 23:523–30.

62. Kobayashi W, Tazaki Y. Effect of the thrombin inhibitor argabatran in acute cerebral thrombosis. Semin Thromb Hemost 1997;23:531–4.

63. Lewis BE, Wallis DE, Leya F, et al. Argabatran anticoagulation in patients with heparin-induced thrombocytopenia. Arch Intern Med 2003;163:1849–56.

64. LaMonte MP, Nash ML, Wang DZ, et al, for the ARGIS-1 Investigators. Argabatran anticoagulation in patients with Acute Ischemic Stroke (ARGIS-1). Stroke 2004;35:1677–82.

65. Fiessinger J-N, Huisman MV, Davidson BL, et al, for the THRIVE Treatment Study Investigators. Ximelagatran vs low-molecular-weight heparin and warfarin for the treatment of deep vein thrombosis: a randomized trial. JAMA 2005;293:681–9.

66. Gurewich V. Ximelagatran – promises and concerns. JAMA 2005;293:736–9.

67. Executive Steering Committee on Behalf of SPORTIF III Investigators. Stroke prevention with the oral direct thrombin inhibitor ximelagatran compared with warfarin in patients with non-valvular atrial fibrillation (SPORTIF III): randomized controlled trial. Lancet 2003;362:1691–8.

68. Craven LL. Experiences with aspirin (acetylsalicylic acid) in the nonspecific prophylaxis of coronary thrombosis. Mississippi Valley Med J 1953;75:38–44.

69. Craven LL. Prevention of coronary and cerebral thrombosis. Mississippi Valley Med J 1956;78:213–15.

70. Mundall J, Quintero P, von Kaulla K, et al. Transient monocular blindness and increased platelet aggregability treated with aspirin – a case report. Neurology 1971;21:402.

71. Harrison MJG, Marshall J, Meadows JC, et al. Effect of aspirin in amaurosis fugax. Lancet 1971;ii:743–4.

72. Fields WS, Lemak N, Frankowski R, et al. Controlled trial of aspirin in cerebral ischemia. Stroke 1977;8:301–6.

73. Barnett HJM. The Canadian Cooperative Study: a randomized trial of aspirin and sulfinpyrazone in threatened stroke. N Engl J Med 1978;299:53–9.

74. Moncada S, Vane J. Arachidonic acid metabolites and the interactions between platelets and blood vessel walls. N Engl J Med 1979;300:1142–7.

75. The Dutch TIA Trial Study Group. A comparison of two doses of aspirin (30 mg vs 283 mg a day) in patients after a transient ischemic attack or minor stroke. N Engl J Med 1991;325:1261–6.

76. Fields WS, Yatsu F, Conomy J, et al. Persantine–aspirin trial in cerebral ischemia: the American–Canadian Cooperative Study group. Stroke 1983;14: 97–103.

77. Bousser MG, Eschwege E, Hagenah M, et al. 'AICLA' controlled trial of aspirin and dipyridamole in the secondary prevention of athero-thrombotic cerebral ischemia. Stroke 1983;14:5–14.

78. ESPS Group. European Stroke Prevention Study (ESPS): principal endpoints. Lancet 1987;ii:1351–4.

79. Diener HC, Cunha L, Forbes C, et al. European Stroke Prevention Study 2. Dipyridamole and acetylsalicylic acid in the secondary prevention of stroke. J Neurol Sci 1996;143:1–13.

80. Hass WK, Easton JD, Adams HP, et al. A randomized trial comparing ticlopidine hydrochloride with aspirin for the prevention of stroke in high-risk patients. N Engl J Med 1989;321:501–7.

81. Gent M, Easton JD, Hachinski V, et al. The Canadian American Ticlopinine Study (CATS) in thromboembolic stroke. Lancet 1989;i:1215–20.

82. CAPRIE Steering Committee. A randomised, blinded, trial of clopidogrel versus aspirin in patients at risk of ischaemic events. Lancet 1996;348:1329–39.

83. Lefkovits J, Plow EF, Topol EJ. Platelet glycoprotein IIb/IIIa receptors in cardiovascular medicine. N Engl J Med 1995;332:1553–9.

84. Wallace RC, Furlan AJ, Moliterno DJ, et al. Basilar artery rethrombosis: successful treatment with platelet glycoprotein IIb/IIIa receptor inhibitor. AJNR Am J Neuroradiol 1997;18:1257–60.

85. Sloan MA. Thrombolysis and stroke, past and future. Arch Neurol 1987;44:748–68.

86. Meyer JS, Gilroy J, Barnhart ME, et al. Anticoagulants plus streptokinase therapy in progressive stroke. JAMA 1964;189:373.

87. Meyer JS, Gilroy J, Barnhart ME, Johnson JF. Therapeutic thrombolysis, in cerebral thrombo-embolism: randomized evaluation of streptokinase. In: Millikan C, Siekert R, Whisnant JP (eds). Cerebral Vascular Disease. Fourth Princeton Conference. New York: Grune & Stratton, 1965:200–13.

88. The Urokinase Pulmonary Embolism Trial: a national cooperative study. Circulation 1973;47(Suppl 2) II1–108.

89. Urokinase–Streptokinase Pulmonary Embolism Trial: phase 2 results, a cooperative study. JAMA 1974;229:1606–13.

90. Van de Werf F, Ludbrook PA, Bergmann SR, et al. Coronary thrombolysis with tissue-type plasminogen activator in patients with evolving myocardial infarction. N Engl J Med 1984;310:609–13.

91. Williams DO, Borer J, Braunwald E, et al. Intravenous recombinant tissue-type plasminogen activator in patients with acute myocardial infarction: a report from the NHLBI Thrombolysis in Myocardial Infarction Trial. Circulation 1986;73:338.

92. DelZoppo GJ. Thrombolytic therapy in cerebrovascular disease. Stroke 1988;19:1174–9.

93. Pessin MS, del Zoppo GJ, Furlan AJ. Thrombolytic treatment in acute stroke: review and update of selected topics. In: Cerebrovascular Diseases, 19th Princeton Conference, 1994. Boston: Butterworth–Heinemann, 1995:409–18.

94. Collen D. On the regulation and control of fibrinolysis: Edward Kowalsky Memorial Lecture. Thromb Haemost 1980;43:77–89.

95. Caplan LR. Caplan's Stroke: A Clinical Approach, 3rd edn. Boston: Butterworth–Heinemann, 2001:124–130.

96. Caplan LR. The case against the present guidelines for stroke thrombolysis. The present guidelines for clinical use should be modified. In: Lyden P (ed). Thrombolytic Therapy for Stroke. Totowa, NJ: Humana, 2001:223–35.

97. Hacke W, Kaste M, Fieschi C, et al. Intravenous thrombolysis with recombinant tissue plasminogen activator for acute hemispheric stroke. The European

Cooperative Acute Stroke Study (ECASS). JAMA 1995;274:1017–25.

98. The National Institute of Neurological Disorders and Stroke rt-PA Study Group. Tissue plasminogen activator for acute ischemic stroke. N Engl J Med 1995;333:1581–7.

99. Adams HP, Brott TG, Furlan AJ, et al. Use of thrombolytic drugs. A supplement to the guidelines for the management of patients with acute ischemic stroke. A statement for health care professionals from a special writing group of the Stroke Council, American Heart Association. Stroke 1996; 27:1711–18.

100. Quality Standards Subcommittee of the American Academy of Neurology, Practice Advisory: Thrombolytic therapy for acute ischemic stroke – summary statement. Neurology 1996;47:835–9.

101. Hacke W, Kaste M, Fieschi C, et al. Randomised double-blind placebo-controlled trial of thrombolytic therapy with intravenous alteplase in acute ischaemic stroke (ECASS II). Lancet 1998;352: 1245–51.

102. Donnan GA, Davis SM, Chambers BR, et al. Trials of streptokinase in severe acute ischemic stroke. Lancet 1995;345:578–9.

103. Multicenter Acute Stroke Trial – Italy (MAST-I) Group. Randomised controlled trial of streptokinase, aspirin, and combination of both in treatment of acute ischaemic stroke. Lancet 1995;346:1509–14.

104. The Multicenter Acute Stroke Trial – Europe Study Group. Thrombolytic therapy with streptokinase in acute ischemic stroke. N Engl J Med 1996;335: 145–50.

105. Furlan AJ, Higashida R, Wechsler L, et al. Intra-arterial prourokinase for acute ischemic stroke. The PROACT II Study: a randomized controlled trial. JAMA 1999;282:2003–11.

106. Kidwell CS, Alger R, Saver JL. Beyond mismatch: evolving paradigms in imaging the ischemic penumbra with multimodal magnetic resonance imaging. Stroke 2003;34:2729–35.

107. Wintermark M, Reichhart M, Thiran JP, et al. Prognostic accuracy of cerebral blood flow measurements by perfusion computed tomography, at the time of emergency room admission in acute stroke patients. Ann Neurol 2002;51:417–32.

108. Schellinger PD, Fiebach JB, Hacke W. Imaging-based decision making in thrombolytic therapy for ischemic stroke: present status. Stroke 2003;34:575–83.

109. Molina CA, Saver JL. Extending reperfusion therapy for acute ischemic stroke. Emerging pharmacological, mechanical, and imaging strategies. Stroke 2005;36:2311–20.

2
Antithrombotic drugs: anticoagulants (heparins)

Ángel Chamorro

Unfractionated heparin (UFH)

Heparins comprise a large group of agents, including sodium and calcium UFH, a large number of low-molecular-weight heparins (LMWH), and heparinoids.[1] Discovered by McLean in 1916,[2] UFH is a sulfated polysaccharide with a molecular weight range of 3–30 kDa (mean 15 kDa). Its major anticoagulant effect results from inactivating thrombin (factor IIa) and activated factor X (factor Xa) through an antithrombin III (ATIII)-dependent mechanism.[3] Heparin binds to ATIII through a high affinity pentasaccharide, which is present on about one-third of heparin molecules.[4,5] As the result of heparin binding, ATIII accelerates its ability to inactivate factors IIa, Xa, and IXa, respectively.[6] Molecules of heparin with fewer than 18 saccharides lack the chain length to bridge between thrombin and ATIII and therefore are unable to inhibit thrombin. In contrast, any heparin fragment that contains the pentasaccharide sequence inhibits factor Xa via ATIII.

By inactivating thrombin, heparin not only prevents fibrin formation but also inhibits thrombin-induced activation of platelets and of factors V and VIII. Heparin binds to platelets, and can induce or inhibit platelet aggregation in vitro.[7] Binding of heparin to von Willebrand factor (vWF) inhibits vWF-dependent platelet function.[8] Heparin prolongs the bleeding time in humans[9] and enhances blood loss from the microvasculature in animals.[10] The interaction of heparin with platelets and endothelial cells may contribute to heparin-induced bleeding by a mechanism independent of its anticoagulant effect.[11] UFH has other actions independent of its anticoagulant activity, including increasing vessel wall permeability, inhibition of the proliferation of vascular smooth muscle cells,[12] and promotion of bone loss.[13] The latter effect has to be remembered in those situations, such as pregnancy, where UFH has to be given for extended periods.

The anticoagulant effects of UFH are partially neutralized because its negative charge renders the molecule highly reactive with several plasma proteins and acute-phase reactants. Therefore, the anticoagulant response of UFH is difficult to predict and variable among patients with thromboembolic disorders. It has been shown that the magnitude of the acute-phase response corresponds well to the extent of brain tissue destruction in patients with ischemic stroke.[14] It is therefore very likely that equivalent anticoagulant doses achieve less anticoagulation activity in patients with larger strokes, as the result of stronger binding of UFH to plasma proteins. Binding to plasma proteins could be the reason for many instances of so-called heparin resistance.[15]

Theoretically, UFH could fail to prevent thrombus formation in clinical practice because the heparin/ATIII complex is unable to inactivate factor Xa in the prothrombinase complex or thrombin bound to fibrin or to subendothelial surfaces. Platelets limit the anticoagulant effect of heparin by protecting surface factor Xa from inhibition by heparin/ATIII,[16] and by secreting platelet factor 4 (PF4).[17] Fibrin limits the anticoagulant effect of heparin by protecting fibrin-bound thrombin from inhibition by heparin/ATIII.[18] Thrombin also binds to subendothelial matrix proteins, where it is protected from inhibition by heparin.

UFH: more than anticoagulation

In the 1970s, the prevailing view regarding the pathogenesis of atherosclerosis and secondary thrombus formation was the response-to-injury hypothesis.[19] Towards the end of that decade, it became clear that the endothelium overlying atherosclerotic lesions could be morphologically intact in many patients, and emphasis soon came to be put on the importance of inflammation in the disease process.[20] Further work demonstrated that the expression on the endothelial surface of vascular cell adhesion molecule 1 (VCAM-1), through interaction with its counterligand very late antigen 4 (VLA-4), causes adhesion of monocytes and T cells to endothelium.[21] The role of oxidative mechanisms, including the possibility that oxygen-derived radicals might be involved in the intracellular signaling events controlling VCAM-1 gene expression, also became centrally important in the cell biology of atherosclerosis. These advances in the understanding of the atherosclerotic process could also be relevant to position the role of antithrombotics for brain protection in acute ischemic stroke.

The contribution of inflammatory processes in brain ischemia is well established,[22,23] and inhibition of inflammation could be a part of the beneficial effects of UFH.[24,25] The inflammatory response is preceded by the expression of several cytokines, including tumor necrosis factor α (TNF-α) and interleukin-1β (IL-1β), resulting in chemotactic cytokine release, leukocyte adhesion molecule upregulation, and conversion of the local endothelium to a prothrombotic state. The latter results from impairment of the normal nonthrombogenicity of the endothelial wall,[26] causing activation of other leukocytes, inducing platelet activation and aggregation, and of certain coagulation factors.[27] Leukocyte–endothelial cell interaction is essentially regulated by cell adhesion molecules, which include the selectins, the immunoglobulin (Ig) superfamily, and the integrin superfamily.[28–30]

Cytokines are the key components in the activation and recruitment of leukocytes into ischemic tissue, and the release of acute-phase reactants, such as C-reactive protein (CRP) and fibrinogen, through the activation of hepatocytes.[31] Most cytokines are upregulated at 1 h post ischemia and have a peak response at 6–12 h.[32–34] Also, mRNA expression of TNF-α and IL-1 has been demonstrated as early as 1 h after focal ischemia, with this expression peaking within 12 h and rapidly decreasing over the next 12–48 h.[35,36] Correspondingly, the expression of selectins and of members of the Ig superfamily is detected as early as 1 h after ischemia and persists for several days.[37,38] Moreover, these findings are more pronounced in central nervous system (CNS) reperfusion models.[39,40]

VCAM-1 is an adhesion factor intensely expressed by human astrocytes and endothelial cells from infarcted tissue[41] that induces tissue factor (TF) expression.[42] Following the release of cytokines, TF is the primary cellular initiator of the coagulation cascade in vivo and represents a hemostatic envelope diffusely expressed in human cortex and cerebral vessels.[43] UFH abrogates the endotoxin-induced increase in TF-positive monocytes in vivo and increases plasma levels of TF pathway inhibitor.[44] UFH decreases high TF plasma levels and monocyte procoagulant activity in unstable angina,[45] and perhaps in acute ischemic stroke.[25]

An exciting new field of research concerns the role of UFH as an anti-inflammatory agent. Indeed, this property of heparin is currently under investigation in inflammatory conditions such as Crohn's disease and ulcerative colitis.[46–48] UFH and LMWH inhibit leukocyte rolling on the vessel wall,[49,50] and evidence has also accumulated that this activity depends on the ability of these agents to block selectins on leukocytes and platelets.[51] Although the expression of adhesion molecules seems to be unaffected by UFH, it binds the leukocyte integrin Mac-1 (CD11b/CD18), thereby interfering with the cellular adhesive interactions between leukocytes and endothelial cells.[52] LMWH seem to reduce leukocyte adherence to endothelial cells to a slightly lesser extent than UFH. In vitro, heparin attenuates in a dose-dependent manner the increase in inducible nitric oxide synthase (iNOS) and NO release after cytokine activation.[53] This suggests that heparin influences the cytokine/membrane interaction or the early steps of signal transduction in inflamed endothelial cells.

Yanaka and colleagues showed in a rat ischemic model that animals receiving UFH showed a significant reduction in leukocyte accumulation, infarct size, and neurological dysfunction 48 h after reperfusion when compared with untreated animals.[54] Further, animals that received UFH showed significantly better results than those that received an equivalent anti-coagulant dose of LMWH. Higher doses of UFH were more effective than lower doses. The investigators concluded from these results that the relative potency of sulfated polysaccharides in the inhibition of leuko-cyte accumulation and the reduction of infarct size depends on their degree of sulfation. The same research group assessed the optimum timing of the administration of heparin.[55] In this study, Yanaka and colleagues compared the extent of leukocyte acti-vation, infarct size, and neurological function of rats subjected to transient middle cerebral artery occlusion and allocated to heparin at 3, 6, or 24 h after reper-fusion. In these experiments, animals treated within 3 h after reperfusion did significantly better than those treated at 6 h after reperfusion. Leukocyte activation, as reflected by myeloperoxidase activity, and infarct size were also significantly reduced in the group of animals treated earlier. These experimental data sug-gest that UFH has more potent anti-inflammatory effects than LMWH and that the effects are dose and time-dependent.

Among stroke patients, total leukocyte count[56] and plasma levels of proinflammatory cytokines[57] were also lower in those who were anticoagulated than in comparable patients treated with aspirin. These effects were associated with greater recovery and less risk of clinical decline. Recovery was also associated with a lower increase in VCAM-1 in patients treated with UFH, but not in those treated with aspirin.[58]

UFH is administered by continuous intravenous infusion if an immediate anticoagulant effect is required, or by subcutaneous route. If the latter route is selected, the initial dose must be sufficient to over-come the lower bioavailability, especially if the drug is prescribed at low or moderate doses.[59,60] Because the anticoagulant response to heparin varies among patients with thromboembolic disorders, it is standard practice to adjust the dose of heparin and monitor its effect by measurement of the activated thromboplastin time (aPTT)[61] or, when very high doses are used, by the activated clotting time (aCT). The value of the aPTT is limited because commercial aPTT reagents vary considerably in responsiveness to heparin. Table 2.1 illustrates marked differences in aPTT results corresponding to equivalent plasma

Table 2.1   aPTT results and aPTT ratios between patients and controls corresponding to equivalent therapeutic heparin levels of 0.3–0.5 IU/ml in three Spanish stroke centers.

Center	aPTT ratio (patient/ control)	aPTT (s)	Heparin (IU/ml)
Hospital Clínic, Barcelona	1.6–2.2	49–66	0.3–0.5
Hospital St Pau, Barcelona	1.7–2.7	54–85	0.3–0.5
Hospital J Trueta, Girona	1.8–3.2	53–96	0.3–0.5

heparin levels in three Spanish tertiary hospitals with stroke centers. The aPTT should be measured 6 h after a bolus dose of heparin, and the continuous intravenous dose should be adjusted according to the result. Various dose-adjustment nomograms have been developed for heparin, but none are applicable to all aPTT reagents, and the therapeutic range must be tailored accordingly.[62] Standardization can be achieved by calibration against plasma heparin concentration by using a therapeutic range of 0.3–0.7 IU/ml, based on an anti-factor Xa chromogenic assay, or a heparin level of 0.2–0.4 IU/ml, by protamine sul-fate titration. The dose of heparin should be reduced when it is used concurrently with fibrinolytic agents or intravenous platelet glycoprotein (GP)IIb/IIIa receptor antagonists.

Low-molecular-weight heparins (LMWH)

These are glycosaminoglycans consisting of chains of alternating residues of D-glucosamine and uronic acid that are produced by controlled enzymatic or chemical depolymerization of UFH yielding chains with a mean molecular weight of about 5 kDa.[63] LMWH also exert their anticoagulant activity through AT-dependent mechanisms.[64] However, as fewer than half of the molecules of LMWH have at least 18 saccharide units, LMWH have greater activity against factor Xa than against thrombin. Nevertheless, the relationship between ex vivo mea-sures of factors IIa and Xa inhibition and clinical antithrombotic and antihemostatic effects remains unsettled in the stroke population.

LMWH offer some advantages over UFH since they have a more predictable anticoagulant response, better bioavailability at low doses, dose-independent clearance mechanisms, and longer half-life.[65,66] These properties of LMWH are consequences of their reduced binding to plasma proteins released from activated platelets or endothelial cells, and to the endothelium and macrophages, and their elimination by a nonsaturable renal mechanism.[67,68] As a result, laboratory monitoring of LMWH is unnecessary except in special circumstances, such as in patients with renal insufficiency or extreme weight.[69] LMWH are also said to cause less bleeding than UFH,[70] although LMWH and UFH have been associated with similar rates of bleeding in reported clinical trials. LMWH may carry a lower risk of osteoporosis than UFH.[71]

LMWH are limited by their inability to inactivate thrombin bound to fibrin or to subendothelial surfaces, which represents an important trigger for clot extension at sites of vascular injury.[72] Additional drawbacks of LMWH are the lack of dose-adjustment guidelines, the lack of any specific antagonist in case of bleeding, and the greater expense than UFH. Moreover, LMWH differ from each other in manufacturing methods and their physicochemical, biological, pharmacokinetic, and biotransformation properties. Thus, the clinical findings associated with a given LMWH preparation cannot be extrapolated to a different one, nor can they be generalized to the whole LMWH family without adequate clinical testing.[73]

Adjustment of the potency of LMWH simply on the basis of anti-factor Xa activity is not appropriate, as the ATIII affinity factors responsible for the anti-factor Xa activity only constitute 20–30% of the agent.[74] The remaining 70–80% includes other properties, such as release of tissue factor pathway inhibitor (TFPI), interaction with heparin cofactor II, inhibition of leukocyte procoagulant activity, promotion of fibrinolysis, and modulation of vascular endothelium.

Heparinoids

Danaparoid sodium is a low-molecular-weight heparinoid composed of a mixture of glycosaminoglycans with a mean molecular weight of 5.5 kDa that is isolated from porcine intestinal mucosa.[75] Its anti-factor Xa activity is attributed to its heparan sulfate component. Like other LMWH, danaparoid sodium is not inactivated by endogenous heparin-neutralizing factors and has virtually no effect on platelet function. In light of these properties, heparinoids are theoretically better suited than UFH for safe administration in acute ischemic stroke. However, these agents have proved to be of limited value in clinical practice.

References

1. Frydman A. Low-molecular-weight heparins: An overview of their pharmacodynamics, pharmacokinetics and metabolism in humans. Haemostasis 1996; 26(Suppl):24–38.
2. McLean J. The thromboplastic action of cephalin. Am J Physiol 1916;41:250–7.
3. Rosenberg RD, Lam L. Correlation between structure and function of heparin. Proc Natl Acad Sci USA 1979;76:1218–22.
4. Choay J, Lormeau JC, Petitou M, et al. Structural studies on a biologically active hexasaccharide obtained from heparin. Ann NY Acad Sci 1981;370:644–9.
5. Andersson LO, Barrowcliffe TW, Holmer E, et al. Anticoagulant properties of heparin fractionated by affinity chromatography on matrix-bound antithrombin III and by gel filtration. Thromb Res 1976;9:575–83.
6. Rosenberg RD, Dumas PS. The purification and mechanism of action of human antithrombin-heparin cofactor. J Biol Chem 1973;248:6490–506.
7. Eika C. Inhibition of thrombin-induced aggregation of human platelets in heparin. Scand J Hematol 1971; 8:216–22.
8. Sobel M, McNeill PM, Carlson PL, et al. Heparin inhibition of von Willebrand factor-dependent platelet

function in vitro and in vivo. J Clin Invest 1991;87: 1787–93.

9. Heiden D, Mielke CH, Rodvien R. Impairment by heparin of primary hemostasis and platelet [^{14}C]5-hydroxytryptamine release. Br J Hematol 1977;36:427–36.

10. Blajchman MA, Young E, Ofosu FA. Effects of unfractionated heparin, dermatan sulfate and low molecular weight heparin on vessel wall permeability in rabbits. Ann NY Acad Sci 1989;556:245–54.

11. Fernandez F, Nguyen P, Van Ryn J, et al. Hemorrhagic doses of heparin and other glycosaminoglycans induce a platelet defect. Thromb Res 1986;43:491–5.

12. Clowes AW, Karnovsky MJ. Suppression by heparin of smooth muscle cell proliferation in injured arteries. Nature 1977;265:625–6.

13. Bhandari M, Hirsh J, Weitz J, et al. The effects of standard and low molecular weight heparin on bone nodule formation in vitro. Thromb Haemost 1998; 80:413–17.

14. Chamorro A, Vila N, Ascaso C, et al. Early prediction of stroke severity. Role of the erythrocyte sedimentation rate. Stroke 1995;26:573–6.

15. Lijnen HR, Hoylaerts M, Collen D. Heparin binding properties of human histidine-rich glycoprotein: mechanism and role in the neutralization of heparin in plasma. J Biol Chem 1983;258:3803–8.

16. Marciniak E. Factor X$_a$ inactivation by antithrombin III: evidence for biological stabilization of factor X$_a$ by factor V–phospholipid complex. Br J Haematol 1973;24:391–400.

17. Lanc DA, Pejler G, Flynn AM, et al. Neutralization of heparin-related saccharides by histidine-rich glycoprotein and platelet factor 4. J Biol Chem 1986;261: 3980–6.

18. Weitz JI, Hudoba M, Massel D, et al. Clot-bound thrombin is protected from inhibition by heparin–antithrombin but is susceptible to inactivation by antithrombin III-independent inhibitors. J Clin Invest 1990;86:385–91.

19. Ross R. Response to injury and atherogenesis. Am J Pathol 1977;86:675–84.

20. Munro JM, Cotran RS. The pathogenesis of atherosclerosis: atherogenesis and inflammation. Lab Invest 1988;58:249–61.

21. Cybulsky MI, Gimbrone MA Jr. Endothelial expression of mononuclear leukocyte adhesion molecule during atherogenesis. Science 1991;251:788–91.

22. Kochanek PM, Hallenbeck JM. Polymorphonuclear leukocytes and monocytes/macrophages in the pathogenesis of cerebral ischemic and stroke. Stroke 1992; 23:1367–79.

23. Feuerstein GZ, Liu T, Barone FC. Cytokines, inflammation and brain injury: role of tumor necrosis α. Cerebrovasc Brain Metab Rev 1994;6:341–60.

24. Ott I, Neumann FJ, Gawaz M, et al. Increased neutrophil–platelet adhesion in patients with unstable angina. Circulation 1996;94:1239–46.

25. Chamorro A. Immediate anticoagulation in acute focal brain ischemia revisited. Gathering the evidence. Stroke 2001;32:577–8.

26. Bevilacqua MP, Pober JS, Majeau GR, et al. Recombinant tumor necrosis factor induces procoagulant activity in cultured human vascular endothelium: characterization and comparisons with the actions of interleukin-1. Proc Natl Acad Sci USA 1986;83:4533–7.

27. van Deventer SJH, Büller HR, ten Cate JW, et al. Experimental endotoxemia in humans: analysis of cytokine release and coagulation, fibrinolytic and complement pathways. Blood 1990;76:2520–6.

28. Kishimoto TK, Rothlein R. Integrins, ICAMs and selectins: role and regulation of adhesion molecules in neutrofil recruitment to inflammatory sites. Adv Pharmacol 1994;25:117–69.

29. Rothlein R. Overview of leukocyte adhesion. Neurology 1997;49(Suppl 4):S3–4.

30. Lasky LA. Selectins: interpreters of cell specific carbohydrate information during inflammation. Science 1992;258:964–9.

31. Gauldie J, Northernmann W, Fey GH. IL-6 functions as an exocrine hormone in inflammation. Hepatocytes undergoing acute phase responses require exogenous IL-6. J Immunol 1990;144:3804–8.

32. Minami M, Kuraishi Y, Yabuuchi K, et al. Induction of interleukin 1β mRNA in a rat brain after transient forebrain ischemia. J Neurochem 1991;59:390–2.

33. Liu T, Clark RK, McDonnell PC, et al. Tumor necrosis factor expression in ischemic neurons. Stroke 1994; 25:1481–8.

34. Tarkowski E, Rosengren L, Blomstrand C, et al. Early intrathecal production of interleukin-6 predicts the size of brain lesion in stroke. Stroke 1995;26:1393–8.

35. Lui T, Clark RK, McDonnell PC, et al. Tumor necrosis factor-α expression in ischemic neurons. Stroke 1994; 25:1481–8.

36. Wang X, Yue TL, Barone FC, et al. Concomitant cortical expression of TNF-α and IL-1β mRNAs follows early response gene expression in transient focal ischemia. Mol Chem Neuropathol 1994;23:103–14.

37. Clark WM, Lauten JD, Lessov N, et al. Time course of ICAM-1 expression and leukocyte subset infiltration in rat forebrain ischemia. Mol Chem Neuropathol 1995;26:213–30.

38. Okada Y, Copeland BR, Mori E, et al. P-selectin and intercellular adhesion molecule-1 expression after focal brain ischemia and reperfusion. Stroke 1994; 25:202–11.

39. Kukielka GL, Smith CW, Manning AM, et al. Induction of interleukin-6 synthesis in the myocardium. Potential role in postreperfusion inflammatory injury. Stroke 1995;92:1866–75.

40. Feuerstein GZ, Wang X, Yue TL, Barone FC. Inflammatory cytokines and stroke: emerging new strategies for stroke therapeutics. In: Moskwitz MA, Caplan LR (eds). Cerebrovascular Disease: Nineteenth Princeton Stroke Conference. Newton, MA: Butterworth–Heinemann, 1995:75–91.

41. Blann A, Kumar P, Krupinski J, et al. Solluble intercellular adhesion molecule-1, E-selectin, vascular cell adhesion molecule-1 and von Willebrand factor in stroke. Blood Coagul Fibrinolysis 1999;10:277–84.

42. McGilvray ID, Lu Z, Bitar R, et al. VLA-4 integrin crosslinking on human monocytic THP-1 cells induces tissue factor expression by a mechanism involving mitogen-activated protein kinase. J Biol Chem 1997; 272:10287–94.

43. Drake TA, Morrissey JH, Edgington TS. Selective cellular expression of tissue factor in human tissues. Implications for disorders of hemostasis and thrombosis. Am J Pathol 1989;134:1087–97.

44. Pernerstorfer T, Hansen JB, Knechtelsdorfer M, et al. Heparin blunts endotoxin-induced coagulation activation. Circulation 1999;100:2485–90.

45. Gori AM, Pepe G, Attanasio M, et al. Tissue factor reduction and tissue factor pathway inhibitor release after heparin administration. Thromb Haemost 1999; 81:589–93.

46. Dupas JL, Brazier F, Yzet T, et al. Treatment of active Crohn's disease with heparin. Gastroenterology 1997; 11:A900.

47. Brazier F, Yzet T, Boruchowicz A, et al. Treatment of ulcerative colitis with heparin. Gastroenterology 1997;11:A872.

48. Dwarakanath AD, Yu LG, Brookes C, et al. Sticky neutrophils, pathergic arthritis, and response to heparin in pyoderma gangrenosum complicating ulcerative colitis. Gut 1995;37:585–8.

49. Tangelder GJ, Arfors KE. Inhibition of leukocyte rolling in venules by protamine and sulfated polysaccharides. Blood 1991;77:1565.

50. Ley K, Cerrito M, Arfors KE. Sulfated polysaccharides inhibit rolling in rabbit mesentery venules. Am J Physiol 1991;260:H1667.

51. Nelson RM, Cecconi O, Roberts WG, et al. Heparin oligosaccharides bind L- and P-selectin and inhibit acute inflammation. Blood 1993;11:3253–8.

52. Kitamura N, Yamaguchi M, Shimabukuro K, et al. Heparin-like glycosaminoglycans inhibit leukocyte adhesion to endotoxin activated human vascular endothelial cells under nonstatic conditions. Eur Surg Res 1996;28:428–35.

53. Bonmann E, Júttler E, Krstel HE, Spranger M. Heparin inhibits induction of nitric oxide synthase by cytokines in rat microvascular endothelial cells. Neurosci Lett 1998;253:95–8.

54. Yanaka K, Spellman SR, McCarthy JB, et al. Reduction of brain injury using heparin to inhibit leukocyte accumulation in a rat model of transient focal cerebral ischemia. I. Protective mechanism. J Neurosurg 1996;85:1102–7.

55. Yanaka K, Spellman R, McCarthy JB, et al. Reduction of brain injury using heparin to inhibit leukocyte accumulation in a rat model of transient focal cerebral ischemia. II. Dose–response effect and the therapeutic window. J Neurosurg 1996;85:1108–12.

56. Chamorro A, Obach V, Vila N, et al. A comparison of the acute-phase response in patients with ischemic stroke treated with high-dose heparin or aspirin. J Neurol Sci 2000;178:18–22.

57. Vila N, Castillo J, Dávalos A, Chamorro A. Proinflammatory cytokines and early stroke progression. Stroke 2000;31:2325–9.

58. Chamorro A, Cervera A, Castillo J, et al. Unfractionated heparin is associated with a lower rise of serum vascular cell adhesion molecule-1 in acute ischemic stroke patients. Neurosci Lett 2002;16(328):229–32.

59. Hull RD, Raskob GE, Hirsh J, et al. Continuous intravenous heparin compared with intermittent subcutaneous heparin in the initial treatment of proximal-vein thrombosis. N Engl J Med 1986;315:1109–14.

60. Turpie AGG, Robinson JG, Doyle DJ, et al. Comparison of high-dose with low-dose subcutaneous heparin to prevent left ventricular mural thrombosis in patients with acute transmural anterior myocardial infarction. N Engl J Med 1989;320:352–7.

61. Basu D, Gallus AS, Hirsh J, Cade J. A prospective study of value of monitoring heparin treatment with the activated partial thromboplastin time. N Engl J Med 1972;287:324–7.

62. Raschke RA, Gollihare B, Peirce JC. The effectiveness of implementing the weight-based heparin nomogram as a practice guideline. Arch Intern Med 1996; 156:1645–9.

63. Holmer E, Matsson C, Nilsson S. Anticoagulant and antithrombotic effects of low molecular weight heparin fragments in rabbits. Thromb Res 1982;25:475–85.

64. Samama MM. Contemporary laboratory monitoring of low molecular weight heparins. Clin Lab Med 1995; 15:119–23.

65. Weitz JI. Low-molecular-weight heparins. N Engl J Med 1997;33:688–98.
66. Bara L, Samama MM. Pharmacokinetics of low molecular weight heparins. Acta Chir Scand 1988;543:65–72.
67. Salzman EW, Rosenberg RD, Smith MH, et al. Effect of heparin and heparin fractions on platelet aggregation. J Clin Invest 1980;65:64–73.
68. Blajchman MA, Young E, Ofosu FA. Effects of unfractionated heparin, dermatan sulfate and low molecular weight heparin on vessel wall permeability in rabbits. Ann NY Acad Sci 1989;556:245–54.
69. Kessler CM, Esparraguera IM, Jacobs HM, et al. Monitoring the anticoagulant effects of a low molecular weight heparin preparation. Am J Clin Pathol 1995;103:642–8.
70. Carter CJ, Kelton JG, Hirsh J, et al. The relationship between the hemorrhagic and antithrombotic properties of low molecular weight heparin in rabbits. Blood 1982;59:1239–45.
71. Bhandari M, Hirsh J, Weitz JI. The effect of heparin and low molecular weight heparin on osteoblastogenesis in vitro. Blood 1998;92:1474 (abst).
72. Weitz JI, Hudoba M, Massel D, et al. Clot-bound thrombin is protected from inhibition by heparin–antithrombin III but is susceptible to inactivation by antithrombin III-independent inhibitors. J Clin Invest 1990;86:385–91.
73. Hull RD, Pineo GF. Therapeutic use of low molecular weight heparins. Haemostasis 1993;23(Suppl 1): 2–9.
74. Fareed J, Jeske W, Hoppensteadt D, et al. Are the available low-molecular-weight heparin preparations the same? Semin Thromb Hemost 1996;2(Suppl 1): 77–91.
75. Bradbrook ID, Magnani HN, Moelker HC, et al. ORG 10172: a low molecular weight heparinoid anticoagulant with a long half life in man. Br J Clin Pharmacol 1987;23:667–75.

3
Fibrinolytic agents

Roger Lijnen, Nobuo Nagai, and Désiré Collen

Introduction

Thrombolysis consists of the pharmacological dissolution of a blood clot by administration of agents that activate the fibrinolytic system. The fibrinolytic system includes a proenzyme, plasminogen, which is converted by plasminogen activators to the active enzyme plasmin, which in turn digests fibrin to soluble degradation products. Inhibition of the fibrinolytic system occurs at the level of the plasminogen activator (by plasminogen activator inhibitors, mainly plasminogen activator inhibitor 1, PAI-1) and at the level of plasmin (by plasmin inhibitors, mainly α_2 antiplasmin). Presently available thrombolytic agents include streptokinase, recombinant tissue-type plasminogen activator (rtPA, alteplase), rtPA derivatives (e.g. reteplase, lanoteplase, monteplase, and tenecteplase), anisoylated plasminogen–streptokinase activator complex (APSAC, anistreplase), two-chain urokinase-type plasminogen activator (tcuPA, urokinase), recombinant single-chain uPA (scuPA, prourokinase, saruplase), and recombinant staphylokinase and derivatives. Fibrin-selective agents (rtPA and derivatives, staphylokinase and derivatives, and to a lesser extent scuPA), which digest the clot in the absence of systemic plasminogen activation are distinguished from non-fibrin-selective agents (streptokinase, tcuPA, and APSAC), which activate systemic and fibrin-bound plasminogen relatively indiscriminately (Figure 3.1).[1,2] Some of these newer derivatives are under clinical investigation, mainly in patients with acute myocardial infarction (AMI), but also in those with deep vein thrombosis, peripheral arterial occlusion, pulmonary embolism, and ischemic stroke. In this chapter, we shall review the main properties of fibrinolytic agents with therapeutic potential.

Physicochemical properties of fibrinolytic agents

tPA and variants

Wild-type recombinant tPA (alteplase) was first obtained as a single-chain serine proteinase of 70 kDa, consisting of 527 amino acids with Ser as the N-terminal amino acid; native tPA actually contains an N-terminal extension of three amino acids, but in general the initial numbering system has been maintained (Figure 3.2). Limited plasmic hydrolysis of the Arg^{275}–Ile^{276} peptide bond converts tPA to a two-chain molecule (the A-chain comprising the N-terminal part and the B-chain comprising the C-terminal part) held together by a single interchain disulfide bond. The tPA molecule contains four domains: (1) an N-terminal region of 47 residues (residues 4–50), which is homologous to the finger domains of fibronectin; (2) residues 50–87, which are homologous to epidermal growth factor (EGF); (3) two kringle regions comprising residues 87–176 and 176–262, which are homologous to the five kringles of plasminogen; and (4) a serine proteinase domain (B-chain, residues 276–527) with active site residues His^{322}, Asp^{371}, and Ser^{478}. There are three potential N-glycosylation sites, at Asn^{117}, Asn^{184}, and Asn^{448}.[3] In contrast to the single-chain precursor form of most serine proteinases, single-chain tPA is enzymatically active. The normal plasma concentration of endogenous tPA is about 5–10 ng/ml, but varies strongly under different physiological and pathological conditions.[2] Alteplase is obtained by expression in Chinese hamster ovary cells.

Structure–function analysis has revealed specific functions for the tPA domains. Thus, high-affinity

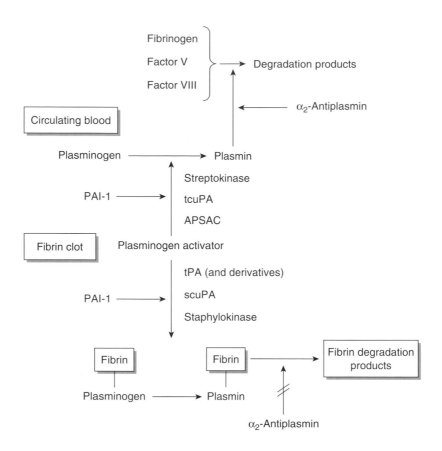

Figure 3.1

Schematic representation of the fibrinolytic system and of molecular interactions determining the fibrin-selectivity of plasminogen activators. The proenzyme plasminogen is activated to the active enzyme plasmin by plasminogen activators. Plasmin degrades fibrin into soluble fibrin degradation products. Inhibition of the fibrinolytic system may occur by plasminogen activator inhibitors (mainly PAI-1) or by plasmin inhibitors (mainly α_2-antiplasmin). Non-fibrin-selective plasminogen activators (streptokinase, tcuPA, and APSAC) activate both plasminogen in the circulating blood and fibrin-associated plasminogen. The generated plasmin is rapidly inactivated by α_2-antiplasmin, and will, after saturation of the inhibitor, degrade other plasma proteins. Fibrin-selective plasminogen activators (tPA, scuPA, and staphylokinase) preferentially activate fibrin-associated plasminogen. The generated plasmin remains associated with fibrin and is protected from rapid inhibition by α_2-antiplasmin.

binding of tPA to fibrin is mediated by the finger and kringle 2 domains; stimulation of its activity by fibrin also involves the finger, kringle 1(?), and kringle 2 domains; in vivo clearance is regulated by the finger and growth factor domains and by the carbohydrate side-chains; rapid inhibition by PAI-1 requires interaction with a positively charged amino acid sequence; and the enzymatic activity resides in the serine proteinase domain.[2] By deletion or substitution of such functional domains, by

site-specific point mutations, and/or by altering the carbohydrate composition, mutant forms of rtPA have been produced with higher fibrin-specificity, more zymogenicity, slower clearance from the circulation, and resistance to plasma proteinase inhibitors.

Reteplase is a single-chain nonglycosylated deletion variant consisting of only the kringle 2 and proteinase domains of human tPA; it contains amino acids 1–3 and 176–527 (deletion of Val^4–Glu^{175}); the

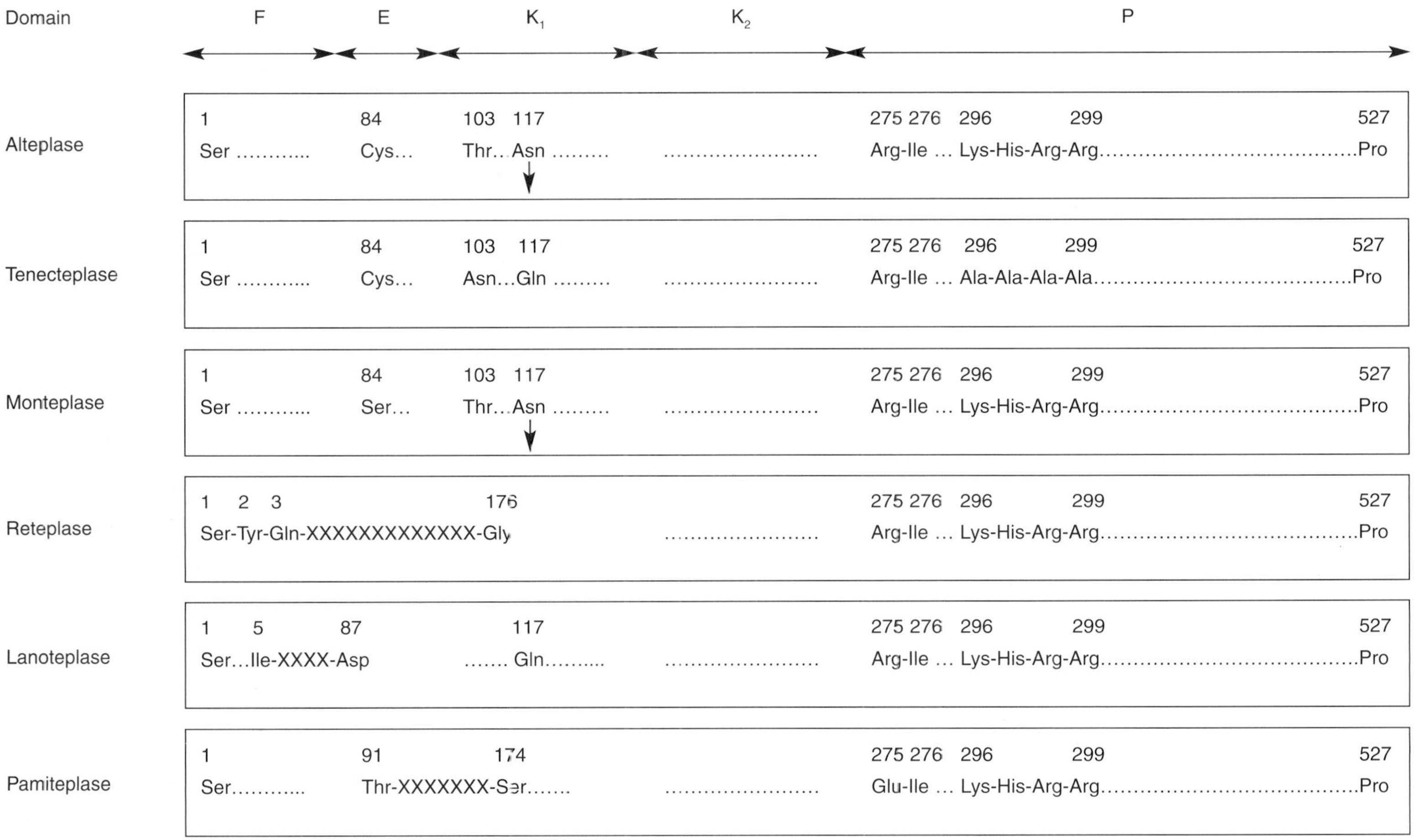

Domain

F   E   K₁   K₂   P

Alteplase

1	84	103 117	275 276	296 299	527
Ser..........	Cys...	Thr...Asn.......→	Arg-Ile ...	Lys-His-Arg-Arg.......	.Pro

Tenecteplase

1	84	103 117	275 276	296 299	527
Ser..........	Cys...	Asn...Gln..........	Arg-Ile ...	Ala-Ala-Ala-Ala.......	.Pro

Monteplase

1	84	103 117	275 276	296 299	527
Ser..........	Ser...	Thr...Asn.......→	Arg-Ile ...	Lys-His-Arg-Arg.......	.Pro

Reteplase

1 2 3	176	275 276	296 299	527
Ser-Tyr-Gln-XXXXXXXXXXXXXX-Gly		Arg-Ile ...	Lys-His-Arg-Arg.......	.Pro

Lanoteplase

1 5 87	117	275 276	296 299	527
Ser..Ile-XXXX-Asp	........Gln..........	Arg-Ile ...	Lys-His-Arg-Arg.......	.Pro

Pamiteplase

1	91 174	275 276	296 299	527
Ser..........	Thr-XXXXXXX-Ser.......	Glu-Ile ...	Lys-His-Arg-Arg.......	.Pro

Figure 3.2

Schematic representation of the structures of wild-type tPA (alteplase), tenecteplase, monteplase, reteplase, lanoteplase, and pamiteplase. F, finger domain; E, growth factor domain; K_1 and K_2, kringle 1 and 2; P, proteinase domain; XXX represents deleted sequences Asn, N-linked glycosylation; (for more details, see text).

Arg^{275}–Ile^{276} plasmin cleavage site is retained.[4] In tenecteplase (TNK-rtPA), replacement of Asn^{117} with Gln (N117Q) deletes the glycosylation site in kringle 1, whereas substitution of Thr^{103} by Asn (T103N) reintroduces a glycosylation site in kringle 1, but at a different locus; these modifications substantially decrease the plasma clearance rate. In addition, the amino acids Lys^{296}–His^{297}–Arg^{298}–Arg^{299} are each replaced with Ala, which confers resistance to inhibition by PAI-1.[5] Lanoteplase is a deletion mutant of rtPA (without the finger and growth factor domains) in which glycosylation at Asn^{117} is lacking.[6] Monteplase has a single amino acid substitution in the growth factor domain (Cys^{84} to Ser);[7] pamiteplase has deletion of the kringle 1 domain and substitution of Arg^{275} to Glu (rendering it resistant to conversion to a two-chain molecule by plasmin).[8] The structures of these rtPA variants are shown schematically in Figure 3.2.

Different molecular forms of the *Desmodus* salivary plasminogen activator (DSPA) have been characterized. Two high-M_r forms, $DSPA\alpha_1$ (desmoteplase, 43 kDa) and $DSPA\alpha_2$ (39 kDa) show about 70–80% structural homology with human tPA, but contain neither a kringle 2 domain nor a plasmin-sensitive cleavage site. $DSPA\beta$ lacks the finger domain and $DSPA\gamma$ lacks the finger and growth factor domains.[9] In several animal models of thrombolysis, $DSPA\alpha_1$ has 2.5-fold greater potency and 4- to 8-fold slower clearance than rtPA.[10,11] In patients with acute ischemic stroke, an elimination half-life of more than 2 h (up to 4.7 h) has been reported, which may have a positive impact on reocclusion rates. Desmoteplase has 70% structural homology to human tPA, but it is a heterologous protein and may be antigenic in humans.

Following intravenous administration of wild-type rtPA, it is cleared from the circulation with an initial half-life of 4–8 min. Clearance is the result of interaction with several receptor systems. Liver endothelial cells have a mannose receptor that recognizes the high-mannose-type carbohydrate side-chain at Asn^{117} in the kringle 1 domain, whereas liver parenchymal cells contain a calcium-dependent receptor that interacts mainly with the growth factor domain of tPA.[12,13] In addition, the low-density lipoprotein receptor-related protein (LRP), expressed in high copy number on hepatocytes, binds free tPA and complexes with PAI-1.[14,15] Several of the rtPA variants have a significantly slower clearance (Table 3.1), allowing bolus administration.

uPA moieties

Urokinase (uPA) is secreted as a 54 kDa single-chain molecule (scuPA, prourokinase) that can be converted to a two-chain form (tcuPA). uPA is a serine proteinase of 411 amino acids, with active site triad His^{204}, Asp^{255}, and Ser^{356} located in the serine proteinase (C-terminal) domain. The molecule contains an N-terminal growth factor domain and one kringle structure homologous to the kringles of plasminogen and tPA;[16] it contains only one N-glycosylation site (at Asn^{302}), and is fucosylated at Thr^{18}. Conversion of scuPA to tcuPA occurs after proteolytic cleavage at position Lys^{158}–Ile^{159} by plasmin, but also by kallikrein, trypsin, cathepsin B, human T-cell-associated serine proteinase 1, and thermolysin. A fully active tcuPA derivative is obtained after additional proteolysis by plasmin at position Lys^{135}–Lys^{136}. A low-M_r form of scuPA is generated by cleavage of the Glu^{143}–Leu^{144} peptide bond. Recombinant scuPA (saruplase) is expressed in *Escherichia coli* and obtained as a 45 kDa non-glycosylated molecule.

Amediplase, a recombinant chimeric plasminogen activator consisting of the kringle 2 domain of the tPA A-chain and the C-terminal region of scuPA, is being evaluated for bolus administration to patients with AMI.[17]

The main mechanism for removal of uPA from the blood is by hepatic clearance. scuPA is taken up in the liver via a recognition site on parenchymal cells and is subsequently degraded in the lysosomes.[18] Following intravenous infusion of recombinant scuPA in AMI patients, a biphasic disappearance was observed, with initial half-life in plasma of 8 min.[19]

Plasmin(ogen) and derivatives

Plasmin, the key enzyme responsible for degradation of fibrin, is generated by activation of the zymogen plasminogen. Human plasminogen is a 92 kDa single-chain glycoprotein, consisting of 791 amino acids; it contains 24 disulfide bonds and 5 homologous

Table 3.1   Properties of fibrinolytic agents

Agent	M_r (kDa)	Plasma $t_{1/2}$ (min)	Fibrin selectivity	Inhibition by PAI-1	Antigenicity
Alteplase	70	4–8	++	Yes	−
Tenecteplase	70	11–20	+++	No	−
Reteplase	39	14–18	+	Yes	−
Lanoteplase	53.5	23–27	+	Yes	−
Monteplase	68	23	++	Yes	−
Pamiteplase	58	30–47	++	Yes	−
Staphylokinase (Sak)	16	3–6	+++	No	++
PEG-Sak	21	15	+++	No	+
Streptokinase	47–50	25[a]	−	No	++
APSAC	≈130	70[a]	±	No	++
Plasmin	85	±840[b]	−	No	−
Microplasmin	29	?	−	No	−

[a]Clearance half-life of the complex with plasminogen.
[b]Clearance of the plasmin–α_2-antiplasmin complex.

kringles.[20] Its normal plasma concentration is 1.5–2.0 μM. It has a half-life of more than 2 days and is cleared via the liver. Native plasminogen has N-terminal glutamic acid ('Glu-plasminogen'), but is easily converted by limited plasmic digestion to modified forms with N-terminal lysine, valine, or methionine, commonly designated 'Lys-plasminogen'. The plasminogen kringles contain lysine-binding sites that mediate the specific binding of plasminogen to fibrin and the interaction of plasmin with α_2-antiplasmin; they play a crucial role in the regulation of fibrinolysis.[21] Conversion to plasmin occurs by cleavage of the Arg^{561}–Val^{562} peptide bond, yielding a two-chain molecule stabilized by two disulfide bonds. Plasmin(ogen) derivatives lacking kringles 1–4 (miniplasmin(ogen)) or consisting only of the proteinase domain (microplasmin(ogen)) have also been characterized.

An engineered plasminogen variant has been constructed with an activation site in which the P3–P1′ residues were substituted by the P7–P1′ residues (Thr^{263}–Ile^{370}) from factor XI. In addition, two mutations were introduced in the proteinase domain, Glu^{606} and Glu^{623} to Lys (BB-10153). The resulting plasminogen moiety is activated by thrombin. It would persist in the blood as a prodrug with long half-life, and be activated to plasmin only at fresh or forming thrombi by localized thrombin. Such an agent could thus be used for bolus administration and may prevent reocclusion by virtue of its long

circulating half-life.[22] It is presently under investigation in animal models.

Staphylokinase and derivatives

Staphylokinase (Sak) is a 135-amino-acid protein (comprising 45 charged amino acids, with no cysteine residues or glycosylation), secreted by Staphylococcus aureus strains after lysogenic conversion or transformation with bacteriophages. The primary structure of Sak shows no homology with that of other plasminogen activators. Staphylokinase folds into a compact ellipsoidal structure in which the core of the protein is composed exclusively of hydrophobic amino acids. It is folded into a mixed five-stranded, slightly twisted β-sheet that wraps around a central α-helix and has two additional short two-stranded β-sheets opposing the central sheet.[23] Recombinant Sak is obtained by expression in E. coli.[24,25]

Being a heterologous protein, Sak is immunogenic in humans. Wild-type Sak contains three immunodominant epitopes. A comprehensive site-directed mutagenesis program resulted in the identification of variants with reduced antigenicity but retained fibrinolytic potency and fibrin-specificity, such as SakSTAR (K35A, E65Q, K74R, E80A, D82A, T90A, E99D, T101S, E108A, K109A, K130T, K135R) (code SY161).[26] Furthermore, SY161 with Ser in position 3 mutated into Cys was derivatized with maleimide-substituted polyethylene glycol (P) with molecular weights of 5 kDa (P5), 10 kDA (P10), or 20 kDa (P20), and characterized in vitro and in vivo.[27] Staphylokinase-related antigen following bolus injection of SY161-P5, SY161-P10, or SY161-P20 in patients disappeared from plasma with initial half-lives of 13, 30, and 120 min and was cleared at rates of 75, 43, and 8 ml/min, respectively, as compared with an initial half-life of 3 min and a clearance of 360 ml/min for wild-type staphylokinase.[27]

Streptokinase and derivatives

Streptokinase is a nonenzyme protein produced by several strains of hemolytic streptococci. It consists of a single polypeptide chain of 47–50 kDa with 414 amino acids.[28] The region comprising amino acids 1–230 shows some homology with trypsin-like serine proteinases, but lacks an active-site serine residue.

APSAC (anistreplase) is an equimolar noncovalent complex between human Lys-plasminogen and streptokinase. The catalytic center is located in the C-terminal region of plasminogen, whereas the lysine-binding sites (with weak fibrin-affinity) are contained within the N-terminal region of the molecule. Specific acylation of the catalytic center in the complex is achieved by the use of a reversible acylating agent, *p*-amidinophenyl-*p'*-anisate hydrochloride. This approach should prevent premature neutralization of the agent in the bloodstream and enable its activation to proceed in a controlled and sustained manner.[29]

Mechanism of action of fibrinolytic agents

tPA and variants

tPA is a poor enzyme in the absence of fibrin, but the presence of fibrin strikingly enhances the activation rate of plasminogen.[30] During fibrinolysis, fibrinogen and fibrin are continuously modified by cleavage with thrombin or plasmin, yielding a diversity of reaction products.[31] Optimal stimulation of tPA is only obtained after early plasmin cleavage in the C-terminal Aα-chain and the N-terminal Bβ-chain of fibrin, yielding fragment X-polymer. Kinetic data support a mechanism in which fibrin provides a surface to which tPA and plasminogen adsorb in a sequential and ordered way, yielding a cyclic ternary complex.[30] Formation of this complex results in an enhanced affinity of tPA for plasminogen, yielding catalytic efficiencies for plasminogen activation up to three orders of magnitude higher. This is mediated at least in part by C-terminal lysine residues generated by plasmin cleavage of fibrin. Plasmin formed at the fibrin surface has both its lysine-binding sites and active site occupied and is thus only slowly inactivated by α_2-antiplasmin (a half-life of about 10–100 s, as compared with about 0.1 s for free plasmin).[21] These molecular interactions mediate the fibrin-specificity of tPA (Figure 3.1).

PAI-1 is the main inhibitor of both tPA and uPA; it is a serpin of 379–381 residues with reactive site peptide bond Arg^{346}–Met^{347}. Rapid inhibition of tPA by PAI-1 involves interaction between a negatively charged region in PAI-1 (residues 350–355) and a positively charged region in tPA (residues 296–304),[32] followed by cleavage of the reactive-site peptide bond and formation of an inactive 1:1 stoichiometric complex.

Reteplase has a similar plasminogenolytic activity as wild-type rtPA in the absence of a stimulator, but its activity in the presence of a stimulator is fourfold lower and its binding to fibrin is fivefold lower. Reteplase and rtPA are inhibited by PAI-1 to a similar degree.[4] Tenecteplase (TNK-rtPA) has a similar ability as wild-type rtPA to bind to fibrin, and lyses fibrin clots in a plasma milieu with enhanced fibrin-specificity and delayed inhibition by PAI-1.[5] DSPAα$_1$ and DSPAα$_2$ exhibit a specific activity in vitro that is equal to or higher than that of rtPA, a relative PAI-1 resistance, and a greatly enhanced fibrin specificity with a strict requirement for polymeric fibrin as a cofactor.[9]

uPA moieties

In contrast to tcuPA, scuPA displays very low activity toward low-molecular-weight chromogenic substrates, but it appears to have some intrinsic plasminogen activating potential, which represents $\leq 0.5\%$ of the catalytic efficiency of tcuPA. In plasma, in the absence of fibrin, scuPA is stable and does not activate plasminogen; however, in the presence of a fibrin clot, scuPA (but not tcuPA) induces fibrin-specific clot lysis.[33,34] This was explained by the finding that scuPA is an inefficient activator of plasminogen bound to internal lysine residues on intact fibrin, but has a higher activity toward plasminogen bound to newly generated C-terminal lysine residues on partially degraded fibrin.[35,36] Rapid inhibition by PAI-1 requires interaction with a positively charged region in uPA (residues 179–184).[37]

Amediplase, containing the tPA kringle 2, displays lower fibrin binding than rtPA, but has higher clot-penetrating potency, similar to that of tcuPA.[38]

Plasmin and derivatives

Plasmin cleaves fibrinogen and fibrin directly, preferentially after Lys and Arg residues. The main plasmin inhibitor is α_2-antiplasmin, a 70 kDa single-chain glycoprotein containing about 13% carbohydrate and 464 amino acids.[39,40] α_2-Antiplasmin is a serpin with reactive site peptide bond Arg^{376}–Met^{377}. Its concentration in normal human plasma is about 7 mg/100 ml (about 1 μM). α_2-Antiplasmin forms an inactive 1:1 stoichiometric complex with plasmin. The inhibition of plasmin (P) by α_2-antiplasmin (A) can be represented by two consecutive reactions: a fast second-order reaction producing a reversible inactive complex (PA), which is followed by a slower first-order transition resulting in an irreversible complex (PA$'$). This model can be represented by P + A $\leftrightarrow$ PA $\rightarrow$ PA$'$. The second-order rate constant of the inhibition of plasmin by α_2-antiplasmin is very high ($2-4 \times 10^7 \, \text{M}^{-1}\text{s}^{-1}$), but this high inhibition rate is dependent both upon the presence of a free lysine-binding site and active site in the plasmin molecule and upon the availability of a plasminogen-binding site and reactive-site peptide bond in the inhibitor.[41] The half-life of plasmin molecules on the fibrin surface, which have both their lysine-binding sites and active site occupied, is estimated to be two to three orders of magnitude longer than that of free plasmin.[42] Also, plasmin moieties lacking the lysine-binding sites

in kringles 1–4 show significantly reduced inhibition rates by α_2-antiplasmin.

Because of the rapid inhibition of plasmin by α_2-antiplasmin and the limited substrate-specificity of excess circulating plasmin, systemic administration of plasmin for thrombolytic therapy is generally not considered to be a valid option. In the 1950s and 1960s, intravenous plasmin for thrombolytic therapy had been investigated in pilot studies in humans. Although plasmin was generally well tolerated, these studies were discontinued, probably because of a lack of understanding of the kinetics of the inhibition of plasmin in plasma (α_2-antiplasmin had not yet been discovered), the unavailability of local catheter delivery, and the lack of adequate methods for the production of stable plasmin devoid of plasminogen activators.[43,44] However, recently, re-examination of local administration of plasmin for arterial and venous thrombolysis has been suggested. This was triggered by a study showing that plasmin induced local thrombolysis without causing hemorrhage in rabbits.[43] Hypothetical advantages of plasmin over plasminogen activators are that (1) no activation is needed; (2) local delivery allows plasmin to attach to and lyse thrombi; and (3) after thrombolysis, circulating plasmin is rapidly neutralized by α_2-antiplasmin. These considerations suggest that local plasmin administration will not cause rebleeding from pre-formed hemostatic plugs and will be efficient and safe for the dissolution of long, retracted blood clots.[45]

The development of adequate methods to produce highly purified and stable natural human plasmin[43] or recombinant human microplasmin[46] preparations has made it possible to reinvestigate the potential of plasmin and its derivatives as fibrinolytic agents. Studies in animal models indicate that plasmin and its derivatives may be useful for the treatment of ischemic stroke. Thus, Nagai et al[47] reported a reduction of infarct size in mice with a permanent ligation of the middle cerebral artery, with a bolus of human plasmin, which was associated with neutralization of plasma α_2-antiplasmin.[48] Microplasmin, lacking the lysine-binding sites, has no affinity for fibrin and is inhibited more slowly by α_2-antiplasmin than intact plasmin; being a truncated molecule, it may be easier to obtain a pharmaceutically useful preparation.[46] In animal models of ischemic stroke and peripheral arterial occlusion, microplasmin was comparable in potency to full-length plasmin. It did not cause a bleeding tendency or hemostatic plug dissolution at distant sites.[46] These data suggest that (micro)-plasmin may be useful for the treatment of arterial thromboembolic disease by local catheter delivery and of ischemic stroke by systemic administration.[43,46]

Staphylokinase and derivatives

Sak forms a 1:1 stoichiometric complex with plasmin. It is not an enzyme, and generation of an active site in its equimolar complex with plasminogen requires conversion of plasminogen to plasmin. In plasma, in the absence of fibrin, no significant amounts of plasmin–Sak complex are generated, because traces of plasmin are inhibited by α_2-antiplasmin. In the presence of fibrin, generation of the active complex is facilitated because traces of fibrin-bound plasmin are protected from α_2-antiplasmin, and inhibition of the complex by α_2-antiplasmin at the clot surface is delayed more than 100-fold. Furthermore, Sak does not bind to a significant extent to plasminogen in circulating plasma, but binds with high affinity to plasmin and to plasminogen that is bound to partially degraded fibrin.[49–51] During the activation process, the 10 N-terminal amino acids of Sak are cleaved off. With SY161-P5, this results in removal of the polyethylene glycol moiety.

Streptokinase and derivatives

Streptokinase activates plasminogen indirectly, following a three-step mechanism.[52] In the first step, streptokinase forms an equimolar complex with plasminogen, which undergoes a conformational change resulting in the exposure of an active site in the plasminogen moiety. In the second step, this active site catalyzes the activation of plasminogen to plasmin. In a third step, plasminogen–streptokinase molecules are converted to plasmin–streptokinase complexes.

The active-site residues in the plasmin–streptokinase complex are the same as those in the plasmin molecule. The main differences between the enzymatic properties of the two moieties are that plasmin, in contrast to its complex with streptokinase, is unable to activate plasminogen, and is rapidly neutralized by α_2-antiplasmin, which does not inhibit the complex. Since streptokinase generates free circulating plasmin when α_2-antiplasmin becomes exhausted, its use is associated with generation of a systemic lytic state.

Reversible blocking of the catalytic site by acylation (APSAC) delays the formation of plasmin but has no influence on the lysine-binding sites involved in binding of the complex to fibrin, although the affinity of plasminogen for fibrin is very weak. Deacylation uncovers the catalytic center, which converts plasminogen to plasmin.[29]

Conclusions

Thrombolytic agents are plasminogen activators that convert the zymogen plasminogen to the active enzyme plasmin, which degrades fibrin. All currently used thrombolytic agents have significant shortcomings, including the need for large therapeutic doses, limited fibrin-specificity and significant associated bleeding tendency and reocclusion. Newly developed thrombolytic agents, mutants, and variants of the serine proteinases tissue-type and urokinase-type plasminogen activators (tPA and uPA) have reduced plasma clearance and lower reactivity with proteinase inhibitors, and maintained or enhanced plasminogen activator potency and/or fibrin-specificity. The nonenzyme bacterial plasminogen activator staphylokinase has also shown promise for fibrin-specific thrombolysis, although neutralizing antibodies are elicited in most patients. Local delivery of plasmin or plasmin derivatives is under investigation for venous and arterial thrombolysis. The therapeutic value of some of these newer agents and approaches remains to be validated.

References

1. Collen D. Thrombolytic therapy. Thromb Haemost 1997;78:742–6.
2. Lijnen HR, Collen D. Tissue-type plasminogen activator. In: Barrett AJ, Rawlings ND, Woessner JF (eds). Handbook of Proteolytic Enzymes. London: Academic Press, 1998:184–90.
3. Pennica D, Holmes WE, Kohr WJ, et al. Cloning and expression of human tissue-type plasminogen activator cDNA in *E. coli*. Nature 1983;301:214–21.
4. Kohnert U, Rudolph R, Verheijen JH, et al. Biochemical properties of the kringle 2 and protease domains are maintained in the refolded t-PA deletion variant BM 06.022. Prot Engineer 1992;5:93–100.
5. Paoni NF, Keyt BA, Refino CJ, et al. A slow clearing, fibrin-specific, PAI-1 resistant variant of t-PA (T103N,KHRR296–299AAAA). Thromb Haemost 1993;70:307–12.
6. Den Heijer P, Vermeer F, Ambrosioni E, et al. Evaluation of a weight-adjusted single-bolus plasminogen activator in patients with myocardial infarction: a double-blind, randomized angiographic trial of lanoteplase versus alteplase. Circulation 1998; 98:2117–25.
7. Suzuki S, Saito M, Suzuki N, et al. Thrombolytic properties of a novel modified human tissue-type plasminogen activator (E6010): a bolus injection of E6010 has equivalent potency of lysing young and aged canine coronary thrombi. J Cardiovasc Pharmacol 1991;17:738–46.
8. Katoh M, Suzuki Y, Miyamoto T. Biochemical and pharmacokinetic properties of YM866, a novel fibrinolytic agent. Thromb Haemost 1991;65:1193 (Abst 1794).
9. Krätzschmar J, Haendler B, Langer G. The plasminogen activator family from the salivary gland of the vampire bat *Desmodus rotundus*: cloning and expression. Gene 1991;105:229–37.
10. Lijnen HR, Collen D. Strategies for the improvement of thrombolytic agents. Thromb Haemost 1991; 66:88–110.
11. Lijnen HR, Collen D. New thrombolytic strategies and agents. Hematologica 2000;85(Suppl 2):106–9.
12. Otter M, Zockova P, Kuiper J, et al. Isolation and characterization of the mannose receptor from human liver potentially involved in the plasma clearance of tissue-type plasminogen activator. Hepatology 1992; 16:54–9.
13. Kuiper J, Van't Hof A, Otter M, et al. Interaction of mutants of tissue-type plasminogen activator with liver cells: effect of domain deletions. Biochem J 1996;313:775–80.
14. Orth K, Madison EL, Gething MJ, et al. Complexes of tissue-type plasminogen activator and its serpin inhibitor plasminogen-activator inhibitor type 1 are internalized by means of the low density lipoprotein receptor-related protein/α_2-macroglobulin receptor. Proc Natl Acad Sci USA 1992;89:7422–6.
15. Bu G, Williams S, Strickland DK, Schwartz AL. Low density lipoprotein receptor-related protein/α_2-macroglobulin receptor is a hepatic receptor for tissue-type plasminogen activator. Proc Natl Acad Sci USA 1992;89:7427–31.
16. Holmes WE, Pennica D, Blaber M, et al. Cloning and expression of the gene for pro-urokinase in *Escherichia coli*. Biotechnology 1985;3:923–9.
17. Amediplase: CGP 42935, K2tu-PA, MEN 9036. BioDrugs 2002;16:378–9.
18. Kuiper J, Rijken DC, de Munk GAW, van Berkel TJ. In vivo and in vitro interaction of high and low molecular weight single-chain urokinase-type plasminogen activator with rat liver cells. J Biol Chem 1992;267:1589–95.
19. Van de Werf F, Vanhaecke J, De Geest H, et al. Coronary thrombolysis with recombinant single-chain urokinase-type plasminogen activator (rscu-PA) in patients with acute myocardial infarction. Circulation 1986; 74:1066–70.
20. Forsgren M, Raden B, Israelsson M, et al. Molecular cloning and characterization of a full-length cDNA clone for human plasminogen. FEBS Lett 1987;213:254–60.
21. Collen D. On the regulation and control of fibrinolysis. Thromb Haemost 1980; 43: 77–89.
22. Dawson KM, Cook A, Devine JM, et al. Plasminogen mutants activated by thrombin: potential thromboselective thrombolytic agents. J Biol Chem 1994;269: 15989–92.
23. Rabijns A, De Bondt HL, De Ranter C. Three-dimensional structure of staphylokinase, a plasminogen activator with therapeutic potential. Nat Struct Biol 1997;4:357–60.
24. Behnke D, Gerlach D. Cloning and expression in *Escherichia coil*, *Bacillus subtilis* and *Streptococcus sanguis* of a gene for staphylokinase: a bacterial plasminogen activator. Mol Gen Genet 1987;210:528–34.
25. Collen D, Zhao ZA, Holvoet P, Marynen P. Primary structure and gene structure of staphylokinase. Fibrinolysis 1992;6:226–31.

26. Laroche Y, Heymans S, Capaert S, et al. Recombinant staphylokinase variants with reduced antigenicity due to elimination of B-lymphocyte epitopes. Blood 2000; 96:1425–32.

27. Collen D, Sinnaeve P, Demarsin E, et al. Polyethylene glycol-derivatized cysteine-substitution variants of recombinant staphylokinase for single-bolus treatment of acute myocardial infarction. Circulation 2000;102:1766–72.

28. Jackson KW, Tang J. Complete amino acid sequence of streptokinase and its homology with serine proteases. Biochemistry 1982;21:6620–5.

29. Smith RAG, Dupe RJ, English PD, Green J. Fibrinolysis with acyl-enzymes: a new approach to thrombolytic therapy. Nature 1981;290:505–8.

30. Hoylaerts M, Rijken DC, Lijnen HR, Collen D. Kinetics of the activation of plasminogen by human tissue plasminogen activator. Role of fibrin. J Biol Chem 1982;257:2912–19.

31. Thorsen S. The mechanism of plasminogen activation and the variability of the fibrin effector during tissue-type plasminogen activator-mediated fibrinolysis. Ann NY Acad Sci 1992;667:52–63.

32. Madison EL, Goldsmith EJ, Gerard RD, et al. Serpin-resistant mutants of human tissue-type plasminogen activator. Nature 1989;339:721–7.

33. Gurewich V, Pannell R, Louie S, et al. Effective and fibrin-specific clot lysis by a zymogen precursor form of urokinase (pro-urokinase). A study in vitro and in two animal species. J Clin Invest 1984;73:1731–9.

34. Lijnen HR, Van Hoef B, Nelles L, Collen D. Plasminogen activation with single-chain urokinase-type plasminogen activator (scu-PA). Studies with active site mutagenized plasminogen (Ser740→Ala) and plasmin-resistant scu-PA (Lys158→Glu). J Biol Chem 1990;265:5232–6.

35. Liu JN, Gurewich V. Fragment E-2 from fibrin substantially enhances pro-urokinase-induced Glu-plasminogen activation. A kinetic study using the plasmin-resistant mutant pro-urokinase Ala-158-rpro-UK. Biochemistry 1992;31:6311–17.

36. Fleury V, Lijnen HR, Anglès-Cano E. Mechanism of the enhanced intrinsic activity of single-chain urokinase-type plasminogen activator during ongoing fibrinolysis. J Biol Chem 1993;268:18554–9.

37. Adams DS, Griffin LA, Nachajko WR, et al. A synthetic DNA encoding a modified human urokinase resistant to inhibition by serum plasminogen activator inhibitor. J Biol Chem 1991;266:8476–82.

38. Rijken DC, Barrett-Bergshoeff MM, Jie AF, et al. Clot penetration and fibrin binding of amediplase, a chimeric plasminogen activator (K2 tu-PA). Thromb Haemost 2004;91:52–60.

39. Holmes WE, Nelles L, Lijnen HR, Collen D. Primary structure of human α_2-antiplasmin, a serine protease inhibitor (serpin). J Biol Chem 1987;262:1659–64.

40. Bangert K, Johnsen AH, Christensen U, Thorsen S. Different N-terminal forms of α_2-plasmin inhibitor in human plasma. Biochem J 1993;291:623–5.

41. Wiman B, Collen D. On the mechanism of the reaction between human α_2-antiplasmin and plasmin. J Biol Chem 1979;254:9291–7.

42. Wiman B, Collen D. On the kinetics of the reaction between human antiplasmin and plasmin. Eur J Biochem 1978;84:573–8.

43. Marder VJ, Landskroner K, Novokhatny V, et al. Plasmin induces local thrombolysis without causing hemorrhage: a comparison with tissue plasminogen activator in the rabbit. Thromb Haemost 2001;86:739–45.

44. Collen D. Revival of plasmin as a therapeutic agent? Thromb Haemost 2001;86:731–2.

45. Novokhatny VV, Jesmok GJ, Landskroner KA, et al. Locally delivered plasmin: why should it be superior to plasminogen activators for direct thrombolysis? Trends in Pharmacol Sci 2004;25:72–5.

46. Nagai N, Demarsin E, Van Hoef B, et al. Recombinant human microplasmin: production and potential therapeutic properties. J Thromb Haemost 2003;1:307–13.

47. Nagai N, De Mol M, Van Hoef B, et al. Depletion of circulating α_2-antiplasmin by intravenous plasmin or immunoneutralization reduces focal cerebral ischemic injury in the absence of arterial recanalization. Hemost Thromb Vasc Biol 2001;97:3086–92.

48. Nagai N, De Mol M, Lijnen HR, et al. Role of plasminogen system components in focal cerebral ischemic infarction. A gene targeting and gene transfer study in mice. Circulation 1999;99:2440–4.

49. Lijnen HR, Collen D. Staphylokinase, a fibrin-specific bacterial plasminogen activator. Fibrinolysis 1996;10:119–26.

50. Collen D. Staphylokinase: a potent, uniquely fibrin-selective thrombolytic agent. Nat Med 1998;4:279–84.

51. Collen D. The plasminogen (fibrinolytic) system. Thromb Haemost 1999;82:259–70.

52. Reddy KNN. Mechanism of activation of human plasminogen by streptokinase. In: Kline DL, Reddy KNN (eds). Fibrinolysis. Boca Raton, FL: CRC Press, 1980:71–94.

4

The vessel wall in thrombosis: relevance to acute stroke therapy

Gerhard F Hamann and Simone Wagner

Interference between vascular walls that have been weakened by ischemic alterations and thrombolytic agents with proteolytic activity is probably the main cause of hemorrhagic complications following acute fibrinolysis in stroke. Hemorrhages are understood as leakage of cellular blood elements in infarcted tissue or as rupture of cerebral arteries. Previous experimental work exaggerated the importance of the cerebral microvasculature vessel wall in generating petechial bleedings leading to confluent hemorrhagic transformation as well as intracerebral hemorrhages. This chapter summarizes the changes in vessel walls following thrombosis and the possible implications for thrombolysis in acute stroke. We shall focus on microvascular changes.

Vessel wall anatomy and physiology

Large arteries consist of endothelium with an underlying internal elastic lamina (together, both are termed the intima), a strong media with elastic fibers and muscle cells for contraction, and, as the last sheet, the adventitia covering the outside of the artery and connecting the arterial wall with the surrounding tissue (Figure 4.1).[1] This pattern is rather uniform in most arteries, but, depending on their location, the content of elastic fibers and of smooth muscle cells may vary substantially.

The cerebral microvasculature is defined by diameter and consists of cerebral precapillary arterioles, capillaries, and the postcapillary venules (vessels < 100 μm

are termed microvessels).[2] Precapillary arterioles lack an internal elastic lamina. Myoendothelial junctions serve as a gateway for endothelial cell influences on the contraction and relaxation of muscle cells.[3] Intradural vessels lack a vasa vasorum and receive their nutritional supply from cerebrospinal fluid.[4]

Unique to the cerebral microvasculature are three major features:

1. Cerebral endothelial cells are connected by tight junctions. These limit transport across the cerebral endothelial barrier. This functionally important border is called the blood–brain barrier (BBB).[5] In addition, the cerebral endothelium has many special functional and growth properties.[6]
2. Cerebral vessels have a very thick and dense basal lamina, which is a specialized part of the extracellular matrix, consisting of two layers connected by entactin. One layer is formed by laminin and the other by collagen type IV. Various other glucosaminoglycans and proteoglycans such as fibronectin and vitronectin are also included in this weblike base for the overlying endothelial cells. Pericytes are incorporated in the basal lamina.[7]
3. Adjacent to the adventitia of the cerebral microvessels is the glia limitans, consisting of astrocyte end-feet. These end-feet may be important for various cell–cell interactions and for the influence of astrocyte changes on microvessels and the influence of microvascular changes on surrounding glial cells.[7]

The unique properties of the cerebral microvasculature are thought to be induced by the close contact

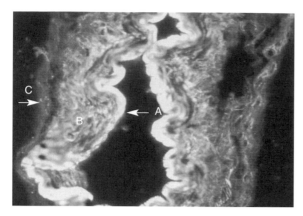

Figure 4.1
Immunofluorescence image of a cerebral artery from the rat stained with collagen type IV and detected by TRITC fluorescence. A, intima; B, media; C, adventitia. Magnification 50x. (See also color plate)

between glial and endothelial cells: cerebral endothelial cells only develop strong BBB functions in the presence of astrocytes. Coculture of these two cell types induces tight junctions, dye exclusion, and antigenic properties such as in vivo brain endothelium.[8] This BBB building effect can also be seen under the influence of soluble factors from astrocytes, which activate endothelial cells to transform to typical cerebral endothelial cells.[9] Brain capillary endothelial barrier function is also influenced by basement membrane proteins. Laminin, collagen type IV, and fibronectin increase the barrier function of cultured primary brain microvessel endothelial cells by 2.3- to 2.9-fold.[10] Laminin seems to be produced by astrocytes under the influence of endothelial cells.[11] This unique presence of specialized endothelial cells, a strong basal lamina, and the surrounding astrocyte sheet are essential for intact barrier function of brain microvessels.

Microvessels form a tree-like branching network in the basal ganglia, and a three-dimensional gridlike web with parallel branching in the cortical regions.[7,12,13] The new technique of 'corrosion casting' permits the angioarchitectural pattern of cerebral vessels to be seen in detail and confirms the previously described pattern of a dense vascular network with many connections in cortical areas.[14] Specific anatomical areas such as hippocampal formations CA1 and CA3 differ

in their capillary density and their ischemic tolerance. The CA1 region is poorly vascularized, and BBB breakdown there is extensive following ischemic insult.[13]

Vessel wall interactions with the coagulation system

In the cerebral endothelium, the reactions with the component of the coagulation system are not completely understood. Endothelial cells produce tissue-type plasminogen activator (tPA), with subsequent activation of the fibrinolytic system by an endogenous pathway.[15] High levels of plasminogen activator inhibitor[1] (PAI-1) are also found on cerebral microvessels.[16,17] The imbalance between fibrinolytic activity and coagulation causes in situ thrombosis in the cerebral vessels. The thrombus can activate various proteolytic pathways, resulting in a severe loss of vessel wall integrity and subsequent brain edema development, as well as extravasation of cellular blood elements. Endothelial pro- and anticoagulatory properties are regulated differently, depending on the vascular territory.[17] The coagulatory properties of the cerebral endothelium are regulated via crosstalk with the surrounding astrocytes. Astrocyte-derived soluble factors regulate tPA and PAI-1 gene transcription and therefore the endothelial coagulation balance.[18] Transforming growth factor β1 (TGF-β1) mediates astrocyte influence on endothelial anticoagulant properties.[19]

Thrombus formation

Thrombus formation always starts with endothelial injury. This endothelial injury might be caused by aggravation of an underlying vessel wall disease (e.g. arteriosclerosis) or by increased shear stress (e.g. trauma induced by intravascular manipulations). The lesion is covered by a few layers of platelets. Release of growth factors activates hyperplasia of the intima and secondary plaque development. Vascular injury with severe endothelial injury (e.g. plaque rupture) may directly activate the intrinsic (by surface activation) or extrinsic (by tissue factor (TF) release) coagulation cascades. In addition, platelets are activated. Growth of the thrombus is regulated by hemodynamic forces, rheologic properties, and activation of the fibrinolytic system; the fibrinolytic system is induced physiologically at the beginning of thrombus formation.[20]

Platelet activation follows a uniform pattern, starting with platelet adhesion, activation, and adherence to the damaged vessel wall. This step is induced by extracellular matrix proteins such as collagen, laminin, fibronectin, and von Willebrand factor (vWF). These proteins interact with specific receptors on the surface of the platelet: collagen with glycoprotein (GP)Ia/IIa and vWF with the GPIb/IX complex. The result of these interactions is adhesion and formation of a monolayer of platelets. Furthermore, these adhesion receptors initiate platelet activation. Binding of vWF or collagen to specific GPs generates outside–in signalling with expression of the GPIIb/IIIa receptor. Interaction of the activated platelets is mediated by binding of fibrinogen to the GPIIb/IIIa receptor. Fibrinogen binds to the receptor on adjacent platelets, ensuring their adhesion. A platelet aggregate is formed, resulting in irreversible deposition at the vessel wall. Platelets may also be activated through activation of different platelet receptors: adenosine diphosphate (ADP), epinephrine, (adrenaline), thrombin, or thromboxane A_2 (TxA$_2$). A platelet plug or white thrombus is often found as a covering of a vessel wall injury. Finally, mixed thrombus forms, when accompanying coagulation processes are activated.

Vessel wall interactions with a thrombus

The development of a thrombus in large arteries is the result of interactions between the vessel wall and the flowing blood. Different mechanisms are involved in this process: a local thrombogenic substrate (e.g. a ruptured plaque with exposure of a thrombogenic intrawall surface with high collagen content), a local flow disturbance with, for example, high-grade stenosis or an ulcerated plaque, and the thrombotic–thrombolytic balance in the circulating blood favoring thrombogenesis by, for example, high fibrinogen content or activated platelets.[21] The thrombogenicity of various vessel wall components varies substantially: physiologically, collagen is a very strongly thrombogenic material, and the lipid core of an arteriosclerotic plaque has a fivefold stronger

capacity to induce a local thrombus.[22] Taking this into account, not only are lipid core plaques very prone to rupture, but are also then very thrombogenic. TF release from the vessel wall or perivascular tissue may also activate the coagulation cascades.[23] A local stenosis activates platelets by shear stress. This shear stress is dependent on the grade of stenosis and the surface of the plaque. High-grade stenosis and rough surfaces induce maximal shear stress, with subsequent strong platelet activation.[24,25] A state of hypercoagulability may occur after infections, as a rebound phenomenon following thrombolysis or inhibition of the coagulation system. It can be due to a defect in the coagulation system with an excess of procoagulatory factors (e.g. fibrinogen or thrombin) or lack of anticoagulatory factors (e.g. protein C or S).

Once a thrombus has been formed, the endothelium undergoes various interactions with its constituents: platelets and leukocytes.[26] The spatiotemporal expression of juxtacrine adhesion and signaling receptors contributes to the coordination of adhesion and inflammatory mechanisms required for prothrombotic imbalanced conditions. MAC-1 (CD11b/CD18) and intercellular adhesion molecule 1 (ICAM-1) act as bridging molecules between leukocytes and fibrinogen and therefore have prothrombotic effects. Leukocytes adherent to the endothelium may induce prothrombotic mechanisms by expressing procoagulatory molecules and promoting thrombin formation. They may induce and activate the expression of coagulation factors by secreted cytokines and proteinases, and activate platelets as well as causing direct damage to the vascular wall by granular secretion products. On the platelet side, these adhesion molecules include P-selectin, which is rapidly translocated from α-granules to the plasma membrane or CD40 ligand. Thrombospondin and fibrinogen serve as bridging factors. These relate to the release of diverse agonists that participate in the amplification of the thrombotic response, such as ADP and platelet-activating factor (PAF).[26]

Microvascular changes in cerebral ischemia

Studies have shown that ischemia and reperfusion initiate related series of pathophysiologic mechanisms.[27,28] Since most studies originally focused on neuronal tissue or glial cells, the changes in cerebral microvessels have only recently become an area of growing interest.[29] There are five different pathophysiologic changes following cerebral ischemia:

1. Loss of BBB function, with subsequent development of edema
2. Change in the patency of microvessels, with secondary changes in microcerebral blood flow (micro-CBF)
3. Expression of endothelial adhesion receptors for immunocompetent blood cells
4. Loss in basal lamina and extracellular matrix antigens, with subsequent hemorrhagic transformation
5. Alterations of cell–matrix adhesion within the microvessels

Loss of BBB function, with subsequent edema development

The barrier function involves three levels: endothelium, basal lamina, and astrocytes. Endothelial changes begin very early following focal cerebral ischemia. As early as 30 min after ischemia, endothelial cell swelling and microvilli formation at the luminal side of the endothelial cells can be observed.[30,31] These findings can be regularly seen after 2 h of ischemia.[32] The endothelial cell nucleus is enlarged and the cell surface is reduced in relation to the volume. Longer periods of ischemia lead to an intense swelling of the cytoplasm, increased number of mitochondria, and activated pinocytosis.[31] The swelling leads to a reduced capillary diameter and may contribute to the so-called no-reflow phenomenon.[33] Studies of endothelial barrier antigen (EBA), a marker for intact cerebral endothelium (but not for tight junctions) showed a loss of about 40–50% of microvessels compared with the nonischemic side.[34] These nonstained vessels may have severe endothelial dysfunction. Later, endothelial cells rupture and expose the subendothelial matrix to the intravasal fluids and cells. The only tight barrier at this stage is the basal lamina, which prevents leakage of blood into the surrounding brain tissue. Changes in the basal lamina will be discussed in detail later.

One consequence of the loss of barrier function is the extravasation of blood components, especially of the large fibrin molecule.[35,36] Fibrin extravasation and platelet accumulation are connected; therefore, the use of GPIIb/IIIa receptor antagonists seems to be advantageous to prevent fibrin/platelet-derived secondary damage. This was proven in a murine middle cerebral artery occlusion (MCA-O) model, which had reduced infarct sizes of 70%.[37] Heparin was also shown to improve outcome after experimental stroke; underlying mechanisms may be variable, and may include increased vascular patency.[38,39]

Change in the patency of microvessels with secondary micro-CBF changes

The occlusion of a proximal cerebral artery causes a reduction in the number of distal patent microvessels. Fragmentation of thrombotic material that has come out of solution of the thrombus is thought to be a major source of reduced microvessel patency. In rats, the injection of emboli leads to an absence of flow in most cerebral microvessels in the territory of the occluded vessel. In cortical areas, after 3 h, all microvessels are reopened; on the other hand, in the basal ganglia, only 50% are reopened.[40] This different pattern of microvascular patency may be responsible for the relative low ischemia tolerance in the striatum. Garcia et al[41] emphasized that the swelling of endothelial cells and astrocytes after induction may contribute substantially to secondary neuronal death, since the time course of the evolving infarct showed early changes in endothelial cells and astrocytes (within 30–60 min), but a peak in neuronal death at 72 h. Similar findings were later reproduced, emphasizing the role in rats of reactive astrocytes as contributors to impaired microvessel perfusion after an embolic stroke.[42,43] Microvascular perfusion may also contribute to the extent to which a penumbra persists after cerebral ischemia. Dawson et al[44] showed that microvessels in the penumbra region display a late (4 h MCA-O) perfusion deficit contributing to the recruitment of the penumbra to the ischemic zone.

Expression of endothelial adhesion receptors for immunocompetent blood cells

Immunocompetent blood-derived cells occluding cerebral microvessels are an attractive concept to explain reduced microvascular patency. This interaction between leukocytes and the vascular wall is mainly

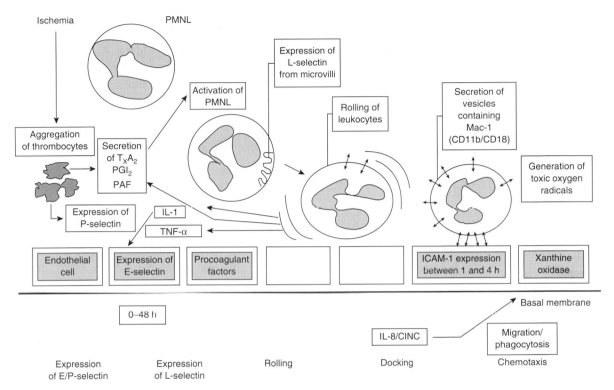

Figure 4.2
Infiltration of leukocytes into the brain in experimental ischemia. CINC, cytokine-induced neutrophil chemoattractant; ICAM-1, intercellular adhesion molecule; IL, interleukin; PAF, platelet-activating factor; PGI_2, prostacyclin; PMNL, polymorphonuclear leukocyte; TNF-α, tumor necrosis factor α; TxA_2, thromboxane A_2.

initiated by the secretion or expression of various adhesion receptors on the endothelium. P-selectin, ICAM-1, and E-selectin are the main players here. They are expressed in a typical pattern after experimental stroke.[45,46] The typical steps in leukocyte recruitment are initial contact (tethering), rolling, firm adhesion and migration (Figure 4.2).

The initial contact can be modulated by P (platelet)- or E (endothelium)-selectin, vascular cell adhesion molecule 1 (VCAM-1), or L (leukocyte)-selectin. The selectins as glycoproteins interact with carbohydrate ligands on activated leukocytes and can be generated by, for example, free radicals or activated coagulation factors.[47] P-selectin is released by preformed storage granules, the so-called Weibel–Palade bodies, in platelets.[48] The selectins and VCAM-1 are also involved in the rolling process. In the next step, cytokine release by astrocytes or endothelial cells, mainly interleukin-1β (IL-1β) and tumor necrosis factor α (TNF-α), leads to the expression of ICAM-1 and also E-selectin on

the endothelial surface.[49] These adhesion molecules and the chemoattractants result in a strong binding and invasion of mainly polymorphonuclear leukocytes (PMNL). ICAM-1 reacts with the β_2 integrins, especially CD11b and CD18, on the leukocyte membrane.[50] Granular enzymes of neutrophils digest parts of the basal lamina and increase microvascular trauma rather than salvaging the threatened tissue.[2]

Loss in basal lamina and extracellular matrix antigens, with subsequent hemorrhagic transformation

Using the 'awake stroke' model in baboons,[51] Hamann et al[52,53] demonstrated that first the cerebral microvessel walls become gradually bleached and lose basal membrane constituents, which are finally destroyed, depending on the duration of ischemia/reperfusion (Figure 4.3). A quantitative analysis of

Cerebral microvessels following ischemia/reperfusion

Normal cerebral microvessels

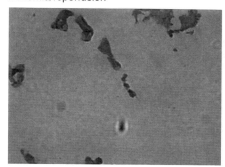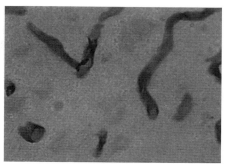

Figure 4.3
Loss in microvascular basal lamina staining following cerebral ischemia/reperfusion: basal ganglia of the rat, anti-collagen IV immunohistochemistry.[60] Magnification 400x. (See also color plate)

immunohistochemically stained vessels within the ischemic basal ganglia and the corresponding regions of the nonischemic side showed a significant reduction of the content of diverse basal lamina antigens (laminin, fibronectin, and collagen type IV). Microvascular basal lamina damage is also important for the BBB disturbances following ischemic stroke.[54–56] Well-known experimental and clinical consequences of these microvessel wall alterations are edema, as a result of endothelial functional deficiency resulting in loss of integrity, as well as leakage of cellular blood elements to form hemorrhages (Figure 4.4).[53,57,58] Research into the proteolytic cascades involved in basal lamina damage and their prevention may in the long term lead to the development of strategies to prevent secondary hemorrhagic complications in stroke patients.[58,59] These results have been reproduced in rats and extended by new findings in cortical microvascular injury.[60]

Alterations of cell–matrix adhesion within the microvessels

Specific receptors link the abluminal side of the endothelium with the basal lamina, and the basal lamina with the astrocytes. It appears that the heterodimeric integrins are the most important cell-to-matrix and matrix-to-cell anchors.[57] Integrin $\alpha_6\beta_4$ seems to connect astrocytes with laminin in the extracellular matrix,[61] whereas integrin $\alpha_1\beta_1$ stabilizes the endothelium by binding to laminin in

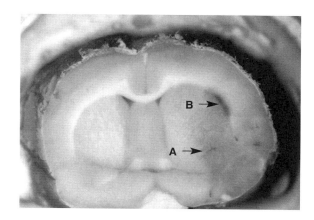

Figure 4.4
Coronal section of an ischemic rat brain: A, petechial bleeding in the infarcted basal ganglia; B, bleeding in the left ventricle. (See also color plate)

the basal lamina.[62] Loss of these structural adhesion complexes occurs very early after experimental ischemia, and is therefore thought to be a prerequisite for the subsequent basal lamina antigen loss.[61]

Mechanisms of microvascular alterations

At least four major proteolytic pathways are induced in ischemic damage:[58,59] the plasminogen–plasmin system, matrix metalloproteinases (MMPs), polymorphonuclear granulocytes, and platelets (Figure 4.5).

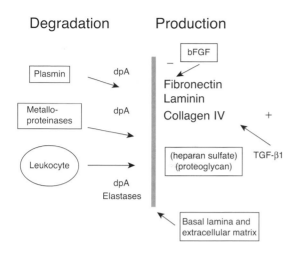

Degradation   Production

Figure 4.5
Pathophysiologic concept of ischemic vessel wall alterations. bFGF, basic fibroblast growth factor; dpA, direct proteolytic activity; TGF-β1, transforming growth factor β1.

The plasminogen–plasmin system

This system is especially interesting, since the first drug licensed for acute stroke treatment was recombinant tPA (rtPA), which has been used in routine clinical stroke treatment following the National Institute of Neurological Disorders and Stroke (NINDS) Study in 1995.[63] The plasminogen–plasmin system is very important for endothelial cells, which produce high levels of tPA. This prevents wall thrombosis and counteracts the antifibrinolytic effects of PAI-1.[17,64] This local balance in this system seems to be relevant for both the occlusion and the reopening of the microvasculature.[2] Unfortunately, the end-product of the plasminogen cascade, plasmin, is a very potent proteinase, able to cleave various components of the extracellular matrix (e.g. laminin).[64,65] The plasminogen–plasmin system cannot directly cleave collagen type IV, but it activates MMPs by transforming inactivated forms into active ones (Figure 4.6).[66,67] Inhibition of MMP activity following the experimental administration of rtPA reduced the frequency of postischemic cerebral hemorrhages in a rabbit stroke model.[68] Administered rtPA results paradoxically in reduced PAI-1 release from the brain endothelium, which might explain the high vulnerability of the brain to the development of hemorrhagic complications

compared with other organs.[69] The difference between administered plasminogen activators and endogenous variants must be emphasized, since it has been shown that tPA deficient mice are more prone to develop microvascular thrombosis compared with wild-type mice.[70] Endogenous tPA has good and bad sides: it prevents local microvascular thrombosis, but in connection with low PAI-1 levels it may digest the vessel wall. Figure 4.7 shows the extent of plasminogen activation from brain sections following different periods of ischemia/reperfusion according to Pfefferkorn et al.[67]

The MMP system

Most of the work in this field is by Rosenberg's group and shows that the appearance of MMPs after ischemia leads to brain edema and hemorrhage.[55,71–74] Rosenberg et al[71] have also shown that the expression of MMPs is related to reperfusion and, interestingly, that the main peak of MMP activity is seen after 12–24 h of reperfusion. A new technique that permits a microscopic analysis of MMP activity shows an increase in gelatine overlay digestion restricted to the ischemic core (Figure 4.8).[75] More detailed insights into the complex MMP system revealed that proMMP-9 (the inactive proform, which is activated by cleavage to MMP-9) is increased in mice from 2 h to 24 h after experimental stroke. Active MMP-9 is seen after 4 h, with subsequent BBB disruption shown by Evans-blue leakage. Tissue inhibitor of matrix metalloproteinase 1 (TIMP-1) expression was not altered at any time, and proMMP-2 levels were elevated after 24 h following the ischemia.[76] Active MMP-2 was not detected. On the other hand, MMP-2 was significantly increased as early as 1 h after ischemia and was associated with neuronal injury in the non-human primate.[77] In this model, MMP-9 was elevated only in animals with hemorrhagic transformation. The therapeutic efficacy of preventing secondary edema by inhibitors of the MMP system has also been established.[78,79] Inhibition of MMPs protects the BBB from postischemic oxidative stress in mice.[80] Whether this positive effect on brain edema formation or BBB function can be directly transferred to neuronal protection has been questioned by a study using MMP-2 gene knockouts.[81] Figure 4.9 summarizes the regulation and interactions of MMPs.

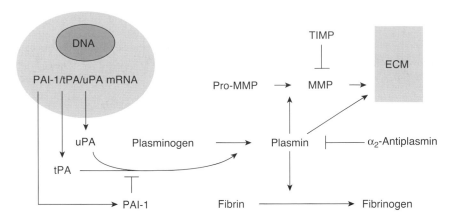

Figure 4.6
The plasminogen–plasmin system and its connection with the matrix metalloproteinase (MMP) system. ECM, extracellular matrix; MMP, matrix metalloproteinase; PAI-1, plasminogen activator inhibitor 1; TIMP, tissue inhibitor of matrix metalloproteinase; tPA, tissue-type plasminogen activator; uPA, urokinase-type plasminogen activator.

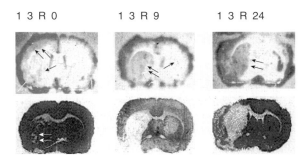

Figure 4.7
Brain section with an overlay containing plasminogen. The plasminogen activators from the underlying brain generate plasmin. Plasmin digests casein in the overlay, and clear lysis zones become visible at the sites of plasminogen activator activity. There is a steady increase in plasminogen activator activity over prolonged periods of ischemia/reperfusion. (See also color plate)

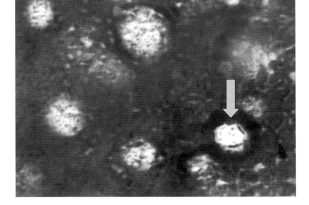

Figure 4.8
High magnification (400x) of a gelatin overlay on brain tissue with an acute infarct. Holes (see arrow) are produced from gelatinolytic activity from the underlying brain.[75] (See also color plate)

Polymorphonuclear granulocytes

These invasive cells are able to secrete digestive enzymes, such as human neutrophil elastase and cathepsin G.[57,82] Elastases are potent enzymes that digest the basal lamina components, especially laminin.[82,83] The invasion of leukocytes starts 12 h after the onset of cerebral ischemia and peaks at 24 h.[84] Even this early leukocyte adhesion results in increased vascular leakage (Figure 4.3).[85] Leukocytes are also known to occlude cerebral vessels resulting in the 'no-reflow' phenomenon.[86] This phenomenon has been described even after 2 hours ischemia and 1 hour reperfusion in rats.[87]

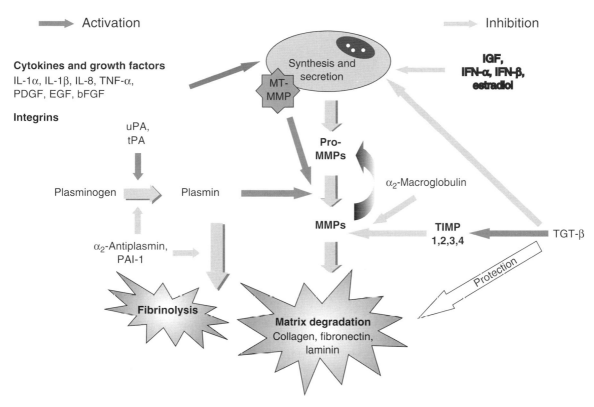

Figure 4.9
Regulation of matrix metalloproteinases (MMPs) and their interactions with various signaling pathways and other proteolytic systems. bFGF, basic fibroblast growth factor; EGF, epidermal growth factor; IFN, interferon; IGF, insulin-like growth factor; IL, interleukin; MT-MMP, membrane-bound MMP; PAI-1, plasminogen activator inhibitor 1; PDGF, platelet-derived growth factor; TGF-β, transforming growth factor β; TIMP, tissue inhibitor of matrix metalloproteinase; TNF-α, tumor necrosis factor α; tPA, tissue-type plasminogen activator; uPA, urokinase-type plasminogen activator.

Platelets

We know much about interactions between vessel walls and platelets in large arteries (see above). In contrast, less is known about platelet behavior in the microvasculature.[88] In an embolic stroke model in the rat, platelet accumulation in the microvasculature was associated with a loss in collagen type IV staining and simultaneous fibrin deposition in the damaged microvessels.[89] Platelet deposition in distal vessels is postulated to be relevant for the thrombolysis resistance that develops over long periods of ischemia and for the loss in vascular integrity with secondary hemorrhages.

Bleeding complications after ischemic stroke

Hemorrhages after ischemic stroke can be either clinically silent hemorrhagic transformations or life-threatening hematomas. Both forms may complicate stroke therapy, especially thrombolysis. Only in rare cases can a large ruptured vessel be implicated – for example, a case of secondary in situ dissection of a cardioembolic occluded middle cerebral artery has been reported.[90] Our current understanding of ischemic stroke-related hemorrhagic complications focuses on the cerebral microvasculature. As discussed above, the gradual bleaching of the microvascular basal lamina[52,60] is a prerequisite for the leakage of cellular blood elements.[53] Loss of microvascular basal lamina is directly associated with the development of petechial hemorrhages, which are the precursors of larger confluating hemorrhages and hematomas.[50,57–59] Clinical observations confirm this theory. Long periods of ischemia and reperfusion foster hemorrhagic complications in both experimental and clinical settings.[53,91] In a rat embolic stroke model, the administration of rtPA after 6 h was associated with hemorrhagic transformation in 50% of cases, whereas no hemorrhagic complications were found following the use of rtPA after 2 hours.[92] Spontaneous intracerebral hematomas may also have a similar pathophysiologic explanation. Small chronic hemorrhages and ischemic lesions are frequently associated with intracerebral hematomas.[93] Acute blood pressure changes and small asymptomatic ischemic lesions may initiate intracerebral hematomas.[58,59]

Present clinical implications

Microvascular damage results in more severe brain edema as well as the development of hemorrhages. Taking this into account, a high-risk population for the development of bleeding complications can be seen in patients with:

- advanced age
- signs of severe microangiopathy (lacunar strokes or confluent white matter lesions)
- severe hypertension and/or diabetes or vasculitis

Several well-known conditions that are aggravated by advancing age, long-term hypertension, and diabetes target the microvasculature and may contribute to a loss of microvascular integrity.[2] These include lipohyalinosis and microangiopathy, which have been classified in three states of damage severity:[94]

1. sclerotic and hyalinotic thickening of the vessel wall with 'onion-skinning', which primarily affects arterioles of 100–200 μm diameter
2. Additional disorganization of the vessel wall and disruption of the internal elastic lamina with occasional foam cells (these changes may be associated with hematoma formation)
3. Additional fibrinoid degeneration of the vessel wall with thrombosis.

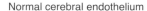

Normal cerebral endothelium

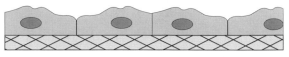

Damaged endothelium after ischemia and reperfusion

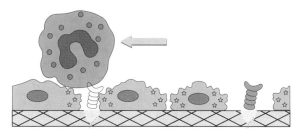

Potential protection

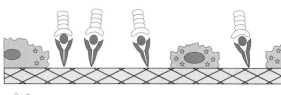

 = Plasmin

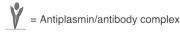 = Antiplasmin/antibody complex

Figure 4.10
Principle of antibody-directed enzyme (pro)drug therapy (ADEPT): normal endothelium in the upper part, damaged endothelium in the middle part, and protection by antiplasmin/antibody complexes in the lower part.[58,59]

The deposition of amyloid in the vessel wall (amyloid angiopathy) also leads to loss of vascular wall integrity, leakage, and later hemorrhagic changes.[95] Most experimental models of focal ischemia do not mimic these age-dependent vascular changes, which may also explain the rare occurrence of large hemorrhages in animal models compared with humans.

Prolonged periods of ischemia/reperfusion lead to more severe microvascular damage. The risk of post-ischemic hemorrhage might be reduced by following strict protocols for therapeutic thrombolysis within the well-known time window (within 3 h). Imaging techniques may help in the future to identify patients at risk and to detect even the earliest stage of hemorrhagic transformation.

Future developments

Strategies to prevent microvascular damage with subsequent hemorrhage include:[58,59]

- definite classification of damaged tissue with high bleeding risk
- laboratory tests of the extent of basal lamina damage
- protection of basal lamina structures

The first strategy is discussed extensively elsewhere in this book. Laboratory tests are still under development. Potentially useful markers include laminin, collagen type IV, and fibronectin breakdown products. These products of proteolytic basal lamina digestion can be determined by enzyme-linked immunosorbent assay (ELISA) or western blotting. However, these techniques take hours to give results. Therefore, they are not suitable for urgent decision making in hyperacute stroke patients. A bedside test for the breakdown products might be helpful, but is not yet available.

Therapeutic protection of the basal lamina deserves more attention, since different approaches may soon be ready for use. A combined therapy of hypothermia and thrombolysis may be more effective in microvascular protection. Hypothermia effectively reduces brain swelling and edema formation.[96,97] New devices with rapid and effective cooling may help to bring clinical trials closer to testing the combined use of hypothermia with thrombolysis. Other pharmacologic strategies such as inhibition of the plasminogen–plasmin system, the MMP system, leukocyte invasion, or platelet accumulation are available. However, they are not specific. General inhibition of the plasmin system might be deleterious, and might even counteract the primary therapeutic goal of recanalization. Also, global MMP, platelet, or leukocyte inhibition might cause susceptibility to severe infections or cause more severe general bleeding. Additionally, the toxicity and relatively low specificity of various MMP antagonists is a problem. These attempts would be much more effective if it were possible to restrict the antiproteolytic effect to the injured microvessel wall. Therefore, we have adopted a strategy of antibody-directed enzyme (pro)drug therapy (ADEPT) and have tested it in a rat model of stroke.[59] An antibody against laminin recognizes the injured endothelium with exposed basal lamina. This antibody is linked with an antiproteolytic agent (e.g. α_2-antiplasmin) and counteracts the local proteolytic effect of the plasminogen–plasmin system (Figure 4.10). This strategy may be used clinically to increase the safety of thrombolysis or to increase its efficacy by allowing higher dosages of thrombolytic agents without the risk of bleeding complications.

References

1. Baker AB, Iannone A. Cerebrovascular disease III: the intracerebrales arterioles. Neurology 1959;9:441–6.
2. del Zoppo GJ. Microvascular changes during cerebral ischemia and reperfusion. Cerebrovasc Brain Metab Rev 1994;6:47–96.
3. Hamann GF, del Zoppo GJ. Leukocyte involvement in vasomotor reactivity of the cerebral vasculature. Stroke 1994;25:2117–19.
4. Liszczak TM, Black PM, Varsos VG, Zervas NT. The microcirculation of cerebral arteries: a morphologic and morphometric examination of the major canine cerebral arteries. Am J Anat 1984;170:223–32.
5. Partridge WM. Introduction to the Blood–Brain Barrier. Cambridge: Cambridge University Press, 1998.
6. Thorin E, Shatos MA, Shreeve SM, et al. Human vascular endothelium heterogeneity. A comparative study of cerebral and peripheral cultured vascular endothelial cells. Stroke 1997;28:375–81.
7. Hodde K, Sercombe R. The anatomy of the brain vasculature. In: Mraovitch S, Sercombe R (eds). Neurophysiological Basis of Cerebral Blood Flow Control: An Introduction. London: John Libbey, 1996.
8. Hurwitz AA, Berman JW, Rashbaum WK, Lyman WD. Human fetal astrocytes induce the expression of

blood–brain barrier specific proteins by autologous endothelial cells. Brain Res 1993;625:238–43.

9. Lobrinus JA, Juillerat-Jeanneret L, Darekar P, et al. Induction of the blood–brain barrier specific HT7 and neurothelin epitopes in endothelial cells of the chick chorioallantoic vessels by a soluble factor derived from astrocytes. Brain Res Dev Brain Res 1992;70:207–11.

10. Tilling T, Korte D, Hoheisel D, Galla HJ. Basement membrane proteins influence brain capillary endothelial barrier function in vitro. J Neurochem 1998;71: 1151–7.

11. Wagner S, Gardner H. Modes of regulation of laminin-5 production by rat astrocytes. Neurosci Lett 2000;284: 105–8.

12. Bär T. Morphometric evaluation of capillaries in different laminae of rat cerebral cortex by automatic image analysis: changes during development and aging. Adv Neurol 1978;20:1–9.

13. Cavaglia M, Dombrowski SM, Drazba J, et al. Regional variation in brain capillary density and vascular response to ischemia. Brain Res 2001;910:81–93.

14. Reina-De La Torre F, Rodriguez-Baeza A, Sahuquillo-Barris J. Morphological characteristics and distribution pattern of the arterial vessels in human cerebral cortex: a scanning electron microscope study. Anat Rec 1998;251:87–96.

15. Zlokovic BV, Wang L, Sun N, et al. Expression of tissue plasminogen activator in cerebral capillaries: possible fibrinolytic function of the blood–brain barrier. Neurosurgery 1995;37:955–61.

16. Fisher M, Francis R. Altered coagulation in cerebral ischemia. Platelet, thrombin, and plasmin activity. Arch Neurol 1990;47:1075–9.

17. Lijnen HR, Collen D. Endothelium in hemostasis and thrombosis. Prog Cardiovasc Dis 1997;39:343–50.

18. Tran ND, Schreiber SS, Fisher M. Astrocyte regulation of endothelial tissue plasminogen activator in a blood–brain barrier model. J Cereb Blood Flow Metab 1998;18:1316–24.

19. Tran ND, Correale J, Schreiber SS, Fisher M. Transforming growth factor-β mediates astrocyte-specific regulation of brain endothelial anticoagulant factors. Stroke 1999;30:1671–8.

20. Badimon L, Badimon JJ, Fuster V. Pathogenesis of thrombosis. In: Verstraete M, Fuster V, Topol EJ (eds). Cardiovascular Thrombosis. Philadelphia: Lippincott–Raven, 1998:23–44.

21. Falk E, Fuster V, Shah PK. Interrelationship between atherosclerosis and thrombosis. In: Verstraete M, Fuster V, Topol EJ (eds). Cardiovascular Thrombosis. Philadelphia: Lippincott–Raven, 1998:45–58.

22. Fernandez-Ortiz A, Badimon JJ, Falk E, et al. Characterization of the relative thrombogenicity of atherosclerotic plaque components: implications for consequences of plaque rupture. J Am Coll Cardiol 1994;23:1562–9.

23. Moreno PR, Bernardi VH, Lopez-Cuellar J, et al. Macrophages, smooth muscle cells, and tissue factor in unstable angina. Implications for cell-mediated thrombogenicity in acute coronary syndromes. Circulation 1996;94:3090–7.

24. Ruggeri ZM. Mechanisms of shear-induced platelet adhesion and aggregation. Thromb Haemost 1993;70: 119–23.

25. de Cesare NB, Ellis SG, Williamson PR, et al. Early reocclusion after successful thrombolysis is related to lesion length and roughness. Coron Artery Dis 1993; 4:159–66.

26. May AE, Neumann FJ, Preissner KT. The relevance of blood cell–vessel wall adhesive interactions for vascular thrombotic disease. Thromb Haemost 1999;82:962–70.

27. Dietrich WD. Neurobiology of stroke. Int Rev Neurobiol 1998;42:55–101.

28. Dirnagl U, Iadecola C, Moskowitz MA. Pathobiology of ischaemic stroke: an integrated view. Trend Neurosci 1999;22:391–7.

29. del Zoppo GJ, Hallenbeck JM. Advances in the vascular pathophysiology of ischemic stroke. Thromb Res 2000;98:73–81.

30. Naganuma Y. Changes of the cerebral microvascular structure and endothelium during the course of permanent ischemia. Keio J Med 1990;39:26–31.

31. Dietrich WD. Morphological manifestations of reperfusion injury in brain. Ann NY Acad Sci 1994;723: 15–24.

32. Okumura Y, Sakaki T, Hiramatsu K, et al. Microvascular changes associated with postischaemic hypoperfusion in rats. Acta Neurochir (Wien) 1997; 139:670–6.

33. Ames A 3rd, Wright RL, Kowada M, et al. Cerebral ischemia. II. The no-reflow phenomenon. Am J Pathol 1968;52:437–53.

34. Lin B, Ginsberg MD. Quantitative assessment of the normal cerebral microvasculature by endothelial barrier antigen (EBA) immunohistochemistry: application to focal cerebral ischemia. Brain Res 2000;865:237–44.

35. Okada Y, Copeland BR, Fitridge R, et al. Fibrin contributes to microvascular obstructions and parenchymal changes during early focal cerebral ischemia and reperfusion. Stroke 1994;25:1847–53.

36. Zhang ZG, Chopp M, Goussev A, et al. Cerebral microvascular obstruction by fibrin is associated with upregulation of PAI-1 acutely after onset of

focal embolic ischemia in rats. J Neurosci 1999;19: 10898–907.

37. Choudhri TF, Hoh BL, Zerwes HG et al. Reduced microvascular thrombosis and improved outcome in acute murine stroke by inhibiting GP IIb/IIIa receptor-mediated platelet aggregation. J Clin Invest 1998;102:1301–10.

38. Li PA, He QP, Siddiqui MM, Shuaib A. Posttreatment with low molecular weight heparin reduces brain edema and infarct volume in rats subjected to thrombotic middle cerebral artery occlusion. Brain Res 1998;801:220–3.

39. Quartermain D, Li Y, Jonas S. Enoxaparin, a low molecular weight heparin, decreases infarct size and improves sensorimotor function in a rat model of focal cerebral ischemia. Neurosci Lett 2000;288:155–8.

40. Wang CX, Todd KG, Yang Y, et al. Patency of cerebral microvessels after focal embolic stroke in the rat. J Cereb Blood Flow Metab 2001;21:413–21.

41. Garcia JH, Liu KF, Yoshida Y, et al. Brain microvessels: factors altering their patency after the occlusion of a middle cerebral artery (Wistar rat). Am J Pathol 1994; 145:728–40.

42. Zhang ZG, Bower L, Zhang RL, et al. Three-dimensional measurement of cerebral microvascular plasma perfusion, glial fibrillary acidic protein and microtubule associated protein-2 immunoreactivity after embolic stroke in rats: a double fluorescent labeled laser-scanning confocal microscopic study. Brain Res 1999;844:55–66.

43. Zhang Z, Davies K, Prostak J, et al. Quantitation of microvascular plasma perfusion and neuronal microtubule-associated protein in ischemic mouse brain by laser-scanning confocal microscopy. J Cereb Blood Flow Metab 1999;19:68–78.

44. Dawson DA, Ruetzler CA, Hallenbeck JM. Temporal impairment of microcirculatory perfusion following focal cerebral ischemia in the spontaneously hypertensive rat. Brain Res 1997;749:200–8.

45. Okada Y, Copeland BR, Mori E, et al. P-selectin and intercellular adhesion molecule-1 expression after focal brain ischemia and reperfusion. Stroke 1994;25: 202–11.

46. Haring HP, Berg EL, Tsurushita N, et al. E-selectin appears in nonischemic tissue during experimental focal cerebral ischemia. Stroke 1996;27:1386–91.

47. Patel KD, Zimmerman GA, Prescott SM, et al. Oxygen radicals induce human endothelial cells to express GMP-140 and bind neutrophils. J Cell Biol 1991;112: 749–59.

48. McEver RP. Selectins: novel receptors that mediate leukocyte adhesion during inflammation. Thromb Haemost 1991;65:223–8.

49. Weller A, Isenmann S, Vestweber D. Cloning of the mouse endothelial selectins. Expression of both E- and P-selectin is inducible by tumor necrosis factor α. J Biol Chem 1992;267:15176–83.

50. Petty MA, Wettstein JG. Elements of cerebral microvascular ischaemia. Brain Res Rev 2001;36:23–34.

51. del Zoppo GJ, Copeland BR, Harker LA, et al. Experimental acute thrombotic stroke in baboons. Stroke 1986;17:1254–65.

52. Hamann GF, Okada Y, Fitridge R, del Zoppo GJ. Microvascular basal lamina antigens disappear during cerebral ischemia and reperfusion. Stroke 1995;26: 2120–6.

53. Hamann GF, Okada Y, del Zoppo GJ. Hemorrhagic transformation and microvascular integrity during focal cerebral ischemia/reperfusion. J Cereb Blood Flow Metab 1996;16:1373–8.

54. Betz AL, Iannotti F, Hoff JT. Brain edema: a classification based on blood–brain barrier integrity. Cerebrovasc Brain Metab Rev 1989;1:133–54.

55. Rosenberg GA. Ischemic brain edema. Prog Cardiovasc Dis 1999;42:209–16.

56. Neuwelt EA, Abbott NJ, Drewes L, et al. Cerebrovascular biology and the various neural barriers: challenges and future directions. Neurosurgery 1999;44:604–8.

57. del Zoppo GJ, von Kummer R, Hamann GF. Ischaemic damage of brain microvessels: inherent risks for thrombolytic treatment in stroke. J Neurol Neurosurg Psychiatr 1998;65:1–9.

58. Hamann GF, del Zoppo GJ, von Kummer R. Hemorrhagic transformation of cerebral infarction – possible mechanisms. Thromb Haemost 1999; 82(Suppl):92–4.

59. Hamann GF, del Zoppo GJ, von Kummer R. Mechanisms for the development of intracranial haemorrhage. Possible implications for thrombolysis in cerebral infarct. Nervenarzt 1999;70:1116–20.

60. Hamann GF, Liebetrau M, Martens H, et al. Microvascular basal lamina injury following experimental focal cerebral ischemia and reperfusion in the rat. J Cereb Blood Flow Metab 2002;22(5):526–33.

61. Wagner S, Tagaya M, Koziol JA, et al. Rapid disruption of an astrocyte interaction with the extracellular matrix mediated by integrin $\alpha_6\beta_4$ during focal cerebral ischemia/reperfusion. Stroke 1997;28:858–65.

62. Haring HP, Akamine BS, Habermann R, et al. Distribution of integrin-like immunoreactivity on primate brain microvasculature. J Neuropathol Exp Neurol 1996;55:236–45.

63. The National Institute of Neurological Disorders and Stroke rt-PA Stroke Study Group. Tissue plasminogen

activator for acute ischemic stroke. N Engl J Med 1995;333:1581–7.

64. Lijnen HR, Van Hoef B, Lupu F, et al. Function of the plasminogen/plasmin and matrix metalloproteinase systems after vascular injury in mice with targeted inactivation of fibrinolytic system genes. Arterioscler Thromb Vasc Biol 1998;18:1035–45.

65. Liotta LA, Goldfarb RH, Terranova VP. Cleavage of laminin by thrombin and plasmin: α thrombin selectively cleaves the β chain of laminin. Thromb Res 1981;21:663–73.

66. Lijnen HR, Luou F, Moons L, et al. Temporal and topographic matrix metalloproteinase expression after vascular injury in mice. Thromb Haemost 1999; 81:799–807.

67. Pfefferkorn T, Staufer B, Liebetrau M, et al. Plasminogen activation in focal cerebral ischemia and reperfusion. J Cereb Blood Flow Metab 2000;20: 337–42.

68. Lapchak PA, Chapman DF, Zivin JA. Metalloproteinase inhibition reduces thrombolytic (tissue plasminogen activator)-induced haemorrhage after thrombo-embolic stroke. Stroke 2000;31:3034–40.

69. Shatos MA, Doherty JM, Penar PL, Sobel BE. Suppression of plasminogen activator inhibitor-1 release from human cerebral endothelium by plasminogen activators. A factor potentially predisposing to intracranial bleeding. Circulation 1996;94:636–42.

70. Tabrizi P, Wang L, Seeds N, et al. Tissue plasminogen activator (tPA) deficiency exacerbates cerebrovascular fibrin deposition and brain injury in a murine stroke model: studies in tPA-deficient mice and wild-type mice on a matched genetic background. Arterioscler Thromb Vasc Biol 1999;19:2801–6.

71. Rosenberg GA, Navratil M, Barone F, Feuerstein G. Proteolytic cascade enzymes increase in focal cerebral ischemia in rat. J Cereb Blood Flow Metab 1996; 16:360–6.

72. Rosenberg GA, Estrada EY, Dencoff JE. Matrix metalloproteinases and TIMPs are associated with blood–brain barrier opening after reperfusion in rat brain. Stroke 1998;29:2189–95.

73. Mun-Bryce S, Rosenberg GA. Matrix metalloproteinases in cerebrovascular disease. J Cereb Blood Flow Metab 1998;18:1163–72.

74. Rosenberg GA, Cunningham LA, Wallace J, et al. Immunohistochemistry of matrix metalloproteinases in reperfusion injury to rat brain: activation of MMP-9 linked to stromelysin-1 and microglia in cell cultures. Brain Res 2001;893:104–12.

75. Loy M, Burggraf D, Martens KH, et al. A gelatin in-situ-overlay technique localizes brain matrix metalloproteinase activity in experimental focal cerebral ischemia. J Neurosci Meth 2002;116:125–33.

76. Gasche Y, Fujimura M, Morita-Fujimura Y, et al. Early appearance of activated matrix metalloproteinase-9 after focal cerebral ischemia in mice: a possible role in blood–brain barrier dysfunction. J Cereb Blood Flow Metab 1999;19:1020–8.

77. Heo JH, Lucero J, Abumiya T, et al. Matrix metalloproteinases increase very early during experimental focal cerebral ischemia. J Cereb Blood Flow Metab 1999;19:624–33.

78. Rosenberg GA, Kornfeld M, Estrada EY, et al. TIMP-2 reduces proteolytic opening of blood–brain barrier by type IV collagenase. Brain Res 1992;576: 203–7.

79. Rosenberg GA, Navratil M. Metalloproteinase inhibition blocks edema in intracerebral haemorrhage in the rat. Neurology 1997;48:921–6.

80. Gasche Y, Copin JC, Sugawara T, et al. Matrix metalloproteinase inhibition prevents oxidative stress-associated blood–brain barrier disruption after transient focal cerebral ischemia. J Cereb Blood Flow Metab 2001;21:1393–400.

81. Asahi M, Sumii T, Fini ME, et al. Matrix metalloproteinase 2 gene knockout has no effect on acute brain injury after focal ischemia. Neuroreport 2001;12:3003–7.

82. Heck LW, Blackburn WD, Irwin MH, Abrahamson DR. Degradation of basement membrane laminin by human neutrophil elastase and cathepsin G. Am J Pathol 1990;136:1267–74.

83. Armao D, Kornfeld EY, Estrada M, et al. Neutral proteases and disruption of the blood–brain barrier in rat. Brain Res 1997;767:259–64.

84. Garcia JH, Liu KF, Yoshida Y, et al. Influx of leukocytes and platelets in an evolving brain infarct (Wistar rat). Am J Pathol 1994;144:188–99.

85. He P, Wang J, Zeng M. Leukocyte adhesion and microvessel permeability. Am J Physiol Heart Circ Physiol 2000;278:H1686–94.

86. Ember JA, del Zoppo GJ, Mori E, et al. Polymorphonuclear leukocyte behavior in a nonhuman primate focal ischemia model. J Cereb Blood Flow Metab 1994;14:1046–54.

87. Ritter LS, Orozco JA, Coull BM, et al. Leukocyte accumulation and hemodynamic changes in the cerebral microcirculation during early reperfusion after stroke. Stroke 2000;31:1153–61.

88. Dietrich WD, Dewanjee S, Prado R, et al. Transient platelet accumulation in the rat brain after common carotid artery thrombosis. An ^{111}In-labeled platelet study. Stroke 1993;24:1534–40.

89. Zhang ZG, Zhang L, Tsang W, et al. Dynamic platelet accumulation at the site of the occluded middle cerebral artery and in downstream microvessels is associated with loss of microvascular integrity after embolic middle cerebral artery occlusion. Brain Res 2001;912:181–94.

90. de Freitas GR, Carruzzo A, Tsiskaridze A, et al. Massive haemorrhagic transformation in cardio-embolic stroke: the role of arterial wall trauma and dissection. J Neurol Neurosurg Psychiatry 2001;70: 672–4.

91. Molina CA, Montaner J, Abilleira S, et al. Timing of spontaneous recanalization and risk of hemorrhagic transformation in acute cardioembolic stroke. Stroke 2001;32:1079–84.

92. Kano T, Katayama Y, Tejima E, Lo EH. Hemorrhagic transformation after fibrinolytic therapy with tissue plasminogen activator in a rat thromboembolic model of stroke. Brain Res 2000;854:245–8.

93. Tanaka A, Ueno Y, Nakayama Y, et al. Small chronic haemorrhages and ischemic lesions in association with spontaneous intracerebral haematomas. Stroke 1999;30:1637–42.

94. Brun A, Fredriksson K, Gustafson L. Pure subcortical atherosclerotic encephalopathy (Binswanger disease): a clinicopathological study. Cerebrovasc Dis 1992;2:87–92.

95. Vinters HV, Wang ZZ, Secor DL. Brain parenchymal and microvascular amyloid in Alzheimer's disease. Brain Pathol 1996;6:179–95.

96. Park CK, Jun SS, Kim MC, Kang JK. Effects of systemic hypothermia and selective brain cooling on ischemic brain damage and swelling. Acta Neurochir Suppl (Wien) 1998;71:225-8.

97. Schwab S, Georgidis D, Berouschot J, et al. Feasibility and safety of moderate hypothermia after massive hemispheric infarction. Stroke 2001; 32: 2033–5.

5

Thrombosis, atherothrombosis, and thromboembolism in the etiology of stroke

Stephen M Davis and Peter J Hand

Introduction

Stroke is estimated to affect 20 million people worldwide each year, with at least 5 million deaths.[1,2] Of these cases, about 80–85% are ischemic in type. Unlike myocardial infarction, the leading cause of death in Western countries, the pathogenesis of ischemic stroke is heterogeneous (Table 5.1). Major subtypes include large-artery atherosclerosis, cardiogenic embolism, small-vessel occlusion involving the deep perforating arteries, stroke due to rarer causes (e.g. arterial dissection, other arteriopathies, and procoagulant states), and a large group in which pathogenesis remains uncertain.[3]

Of these subtypes, atherosclerotic disease affecting the major extracranial arteries has traditionally been regarded as the most common pathogenesis. However, intracranial atherosclerosis is more common in some racial groups, such as African-Americans and Asians. The description by Fisher and colleagues of lacunar syndromes, due to small-vessel disease, led to the delineation of these very common infarct types, using clinical and neuroimaging techniques.[4] Complex atheroma in the aortic arch has more recently been recognized as an important, independent risk factor for stroke.[5,6] Of a variety of cardioembolic sources, nonvalvular atrial fibrillation remains the most important. In recent years, the increasing use of

Table 5.1   Pathogenetic subtypes of ischemic stroke[3]

Subtypes	Comments
1. Large-artery atherosclerosis	• The most common subtype worldwide • Usually due to thromboembolism • Typically extracranial in Caucasians; often intracranial in African-Americans and Asians
2. Cardioembolism	• Most commonly due to nonvalvular atrial fibrillation • Uncertain management for rarer causes (e.g. patent foramen ovale)
3. Small-vessel occlusion	• A common stroke subtype, particularly in Asians • Usually due to in situ thrombosis, but may be embolic
4. Stroke of other determined etiology	• More prevalent in young adult stroke patients • Includes rarer causes, such as dissection, prothrombotic states, and vasculitis
5. Stroke of undetermined etiology	• Despite adequate investigation, 20% of strokes remain cryptogenic

transesophageal echocardiography (TEE) has led to a great deal of interest in alternative cardiac sources such as patent foramen ovale and atrial septal aneurysm.

Although most ischemic strokes in Caucasians are due to thromboembolism to intracranial vessels from an extracranial source, prothrombotic causes of in situ intracerebral thrombosis are also important in younger patients. When considering the use of antithrombotic and thrombolytic therapies for stroke, understanding of the specific pathogenesis is likely to be important. For the rational selection of secondary prevention techniques, it is essential.

Atherosclerosis and stroke

The major complication of atherosclerosis is thrombosis, with local thrombotic occlusion or distal thromboembolism.[7] It accounts for at least 20% of all strokes, diagnostic criteria including evidence of relevant arterial stenosis and exclusion of other causes.[7,8] Wepfer first recognized the significance of carotid occlusion in 1658 and its relationship to underlying 'fibrous masses' (atherosclerosis) and thrombus.[9] Willis[10] related carotid occlusion to the risk of apoplexy. In the 19th century, Virchow and others related carotid occlusive disease to cerebral ischemic symptoms.[9] Chiari[11] described thrombo-embolism from carotid atherosclerosis to intracranial vessels in 1905. In 1914, Hunt[12] urged pathological examination of the major extracranial arteries in ischemic stroke – frequently overlooked in previous clinical and pathological studies. The importance of carotid occlusion was again highlighted by the intro-duction of arteriography by Moniz et al.[13] Despite these earlier publications, there was still a prevailing view in the early 1950s that most ischemic strokes were due to intracerebral artery thrombosis.

Carotid atherosclerosis

The work of Fisher[14] in the early 1950s and a number of autopsy studies[15–24] changed this per-ception, demonstrating that the predominant site for atherosclerosis was the extracranial internal carotid artery at the carotid bifurcation (Figures 5.1 and 5.2). Other sites were the carotid siphon, the proximal and

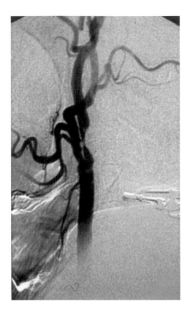

Figure 5.1
Carotid angiogram demonstrating severe internal carotid stenosis.

distal vertebral arteries, and the midbasilar artery (Table 5.2). In contrast, intracranial lesions were found to be very rare. These, and more recent patho-logical studies,[25] indicated that the thrombus often found at autopsy in intracranial vessels emanated from extracranial atherosclerotic lesions. Fisher[21] reported a 9.5% incidence of near or total occlusion of at least one extracranial carotid artery in 432 con-secutive adult autopsies. Adams and Vander Eecken[15] pointed out that fatty streaks in the aorta occurred in 95% of subjects by the age of 16 years, the cerebral arteries being affected later. Hutchinson and Yates[16] also emphasized that extracranial atherosclerosis was the major cause of cerebral infarction. Martin et al[18] confirmed that the maximal degree of carotid athero-sclerosis was present at the carotid bifurcation and in the proximal 2 cm of the internal carotid artery. In those with cerebral ischemia, most had greater than 50% stenosis of at least one major extracranial artery.[26]

There were no sex differences in distribution or severity (although this has since been refuted).[27,28] Fisher et al[26] found that the degree of atherosclerosis increased with age. Fisher emphasized that these lesions were frequently asymptomatic and that intracranial atherosclerosis was less common.

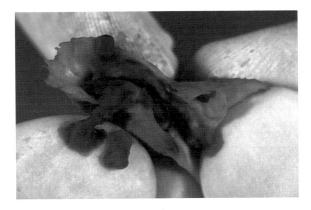

Figure 5.2
Endarterectomy specimen showing thrombus in the internal carotid artery. (See also color plate)

Table 5.2   Racial differences in cerebrovascular atherosclerosis

Population group	Distribution of atherosclerosis
Caucasians	• Predominantly extracranial disease • Common carotid bifurcation • Vertebral artery origins and distal sites • Basilar artery • Aortic arch
African-Americans	• Predominantly intracranial disease • Supraclinoid internal carotid artery, middle cerebral stem • Distal basilar, intracranial posterior circulation
Asians	• Predominantly distal intracranial atherosclerosis • Middle cerebral stenosis and lacunes common

Blackwood et al[23] found a good correlation between atheromatous internal carotid obstruction and intracranial occlusion, and that in situ middle cerebral artery thrombosis was very uncommon. They also emphasized the importance of cardiogenic brain embolism.[23] Lhermitte et al[22] and Castaigne et al,[30] studying patients with cerebral ischemia, found that atherosclerotic internal carotid artery occlusion with superimposed thrombosis was common. Recent and old emboli in the intracranial distribution and anterograde thrombus from the site of the occlusive thrombosis into the brain were frequent findings.

Following these autopsy studies, carotid ultrasound studies demonstrated the prevalence of extracranial atherosclerosis in larger cohorts. Josse et al[31] found that in men aged 75–84 years, 6.1% had greater than 50% stenosis. Prati et al[32] found a 25% prevalence of carotid atherosclerosis, both intimal–medial thickening and frank plaque formation. Hennerici et al[33] studied 2009 asymptomatic patients with severe peripheral or coronary heart disease or with multiple risk factors. They found a particularly high correlation between carotid disease and peripheral atherosclerosis. Colgan et al[34] found that only 4% of unselected volunteers had greater than 50% carotid stenosis. Li et al[35] insonated the extracranial carotid arteries in 14 046 individuals in a community-based study and showed correlations between plaque development, age, Caucasian race, and male gender. Even in young adult strokes, atherosclerosis still accounts for between 15%[36] and 30%[37,38] of ischemic strokes in adults younger than 50 years.

Vertebrobasilar atherosclerosis

Hutchinson and Yates[16,39] found that proximal vertebral atherosclerosis was common in stroke patients, contrasting with the less affected intracerebral arteries. However, Fisher et al[29] found that all symptomatic vertebrobasilar occlusions were intracranial, and that cervical occlusions tended to be asymptomatic. Various authors[19] found that vertebral atherosclerosis was less common and severe than carotid disease. Castaigne et al[30] found that the distal vertebral artery was more commonly affected by thrombosis than the proximal vessel, while nearly all basilar artery occlusions were due to localized atherosclerosis, rather than embolism from a proximal source (Figure 5.3).

Intracranial atherosclerosis and racial differences

Caplan pointed out that most autopsy and angiographic studies had been performed on White, predominantly male subjects and that intracranial atherosclerosis is more common in Blacks, Asians,

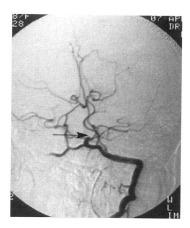

Figure 5.3
Vertebral digital subtraction angiogram showing severe basilar atherosclerosis (arrow).

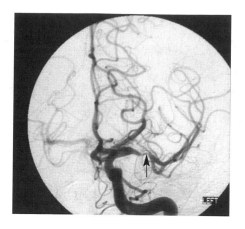

Figure 5.4
Carotid angiogram showing advanced middle cerebral artery atherosclerosis.

women, and diabetic patients[40–42] (Figure 5.4). The Joint Study of Extracranial Arterial Occlusion[38] reported that Blacks had more occlusive, intracranial disease. Other investigators[40,44–47] also showed that African-Americans had more atherosclerotic lesions of the supraclinoid internal carotid artery and the middle cerebral artery stem, contrasting with the extracranial predominance in Whites, and that these differences could not be explained by variations in risk factors. Caplan's group[40,48] found that while White patients had more lesions of the vertebral origins, Blacks had more lesions in the distal basilar and intracranial posterior circulation vessels. Diabetes was also associated with intracranial arterial disease.

The pattern of predominant intracranial atherosclerosis in African-Americans appears to be similar to findings in Asian populations, both exhibiting intracranial lesions in the large arteries, as well as a greater rate of small-vessel disease and lacunar infarction.[49–51]

Aortic arch atheroma

Earlier investigators had pointed out that the aortic arch is a prominent site for the formation of atherosclerosis,[18,29] but the importance of aortic arch atheroma in the pathogenesis of cerebral ischemia has been highlighted more recently as an important independent risk factor for ischemic stroke, presumably as an embolic nidus.[52] Using an autopsy databank, Amarenco et al[53] found that complex

aortic arch plaques occurred in 28% of patients with cerebral infarction. In a case–control study using TEE,[5] atherosclerotic plaques of thickness greater than 4 mm were found in 14.4% of patients with ischemic stroke, but in only 2% of controls, such plaques being most common in patients without a known cause of stroke (Figure 5.5). Jones et al[6] also found that aortic arch atheroma was an independent risk factor, with an increased odds of 7.1 for complex atheroma. A recent study suggested that both thickness and extent of aortic atheroma predicted recurrence of ischemic stroke.[54] Davila-Roman et al[55] used intraoperative aortic ultrasound on 12 000 patients undergoing cardiac surgery, finding aortic arch atheroma in 19.3% of patients, independently correlating with a history of cerebral ischemia, age, smoking, or coronary or peripheral vascular disease. Management is quite uncertain,[56] and aortic arch endarterectomy has been associated with a high stroke rate.[57]

Mechanisms of cerebral ischemia due to atherosclerosis

Hemodynamic and embolic mechanisms

Early workers emphasized the importance of hemodynamic mechanisms in transient or sustained cerebral ischemia. For instance, Denny-Brown[58,59]

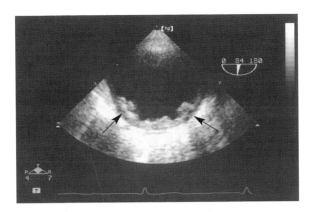

Figure 5.5
Transesophageal echocardiogram showing protruberent atheromatous plaques in the aortic arch
(arrows). (See also color plate)

considered that internal carotid stenosis could
produce a state of 'episodic insufficiency' in the circle
of Willis, whereby a hemodynamic crisis could be
produced by systemic hypotension. Meyer et al[60] also
described 'cerebral hemodynamic crises'.

In 1948, Pickering[61] first proposed an embolic
basis for transient ischemic attacks (TIAs). He
suggested that they were due to transient obstruction
of a cerebral artery or arteriole. Fisher[14,21] coined the
term 'transient attacks' and linked them to extracranial occlusive disease. He later reported the efficacy
of anticoagulants in their prevention, favoring
embolism as a cause rather than a hemodynamic
mechanism.[62] Detailed observations of the retinal
circulation by Fisher[63] and Russell,[64] recording
microemboli during amaurosis fugax, supported the
embolic hypothesis. Gunning et al[65] reported a series
of TIAs and ischemic strokes associated with ipsilateral mural thrombus in the extracranial carotid
artery. However, Fisher[66] and Duncan et al[67] claimed
that hemodynamic factors were a more likely explanation than microemboli in those patients with frequent, brief, stereotyped, transient ischemic attacks.

Hemodynamic effects
of carotid stenosis

The hemodynamic effects of carotid stenosis
have been well studied.[68–71] Brice et al[69] found that
a stenosis would reduce arterial blood flow if the
cross-sectional area were less than $2\,mm^2$, but
the effect of stenosis also depended on configuration,
length and the number in series. Deweese et al[70] found
that a residual lumen of less than 1mm in diameter
(approximately 63% diameter restriction) always produced a hemodynamic change, while a residual lumen
of greater than 3mm (47% narrowing) was never
significant. Spencer and Reid,[72] using Doppler techniques, found that carotid flow would not be reduced
until the luminal diameter was less than 1.5mm.

Many workers have reported impaired cerebral
hemodynamics that improved following carotid
endarterectomy, supporting a significant hemodynamic role in cerebral ischemia.[73–76] Similar benefits were reported following extracranial–intracranial
(EC/IC) bypass surgery,[77–79] but the hemodynamic
hypothesis of cerebral ischemia received a severe
setback when EC/IC bypass anastomosis was shown
to produce no improvement over medical therapy.[80]
One study[81] found that patients with ischemic symptoms and abnormal cerebral hemodynamics on
positron emission tomography (PET) did not neces
sarily have an increased stroke risk at follow-up.

Large-artery disease, atherothrombosis,
and thromboembolism

Large-artery atherothrombosis with thromboembolism is considered to be the major pathological
determinant of ischemic stroke, due to extracranial
and intracranial atherosclerosis.[7,24] Van Damme
et al[82] histologically examined a series of carotid
plaques, showing combinations of intraplaque
hemorrhage, ulceration, and fresh and recanalized
thrombus. The presence of fresh thrombus was the
only significant clinicopathological correlation in
symptomatic carotid disease.

Fisher et al[83] found that patients with intraluminal
thrombosis at endarterectomy had arteriographic evidence of severe carotid stenosis. Torvik et al[20] found
that severe atherosclerotic stenosis was frequent, but
was not a prerequisite for thrombus formation, since
occluding thrombi in carotid vessels could be seen
without hemodynamic stenosis.[20] Ogata et al[84] suggested that the mechanism of carotid occlusion producing stroke was a rupture of the fibrous lining of the
arterial wall over the nidus of bifurcation atheroma,
producing tight luminal stenosis and thrombosis.

The detection of angiographic thrombus in ischemic stroke is likely to be related to the timing of the study. Hence, Buchan et al[85] noted that angiographic evidence of intraluminal carotid thrombus was rare, being identified in only 1.5% of angiograms performed for ischemic symptoms over 10 years, and generally associated with severe plaques. In contrast, Bladin[86] demonstrated a high frequency of both carotid occlusion and distal embolism on acute angiography of stroke patients. Fieschi et al[87] also found that a high proportion of ischemic stroke patients had intracranial vascular occlusions on acute angiography, performed within 6 hours of stroke onset. These could be attributed to thromboembolism, since most arteries subsequently recanalized. A significant minority of patients had ipsilateral internal carotid occlusions.

Hence, the underlying pathology in most strokes is arterial thrombosis, involving a combination of platelet adhesion, activation, and aggregation, and is therefore similar to that in acute myocardial infarction.[88]

Atheromatous embolism

The frequent finding of ulceration in carotid plaques at endarterectomy, and the observation of cholesterol emboli in the retinal vessels of some patients with amaurosis fugax, have supported the mechanism of artery-to-artery embolism in cerebral ischemia. However, atheromatous or cholesterol embolism has been less frequently documented than platelet–fibrin thromboembolism. Beal et al[89] reported the autopsy of a patient who died after multiple TIAs, in which many small cerebral arteries were occluded by cholesterol emboli, producing multiple small infarcts in both hemispheres. Masuda et al[90] reported 15 autopsy cases of cerebral atheromatous embolism. The emboli were composed mostly of cholesterol crystals, occluding arteries from 50 to 300 µm in diameter, producing border-zone infarcts or arterial territorial infarcts if the emboli were larger due to fibrin association.

Microembolic signals detected by transcranial Doppler ultrasound have received much attention and appear to be a marker of risk related to disease activity. They are frequently present in a variety of stroke subtypes, and their detection could be helpful in determination of stroke pathogenesis.[91] The number of microembolic signals may be modified by therapy.[92, 93]

Hemodynamic strokes – border-zone infarction

Although most nonlacunar cerebral infarcts are considered to have a thromboembolic pathogenesis, hemodynamic strokes involving external or internal border zones (watershed regions) have now been well documented. Hemodynamic infarcts can occur due to systemic hypotension, severe extracranial vascular disease, or a combination of these determinants.[94,95] Because of the topographic variability of the major cerebral arteries,[96,97] precise diagnosis of the arterial border zones on computed tomography (CT) or magnetic resonance imaging (MRI) scans can be difficult. This variability in territorial volumes is related to normal differences in the arterial diameters of the anterior, middle, and posterior cerebral arteries.[97] The location of the border zones may also be affected by the development of occlusive cerebrovascular disease.[97]

Bogousslavsky and Regli[94] studied watershed infarcts occurring in the anterior and posterior border zones as well as the subcortical watershed region, delineated by CT scans. Syncope at onset and focal limb shaking were frequent. A high proportion of patients had hemodynamic internal carotid obstruction associated with a systemic precipitant, such as hypotension or increased hematocrit, that would contribute to impaired cerebral perfusion.[94] In patients with bilateral internal carotid occlusions, some patients have vertebrobasilar or presyncopal episodes due to hemodynamic insufficiency.[98]

In a series of 300 consecutive patients with ischemic stroke, nearly 10% had hypotension at stroke onset, most of these having border-zone infarcts on CT scan.[95] Most strokes were related to underlying cardiac disease or hypotension due to autonomic failure or antihypertensive therapy. Two-thirds of patients had associated moderate or severe carotid stenosis or occlusion. However, although border-zone infarcts are typically precipitated by hypotensive episodes, they can also be caused by microemboli, which can lodge preferentially in the cerebral watershed areas.[99, 100]

In contrast to embolic stroke, a hemodynamic stroke is often slowly progressive over several hours to days.[101] Based on CT findings, Ringelstein et al[101] attempted to differentiate hemodynamic infarctions in border-zone regions affecting either the cortex or subcortical 'terminal zone' infarcts from embolic

Table 5.3   Plaque morphology

Characteristic	Relationship to ischemic symptoms
Stenosis	• Strong relationship between degree of stenosis and ischemia in both symptomatic and asymptomatic patients
Ulceration	• Angiographic ulceration correlates with increased risk in severe stenosis • Uncertain risk in mild to moderate stenosis
Hemorrhage	• Common finding: complicated plaque • Controversial role in precipitation of cerebral ischemia
Progression and regression	• Progression correlates with both risk factors and development of ischemic symptoms • Regression occurs in a minority of patients

infarctions. Bladin et al[102] identified confluent and partial internal watershed infarctions on CT scan, accounting for 6% of acute stroke admissions. Severe carotid occlusive disease and transiently impaired cardiac output were common in these patients. Hemodynamic stroke tends to have a poor prognosis.[95] In an analysis of the NASCET (North American Symptomatic Carotid Endarterectomy Trial) dataset, subcortical internal border-zone infarcts were associated with higher degrees of arterial stenosis than perforating artery infarcts.[103]

Hemodynamic cerebral infarcts may also be delineated by cerebral blood flow techniques such as single photon emission computed tomography (SPECT), positron emission tomography (PET) and transcranial Doppler with testing of vascular reserve.[100,104] Perfusion reserve and vasomotor reactivity were reduced in one study in patients with low-flow infarcts defined on CT and MRI, and yet were normal in patients with embolic territorial infarcts.[104] Unilateral border-zone infarcts were typically associated with internal carotid artery occlusion.[104] Diffusion and perfusion MRI are also helpful in determining embolic versus hypoperfusion substrates for border-zone infarction.[100,105]

Does plaque morphology and progression relate to atherothrombosis?

Based on the pathological examination of carotid plaques obtained at endarterectomy, and abnormalities in vessel imaging using angiography and Doppler

ultrasound, differing manifestations of atherosclerosis have been linked to the development of ischemic symptoms (Table 5.3). These include vessel stenosis, wall thickness, ulceration, and intraplaque hemorrhage. In addition, dynamic changes in atherosclerotic plaques, notably progression, have been correlated with the development of ischemic symptoms.[106]

Of the various parameters of cerebrovascular atherosclerosis, the degree of plaque stenosis bears the clearest relationship with ischemic symptoms. In NASCET,[107] the risk reduction ranged from 12% for ipsilateral stroke at 2 years in those with 70–79% stenosis, up to 26% for 90–99% stenosis. The European Carotid Surgery Trial[108] showed that patients with mild carotid stenosis (<30%) were at very low risk for cerebral ischemia.

Fisher and Ojemann[109] serially sectioned carotid endarterectomy plaques, and found that neurological deficits correlated best with carotid occlusion or severe stenosis. Similarly, studies of the natural history of asymptomatic carotid disease have shown a strong correlation between the degree of stenosis and the risk of stroke, particularly with high-grade stenosis.[110–113]

Carotid plaque ulceration has long been cited as an important factor in the development of artery-to-artery embolism[114–119] (Figures 5.6 and 5.7). Other authors, however, have questioned the relevance of plaque ulceration in the causation of ischemic symptoms, pointing out that ulceration is usually associated with major stenosis.[120] In NASCET[121] and ECST[109] the presence of ulceration substantially increased the risk of stroke for all degrees of stenosis.

Intraplaque hemorrhages are common in patients with stenotic atherosclerotic plaques, but their

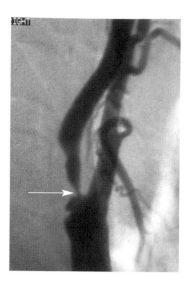

Figure 5.6
Carotid angiogram showing moderate internal carotid stenosis and a large ulcer (arrow).

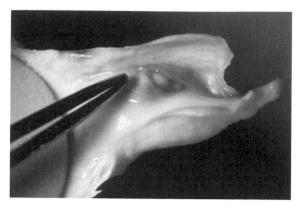

Figure 5.7
Endarterectomy specimen showing an ulcerated plaque. (See also color plate)

relationship to the development of cerebral ischemic symptoms is controversial, with conflicting reports from a large number of studies. Some studies concluded that intramural hemorrhage was important[83,122–126] and correlated with ischemic symptoms. In contrast, others found no correlation between intraplaque hemorrhage and cerebral ischemia[127,128] (Figure 5.8).

Changes in plaque size over time have been investigated using serial Doppler examinations and also in follow-up studies after either carotid endarterectomy or angioplasty. Progression has been correlated with the development of cerebral ischemic symptoms.[112,129]

Lacunar infarcts – usually in situ thrombosis, but is embolism relevant?

Fisher[4,29,130] defined the clinicopathological syndrome of lacunar infarction, caused by a combination of hypertensive and atherosclerotic occlusion of small penetrating arteries. He demonstrated the small-vessel, arterial lesions typically underlying lacunar infarcts and defined the five classical lacunar syndromes (pure motor hemiparesis, pure sensory syndrome, sensorimotor syndrome, ataxic–hemiparesis, and dysarthria–clumsy hand syndrome) in the 1960s.[9,22–24,26,131] The term 'lacunar infarct' implied both the pathological features and underlying etiology (typically small-vessel disease, rather than embolism), based on the clinical syndromes. Fisher found atheromatous plaques at the origin of deep penetrating arteries, as well as small, stenosing plaques. Superimposed thrombus was sometimes present, in addition to the hypertension-induced lipohyalinosis in other lacunar infarcts.[130] Caplan also emphasized the importance of atheromatous branch disease affecting the vessel orifice of the deep, penetrating arteries.[132] The microatheroma in the perforating arteries in patients with lacunar infarcts and deep white matter ischemic lesions has some pathological features distinguishing it from large-artery atherosclerosis.[130,133]

With the introduction of CT scanning, radiological confirmation of lacunar syndromes became possible. Studies were performed to test the first part of the hypothesis that the five lacunar syndromes were associated with radiological evidence of lacunar infarcts. To test the second part of the hypothesis, namely that lacunar syndromes were due to small-vessel vasculopathy, rather than embolism from proximal sources, studies were performed using brain imaging, cardiac investigation with echocardiography, and large-vessel investigation with duplex Doppler and digital subtraction angiography.[15,16,131]

Newer MRI techniques are contributing to a modification of the lacunar hypothesis. There is

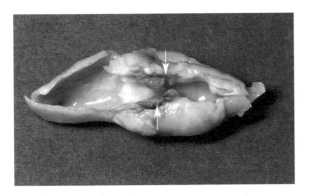

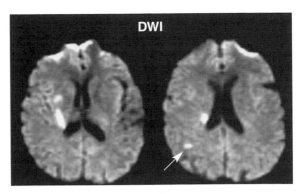

Figure 5.8
Endarterectomy specimen showing intraplaque hemorrhage (arrows). (See also color plate)

Figure 5.9
Multiple acute infarcts on diffusion weighted magnetic resonance imaging in a patient with a lacunar syndrome.

accumulating evidence that acute diffusion-weighted imaging (DWI) identifies a subset of patients presenting with typical lacunar syndromes who have a pattern of lesions suggesting an embolic pathogenesis (Figure 5.9). One DWI study aimed to determine whether clinical lacunar syndromes predicted lacunar infarcts.[5] Although most patients had small subcortical infarcts compatible with single-penetrator occlusion, a small number had cortical involvement.

Other reports have confirmed that multiple acute lesions are evident on DWI in some patients presenting with classical lacunar syndromes, implying embolism in some patients[131,134] (Figure 5.9). Our group[135] has found that of 16 patients with clinical presentations of subcortical infarcts, 10 had some evidence to suggest an embolic etiology, indicated by a pattern of multiple acute lesions in more than one single small-vessel territory. In this series, some patients also had perfusion lesions larger than expected for single-penetrator occlusion, suggesting that in situ small-vessel disease was not the source of infarction.[135]

Cardiac causes of stroke

Concurrent cerebral atherosclerosis and coronary artery disease

Fisher et al[29] emphasized the association between extracranial cerebrovascular disease and coronary artery disease in a large autopsy study. Myocardial infarction was much more common in patients with stenosis or occlusion of cervical carotid arteries. Many other studies have confirmed this relationship, including a link between coronary atherosclerosis and silent cerebral infarction. One study[136] also showed a correlation between progression of coronary and carotid atherosclerosis on ultrasound. Tanaka et al[137] evaluated both coronary and cerebrovascular atherosclerosis in patients with ischemic heart disease. They found that patients with silent cerebral infarctions were older and had a greater extent of coronary atherosclerosis. There is also a strong association between TIAs and coronary artery disease.[138] Salonen and Salonen[139] studied intimal–medial thickness (IMT) with B-mode ultrasound and found that for each 0.1mm of common carotid IMT, the risk of myocardial infarction increased by 11%.

Cardiogenic thromboembolism and brain infarction

A variety of cardiac diseases affecting the cardiac walls, valves or chambers can lead to cerebal embolism. Well-recognized causes include:[140]

- non-valvular atrial fibrillation
- valvular heart disease
- myocardial infarction with ventricular thrombus formation
- postcardiac surgery (either valvular surgery or coronary artery bypass grafts)
- prosthetic cardiac valves

- infective endocarditis
- atrial myxoma
- cardiomyopathy
- septal defect with paradoxical embolism

The first five cardiac pathologies here are the most common causes of cerebral embolism. More sensitive cardiac imaging, particularly TEE, facilitates diagnosis of more recently recognized embolic sources, such as patent foramen ovale, atrial septal aneurysm, and major aortic atherosclerosis (see above). Many studies have shown the superiority of TEE over transthoracic echocardiography.[141] It is now recognized that occlusion of cerebral vessels from these embolic sources is often clinically silent. Cerebral infarction due to cardiogenic embolism is more likely to be hemorrhagic than is infarction due to extracranial atherosclerosis. Mortality rates tend to be higher with atrial fibrillation and stroke, compared with large-vessel atherothrombosis.[142] Diagnostic predictors favoring cardioembolic stroke include a sudden onset and valvular heart disease, whereas subacute onset, hypertension, hypercholesterolemia, TIA, ischemic heart disease, and diabetes favour large-vessel stroke.[142]

Atrial fibrillation is associated with a sixfold increased risk of ischemic stroke, and substantial evidence now exists to allow rational selection of antithrombotic therapy in prophylaxis.[143] Paroxysmal atrial fibrillation is common, occurring in up to 62% of cases of atrial fibrillation, with similar causes and natural history.[144] It is an important cause of stroke in older patients.[145] The role of echocardiography in risk stratification in atrial fibrillation remains somewhat uncertain, although studies have indicated that TEE may well be useful.[146,147] Markers of high stroke risk include dense spontaneous echo contrast, appendage thrombus, and complex aortic plaque.[147]

Patent foramen ovale (PFO) has received particular attention as an important cause of stroke in young adults, particularly when no other cause is identified.[148] The autopsy incidence is approximately 27% (6% for large defects measuring 0.6–1.0 cm).[149] These lesions are often associated with atrial septal aneurysms, which are also a recognized cause of cardiogenic embolism. Indeed, atrial septal aneuryms have been associated with a 69% rate of concurrent PFOs.[150] In a large prospective study, the risk of recurrent stroke was only 2.3% over 4 years in patients with PFO alone (no higher than in controls), but increased to 15.2% in those with combined PFO and atrial septal aneurysm.[151] Larger defects and those with resting shunts convey higher risk.[149,152] Overall, the data indicate that PFO is not associated with an increased risk of subsequent stroke or death in medically treated patients with cryptogenic stroke (warfarin or aspirin). There is currently insufficient evidence to evaluate the efficacy of surgical or endovascular closure, although randomized controlled trials are underway.[148,153]

Prothrombotic states and cerebral thrombosis

In young adults with stroke, an underlying prothrombotic abnormality is often detected, although a causal relationship is often difficult to define.[154,155] A case–control study found that these abnormalities occurred in stroke patients and controls to a similar degree, so that the finding is often coincidental.[156] Examples include: (1) congenital deficiencies of the inhibitors of blood coagulation (antithrombin III, protein C, protein S, and heparin cofactor II), activated protein C resistance; (2) hereditary abnormalities of fibrinolysis (such as hereditary plasminogen deficiency and plasminogen activator deficiency); (3) erythrocyte disorders such as polycythemia rubra vera and sickle cell anemia; (4) thrombocytosis and other platelet abnormalities; (5) underlying cancer, with or without an associated nonbacterial thrombotic endocarditis; and (6) a range of autoantibody syndromes, including lupus anticoagulants.[154,155,157–159]

Lupus anticoagulants are acquired immunoglobulins that are prothrombotic[154] and are antiphospholipid antibodies. Many of the reported cases of stroke in the setting of antiphospholipid antibodies have had an additional possible contributing factor, such as nonbacterial thrombotic endocarditis. The presence of the lupus anticoagulant has been linked to defective fibrinolysis caused by higher levels of plasminogen activator inhibitor.[160] The optimal prophylactic treatment remains poorly defined.[159]

Although ischemic stroke has been linked to the estrogen content in the oral contraceptive pill, a recent systematic review found that the current low dose estrogen preparations were not associated with significant hazard.[161]

Hyperhomocysteinemia (homocystinuria) is another prothrombotic state, related to deficient synthesis of coagulation factors caused by defective amino acid metabolism. Therapy with folate and pyridoxine can normalize these amino acid levels and prevent thrombotic events.[162] A large, randomized controlled trial is underway to evaluate homocystine-lowering multivitamin therapy in patients with TIA or stroke.[163]

Activated protein C resistance is due to a mutation in coagulation factor V termed the Leiden V mutation, and has been particularly associated with venous rather than arterial thrombosis.[164–166] It occurs in a similar frequency in patients with ischemic stroke and healthy volunteers, but is a well-recognized association of cerebral vein thrombosis.[167]

Conclusions

There have been important changes in the understanding of the pathogenesis of ischemic stroke since the 1950s, when Fisher showed that most cerebral infarcts were related to thromboembolism from extracranial, atherosclerotic plaques, rather than in situ thrombosis in intracranial vessels. Intracranial disease is common in Asians and Africans, and stroke is a disease of epidemic proportions in developing countries. To date, most therapeutic trials have been conducted in First World Caucasian subjects. Although the risk of embolism from atherosclerotic plaques most clearly relates to the degree of stenosis, there is uncertainty about the pathological importance of other parameters, such as ulceration, intraplaque hemorrhage, and plaque progression.

Fisher also defined the syndrome of lacunar infarction, usually due to small-vessel thrombosis, but recent MRI studies have confirmed earlier suspicions that a proportion of lacunar infarcts are indeed embolic. With advances in cardiac investigation, particularly TEE, newly recognized cardiac causes of cerebral embolism have been delineated, particularly PFO. There remains uncertainty, however, about the natural history of this condition and no trial evidence of optimal therapy for stroke prophylaxis.

Finally, prothrombotic states are prevalent in series of young adult strokes, although they are more closely linked to cerebral venous thrombosis than arterial thromboembolism. There is particular interest in the role of hyperhomocysteinemia and the potential for modification of risk with vitamins such as folate and pyridoxine.

References

1. World Health Report. Geneva: WHO. 1999.
2. Bonita R. Epidemiology of stroke. Lancet 1992;339: 342–4.
3. Adams HP Jr, Bendixen BH, Kappelle LJ, et al. Classification of subtype of acute ischemic stroke. Definitions for use in a multicenter clinical trial. TOAST. Trial of Org 10172 in Acute Stroke Treatment. Stroke 1993;24:35–41.
4. Fisher C. Lacunes – small, deep cerebral infarcts. Neurology 1998;50:841–52.
5. Amarenco P, Cohen A, Tzourio C, et al. Atherosclerotic disease of the aortic arch and the risk of ischemic stroke. N Engl J Med 1994;331:1474–9.
6. Jones EF, Kalman JM, Calafiore P, et al. Proximal aortic atheroma. An independent risk factor for cerebral ischemia. Stroke 1995;26:218–24.
7. Leys D. Atherothrombosis: a major health burden. Cerebrovasc Dis 2001;11:1–4.
8. MacKenzie JM. Are all cardio-embolic strokes embolic? An autopsy study of 100 consecutive acute ischaemic strokes. Cerebrovasc Dis 2000;10:289–92.
9. Gurdjian ES. History of occlusive cerebrovascular disease. I. From Wepfer to Moniz. Arch Neurol 1979; 36:340–3.
10. Willis T. Cerebri Anatome: cui accessit nervorum descriptio et usus. London, 1664.

11. Chiari H. Uber das verhalten des teilungswinkels der carotis communis bei der endarteriitis chronica deformans. Verh dtsch path Ges 1905;9:326–30.

12. Hunt JR. The role of the carotid arteries, in the causation of vascular lesions of the brain, with remarks on certain special features of the symptomatology. Am J Med Sci 1914;147:704–13.

13. Moniz R, Lima A, de Lacerda R. Hemiplegies par thrombose de la carotide interne. Presse Med 1937;45:977–80.

14. Fisher M. Occlusion of the internal carotid artery. AMA Arch Neurol Psychiat 1951;65:346–77.

15. Adams RD, Vander Eecken HM. Vascular diseases of the brain. Annu Rev Med 1953;4:213–52.

16. Hutchinson EC, Yates PO. Carotico-vertebral stenosis. Lancet 1957;i:2–8.

17. Baker AB, Iannone A. Cerebrovascular disease. The large arteries of the circle of Willis. Neurology 1959;9:321–32.

18. Martin MJ, Whisnant JP, Sayre GP. Occlusive vascular disease in the extracranial cerebral circulation. Arch Neurol 1960;5:530–8.

19. Schwartz CJ, Mitchell JRA. Atheroma of the carotid and vertebral arterial systems. BMJ 1961;ii:1057–63.

20. Torvik A, Svindland A, Lindboe CF. Pathogenesis of carotid thrombosis. Stroke 1989;20:1477–83.

21. Fisher M. Occlusion of the carotid arteries. Further experiences. AMA Arch Neurol Psychiatry 1954;72:187–204.

22. Lhermitte F, Gautier JC, Derouesne C, Guiraud B. Ischemic accidents in the middle cerebral artery territory: a study of causes of 122 cases. Arch Neurol 1968;19:248–56.

23. Blackwood W, Hallpike JF, Kocen RS, Mair WGP. Atheromatous disease of the carotid arterial system and embolism from the heart in cerebral infarction: a morbid anatomical study. Brain 1969;92:897–910.

24. Castaigne P, Lhermitte F, Gautier JC, et al. Internal carotid artery occlusion. A study of 61 instances in 50 patients with post-mortem data. Brain 1970;93:231–58.

25. Lammie GA, Sandercock PAG, Dennis MS. Recently occluded intracranial and extracranial carotid arteries. Relevance of the unstable atherosclerotic plaque. Stroke 1999;30:1319–1325.

26. Whisnant JP, Martin MJ, Sayre GP. Atherosclerotic stenosis of cervical arteries. Arch Neurol 1961;5:429–432.

27. Schulz UGR, Rothwell PM. Sex differences in carotid bifurcation anatomy and the distribution of atherosclerotic plaque. Stroke 2001;32:1525–31.

28. Iemolo F, Martiniuk A, Steinman DA, Spence JD. Sex differences in carotid plaque and stenosis. Stroke 2004;35:477–81.

29. Fisher CM, Gore I, Okabe N, White PD. Atherosclerosis of the carotid and vertebral arteries – extracranial and intracranial. J Neuropathol Exp Neurol 1965;24:455–476.

30. Castaigne P, Lhermitte F, Gautier JC, et al. Arterial occlusions in the vertebral–basilar system. A study of 44 patients with postmortem data. Brain 1973;96:133–54.

31. Josse MO, Touboul PJ, Mas JL, Laplane D, Bousser MG. Prevalence of asymptomatic internal carotid artery stenosis. Neuroepidemiology 1987;6:150–2.

32. Prati P, Vanuzzo D, Casaroli M, et al. Prevalence and determinants of carotid atherosclerosis in a general population. Stroke 1992;23:1705–11.

33. Hennerici M, Aulich A, Sandmann W, Freund HJ. Incidence of asymptomatic extracranial arterial disease. Stroke 1981;12:750–8.

34. Colgan MP, Strode GR, Sommer JD, et al. Prevalence of asymptomatic carotid disease: results of duplex scanning in 348 unselected volunteers. J Vasc Surg 1988;8:674–8.

35. Li R, Duncan BB, Metcalf PA, et al. B-mode-detected carotid artery plaque in a general population. Atherosclerosis Risk in Communities (ARIC) Study Investigators. Stroke 1994;25:2377–83.

36. Marini C, Totaro R, Carolei A. Long-term prognosis of cerebral ischemia in young adults. Stroke 1999;30:2320–5.

37. Lanzino G, Andreoli A, Di Pasquale G, et al. Etiopathogenesis and prognosis of cerebral ischemia in young adults. A survey of 155 treated patients. Acta Neurol Scand 1991;84:321–5.

38. Naess J, Waje-Andreassen U, Thomassen L, et al. Do all young ischemic stroke patients need long-term secondary preventive medication? Neurology 2005;65:609–11.

39. Hutchinson EC, Yates PO. The cervical portion of the vertebral artery: a clinico-pathological study. Brain 1956;79:319–31.

40. Caplan LR, Gorelick PB, Hier DB. Race, sex and occlusive cerebrovascular disease: a review. Stroke 1986;17:648–55.

41. Caplan LR. Intracranial branch atheromatous disease: a neglected, understudied, and underused concept. Neurology 1989;39:1246–50.

42. Caplan L, Babikian V, Helgason C, et al. Occlusive disease of the middle cerebral artery. Neurology 1985;35:975–82.

43. Heyman A, Fields WS, Keating RD. Joint Study of Extracranial Arterial Occlusion. VI. Racial differences in hospitalized patients with ischemic stroke. JAMA 1972;222:285–9.

44. Gorelick PB, Caplan LR, Hier DB, et al. Racial differences in the distribution of anterior circulation occlusive disease. Neurology 1984;34:54–57.

45. McGarry P, Solberg LA, Guzman MA, Strong JP. Cerebral atherosclerosis in New Orleans. Comparisons of lesions by age, sex, and race. Lab Invest 1985;52: 533–9.

46. Gil-Peralta A, Alter M, Lai SM, et al. Duplex Doppler and spectral flow analysis of racial differences in cerebrovascular atherosclerosis. Stroke 1990;21: 740–4.

47. Ryu JE, Murros K, Espeland MA, et al. Extracranial carotid atherosclerosis in black and white patients with transient ischemic attacks. Stroke 1989;20: 1133–7.

48. Gorelick PB, Caplan LR, Hier DB, et al. Racial differences in the distribution of posterior circulation occlusive disease. Stroke 1985;16:785–90.

49. Mitsuyama Y, Thompson LR, Hayashi T, et al. Autopsy study of cerebrovascular disease in Japanese men who lived in Hiroshima, Japan, and Honolulu, Hawaii. Stroke 1979;10:389–95.

50. Reed D, Jacobs DR Jr, Hayashi T, et al. A comparison of lesions in small intracerebral arteries among Japanese men in Hawaii and Japan. Stroke 1994; 25:60–5.

51. Leung SY, Ng TH, Yuen ST, Lauder IJ, Ho FC. Pattern of cerebral atherosclerosis in Hong Kong Chinese. Severity in intracranial and extracranial vessels. Stroke 1993;24:779–86.

52. Tunick PA, Perez JL, Kronzon I. Protruding atheromas in the thoracic aorta and systemic embolization. Ann Intern Med 1991;115:423–7.

53. Amarenco P, Duyckaerts C, Tzourio C, et al. The prevalence of ulcerated plaques in the aortic arch in patients with stroke. N Engl J Med 1992;326:221–5.

54. Fujimoto S, Yasaka M, Otsubo R, et al. Aortic arch atherosclerotic lesions and the recurrence of ischemic stroke. Stroke 2004;35:1426–9.

55. Davila-Roman VG, Barzilai B, Wareing TH, et al. Atherosclerosis of the ascending aorta. Prevalence and role as an independent predictor of cerebrovascular events in cardiac patients. Stroke 1994;25:2010–6.

56. Macleod MR, Amarenco P, Davis SM, Donnan GA. Atheroma of the aortic arch: an important and poorly recognised factor in the aetiology of stroke. Lancet Neurol 2004;3:408–14.

57. Stern A, Tunick PA, Culliford AT, et al. I. Protruding aortic arch atheromas: risk of stroke during heart surgery with and without aortic arch endarterectomy. Am Heart J 1999;138:746–52.

58. Denny-Brown D. The treatment of recurrent cerebrovascular symptoms and the question of 'vasospasm'. Med Clin North Am 1951;35:1457–74.

59. Denny-Brown D. Recurrent cerebrovascular episodes. Arch Neurol 1960;2:194–210.

60. Meyer JS, Leiderman H, Denny-Brown D. Electroencephalographic study of insufficiency of the basilar and carotid arteries in man. Neurology 1956;6:455–77.

61. Pickering GW. Transient cerebral paralysis in hypertension and in cerebral embolism. JAMA 1948;137:423–30.

62. Fisher CM. The use of anticoagulants in cerebral thrombosis. Neurology 1958;8:311–32.

63. Fisher CM. Observations of the fundus oculi in transient monocular blindness. Neurology 1959;9:333–47.

64. Russell R. Observations on the retinal blood vessels in monocular blindness. Lancet 1961;ii:1422–8.

65. Gunning AJ, Pickering GW, Robb-Smith AHT, Ross R. Mural thrombosis of the internal carotid artery and subsequent embolism. Q J Med 1964;33:155–95.

66. Fisher CM. Transient ischemic attacks. Discussion. In: Scheinberg P (ed). 10th Research (Princeton) Conference. New York: Raven Press, 1976:50–3.

67. Duncan GW, Pessin MS, Mohr JP, Adams RD. Transient cerebral ischemic attacks. Adv Intern Med 1976;21:1–20.

68. Crawford ES, Wukasch DW, DeBakey ME. Hemodynamic changes associated with carotid artery occlusion: an experimental and clinical study. Cardiovasc Res Cent Bull 1962;1:3–10.

69. Brice JG, Dowsett DJ, Lowe RD. Haemodynamic effects of carotid artery stenosis. BMJ 1964;ii:1363–1366.

70. Deweese JA, May AG, Lipchik EO, Rob CG. Anatomic and hemodynamic correlations in carotid artery stenosis. Stroke 1970;1:149–57.

71. Grady PA. Pathophysiology of extracranial cerebral arterial stenosis – a critical review. Stroke 1984;15: 224–36.

72. Spencer MP, Reid JM. Quantitation of carotid stenosis with continuous-wave (C-W) Doppler ultrasound. Stroke 1979;10:326–30.

73. Obrist WD, Silver D, Wilkinson WE, et al. The ^{133}Xe inhalation method: assessment of rCBF in carotid endarterectomy. New York: Springer-Verlag, 1975.

74. Takagi Y, Hata T, Ishitobi K, Kitagawa Y. Cerebral blood flow and CO_2 reactivity before and after carotid endarterectomy. Acta Neurol Scand 1979;60:506–7.

75. Jones FH, Dyken ML, King R. Cerebral blood flow, metabolism and mean arterial pressure changes following unilateral internal carotid endarterectomy: cerebral ischemia and elevated systemic arterial pressure. Stroke 1972;3:441–5.

76. Engell HC, Boysen G, Ladegaard-Pedersen HJ, Henriksen H. Cerebral blood flow before and after carotid endarterectomy. Vasc Surg 1972;6:14–19.

77. Meyer JS, Nakajima S, Okabe T, et al. Redistribution of cerebral blood flow following STA-MCA by-pass in patients with hemispheric ischemia. Stroke 1982;13: 774–84.

78. Halsey JHJ, Morawetz RB, Blauenstein UW. The hemodynamic effect of STA-MCA bypass. Stroke 1982;13:163–6.

79. Baron JC, Bousser MG, Comar D, et al. Noninvasive tomographic study of cerebral blood flow and oxygen metabolism in vivo. Potentials, limitations, and clinical applications in cerebral ischemic disorders. Eur Neurol 1981;20:273–84.

80. EC/IC, Bypass, Group S. Failure of extracranial–intracranial arterial bypass to reduce the risk of ischemic stroke. Results of an international randomized trial. The EC/IC Bypass Study Group. N Engl J Med 1985;313:1191–200.

81. Powers WJ, Tempel LW, Grubb RL Jr. Influence of cerebral hemodynamics on stroke risk: one-year follow-up of 30 medically treated patients. Ann Neurol 1989; 25:325–30.

82. Van Damme H, Demoulin JC, Zicot M, et al. Pathological aspects of carotid plaques. Surgical and clinical significance. J Cardiovasc Surge (Torino) 1992;33:46–53.

83. Fisher M, Sacoolidge JC, Taylor CR. Patterns of fibrin deposits in carotid artery plaques. Angiology 1987; 38:393–9.

84. Ogata J, Masuda J, Yutani C, Yamaguchi T. Rupture of atheromatous plaque as a cause of thrombotic occlusion of stenotic internal carotid artery. Stroke 1990; 21:1740–5.

85. Buchan A, Gates P, Pelz D, Barnett HJ. Intraluminal thrombus in the cerebral circulation. Implications for surgical management. Stroke 1988;19:681–7.

86. Bladin PF. A radiologic and pathologic study of embolism of the internal carotid–middle cerebral arterial axis. Radiology 1964;82:615–25.

87. Fieschi C, Argentino C, Lenzi GL, et al. Clinical and instrumental evaluation of patients with ischemic stroke within the first six hours. J Neurol Sci 1989;91:311–22.

88. Fitzgerald DJ. Vascular biology of thrombosis: the role of platelet–vessel wall adhesion. Neurology 2001;57: S1–4.

89. Beal MF, Williams RS, Richardson EP Jr, Fisher CM. Cholesterol embolism as a cause of transient ischemic attacks and cerebral infarction. Neurology 1981;31:860–5.

90. Masuda J, Yutani C, Ogata J, et al. Atheromatous embolism in the brain: a clinicopathologic analysis of 15 autopsy cases. Neurology 1994;44:1231–7.

91. Lund C, Rygh J, Stensrod B, et al. Cerebral microembolus detection in an unselected acute ischemic stroke population. Cerebrovasc Dis 2000;10:403–8.

92. Markus HS, Droste DW, Kaps M, et al. Dual antiplatelet therapy with clopidogrel and aspirin in symptomatic carotid stenosis evaluated using doppler embolic signal detection. The clopidogrel and aspirin for reduction of emboli in symptomatic carotid stenosis (CARESS) trial. Circulation 2005;111:2233–40.

93. Infeld B, Bowser DN, Gerraty RP, et al. Cerebral microemboli in atrial fibrillation detected by transcranial Doppler ultrasonography. Cerebrovasc Dis 1996;6:339–45.

94. Bogousslavsky J, Regli F. Unilateral watershed cerebral infarcts. Neurology 1986;36:373–7.

95. Bladin CF, Chambers BR. Frequency and pathogenesis of hemodynamic stroke. Stroke 1994;25:2179–82.

96. van der Zwan A, Hellen B. Review of the variability of the territories of the major cerebral arteries. Stroke 1991;22:1078–84.

97. van der Zwan A, Hellen B, Tulleken CAF, Dujovny M. A quantitative investigation of the variability of the major cerebral arterial territories. Stroke 1993; 24:1951–9.

98. Wade JP, Wong W, Barnett HJ, Vandervoort P. Bilateral occlusion of the internal carotid arteries. Presenting symptoms in 74 patients and a prospective study of 34 medically treated patients. Brain 1987;110:667–82.

99. Torvik A, Skullerud K. Watershed infarcts in the brain caused by microemboli. Clin Neuropathol 1982;1:99–105.

100. Momjian-Mayor I, Baron JC. The pathophysiology of watershed infarction in internal carotid artery disease. Review of cerebral perfusion studies. Stroke 2005;36: 567–77.

101. Ringelstein EB, Zeumer H, Angelou D. The pathogenesis of strokes from internal carotid artery occlusion. Diagnostic and therapeutical implications. Stroke 1983;14:867–75.

102. Bladin CF, Chambers BR. Clinical features, pathogenesis, and computed tomographic characteristics of internal watershed infarction. Stroke 1993;24:1925–32.

103. Del Sette M, Eliasziw M, Streifler JY, et al. Internal borderzone infarction: a marker for severe stenosis in patients with symptomatic internal carotid artery disease. For the North American Symptomatic Carotid Endarterectomy (NASCET) Group. Stroke 2000;31:631–6.

104. Weiller C, Ringelstein EB, Reiche W, Buell U. Clinical and hemodynamic aspects of low-flow infarcts. Stroke 1991;22:1117–23.

105. Chaves CJ, Silver B, Schlaug G, et al. Diffusion- and perfusion-weighted MRI patterns in borderzone infarcts. Stroke 2000;31:1090–6.

106. Touboul P. Evolving thrombotic and embolic potentials of atherosclerotic lesions. Cerebrovasc Dis 1994; 4(Suppl 4):8–11.

107. North American Symptomatic Carotid Endarterectomy Trial Collaborators. Beneficial effect of carotid endarterectomy in symptomatic patients with high-grade carotid stenosis. N Engl J Med 1991;325:445–53.

108. European Carotid Surgery Triallists' Collaborative Group. MRC European Carotid Surgery Trial: interim results for symptomatic patients with severe (70–99%) or with mild (0–29%) carotid stenosis. Lancet 1991;337:1235–43.

109. Fisher CM, Ojemann RG. A clinico-pathologic study of carotid endarterectomy plaques. Rev Neurol 1986;142:573–89.

110. O'Holleran LW, Kennelly MM, McClurken M, Johnson JM. Natural history of asymptomatic carotid plaque. Five year follow-up study. Am J Surg 1987;154:659–62.

111. Johnson JM, Kennelly MM, Decesare D, et al. Natural history of asymptomatic carotid plaque. Arch Surg 1985;120:1010–2.

112. Chambers BR, Norris JW. Outcome in patients with asymptomatic neck bruits. N Engl J Med 1986; 315:886–8.

113. Bogousslavsky J, Despland PA, Regli F. Asymptomatic tight stenosis of the internal carotid artery: long-term prognosis. Neurology 1986;36:861–3.

114. Gomez CR. Carotid plaque morphology and risk for stroke. Stroke 1990;21:148–51.

115. Bartynski WS, Darbouze P, Nemir P Jr. Significance of ulcerated plaque in transient cerebral ischemia. Am J Surg 1981;141:353–7.

116. Imparato AM, Riles TS, Mintzer R, Baumann FG. The importance of hemorrhage in the relationship between gross morphologic characteristics and cerebral symptoms in 376 carotid artery plaques. Ann Surg 1982;2:195–203.

117. Rothwell PM, Gibson R, Warlow CP. Interrelation between plaque surface morphology and degree stenosis on carotid angiograms and the risk of ischemic stroke in patients with symptomatic carotid stenosis. Stroke 2000;31:615–21.

118. Perez-Burkhardt JL, Gonzalez-Fajardo JA, et al. Amaurosis fugax as a symptom of carotid artery stenosis. Its relationship with ulcerated plaque. J Cardiovasc Surg (Torino) 1994;35:15–18.

119. Zukowski AJ, Nicolaides AN, Lewis RT, et al. The correlation between carotid plaque ulceration and cerebral infarction seen on CT scan. J Vasc Surg 1984;1:782–6.

120. Wechsler LR. Ulceration and carotid artery disease. Stroke 1988;19:650–3.

121. Eliasziw M, Streifler JY, Fox AJ, et al. Significance of plaque ulceration in symptomatic patients with high-grade carotid stenosis. North American Symptomatic Carotid Endarterectomy Trial. Stroke 1994;25:304–8.

122. Imparato AM, Riles TS, Gorstein F. The carotid bifurcation plaque: pathologic findings associated with cerebral ischemia. Stroke 1979;10:238–45.

123. Lusby RJ, Ferrell LD, Ehrenfeld WK, et al. Carotid plaque hemorrhage. Its role in production of cerebral ischemia. Arch Surg 1982;117:1479–88.

124. Persson AV, Robichaux WT, Silverman M. The natural history of carotid plaque development. Arch Surg 1983;118:1048–1052.

125. Langsfeld M, Gray-Weale AC, Lusby RJ. The role of plaque morphology and diameter reduction in the development of new symptoms in asymptomatic carotid arteries. J Vasc Surg 1989;9:548–57.

126. Ammar AD, Ernst RL, Lin JJ, Travers H. The influence of repeated carotid plaque hemorrhages on the production of cerebrovascular symptoms. J Vasc Surg 1986;3:857–9.

127. von Maravic C, Kessler C, von Maravic M, et al. Clinical relevance of intraplaque hemorrhage in the internal carotid artery. Eur J Surg 1991;157:185–8.

128. Lennihan L, Kupsky WJ, Mohr JP, et al. Lack of association between carotid plaque hematoma and ischemic cerebral symptoms. Stroke 1987;18: 879–81.

129. Bornstein NM, Norris JW. The unstable carotid plaque. Stroke 1989;20:1104–6.

130. Fisher CM. Capsular infarcts: the underlying vascular lesions. Arch Neurol 1979;36:65–73.

131. Davis SM, Parsons MW. MRI and Other Neuroimaging Modalities for Subcortical Stroke. Oxford: Oxford Medical Publications, 2002.

132. Raju S, Fredericks RK. Carotid siphon stenosis. J Cardiovasc Surg (Torino) 1987;28:671–7.

133. Furuta A, Ishii N, Nishihara Y, Horie A. Medullary arteries in aging and dementia. Stroke 1991;22:442–6.

134. Wessels T, Rottger C, Jauss M, et al. Identification of embolic stroke patterns by diffusion-weighted MRI in clinically defined lacunar stroke syndromes. Stroke 2005;36:757–61.

135. Gerraty RP, Parsons MW, Barber PA, et al. Examining the lacunar hypothesis with diffusion and perfusion MRI. Stroke 2002;33:2019–24.

136. Nishino M, Sueyoshi K, Yasuno M, et al. Risk factors for carotid atherosclerosis and silent cerebral infarction in patients with coronary heart disease. Angiology 1993;44:432–40.

137. Tanaka H, Sueyoshi K, Nishino M, et al. Silent brain infarction and coronary artery disease in Japanese patients. Arch Neurol 1993;50:706–9.

138. Scheinberg P. Transient ischemic attacks: an update. J Neurol Sci 1991;101:133–40.

139. Salonen JT, Salonen R. Ultrasound B-mode imaging in observational studies of atherosclerotic progression. Circulation 1993;56–65.

140. Di Tullio MR, Homma S. Mechanisms of cardioembolic stroke. Curr Cardiol Rep 2002;4:141–8.

141. Palazzuoli A, Ricci D, Lenzi C, et al. Transesophageal echocardiography for identifying potential cardiac sources of embolism in patients with stroke. Neurol Sci 2000;21:195–202.

142. Arboix A, Garcia-Eroles L, Massons JB, et al. Atrial fibrillation and stroke: clinical presentation of cardioembolic versus atherothrombotic infarction. Int J Cardiol 2000;73:33–42.

143. Hart RG, Halperin JL, Pearce LA, et al. Lessons from the Stroke Prevention in Atrial Fibrillation trials. Ann Intern Med. 2003;138:831–8.

144. Lip GY, Hee FL. Paroxysmal atrial fibrillation. Q J Med 2001;94:665–78.

145. Yamanouchi H, Mizutani T, Matsushita S, Esaki Y. Paroxysmal atrial fibrillation: high frequency of embolic brain infarction in elderly autopsy patients. Neurology 1997;49:1691–4.

146. Shinokawa N, Hirai T, Takashima S, et al. Relation of transesophageal echocardiographic findings to subtypes of cerebral infarction in patients with atrial fibrillation. Clin Cardiol 2000;23:517–22.

147. The Stroke Prevention in Atrial Fibrillation Investigators Committee on Echocardiography. Transesophageal echocardiographic correlates of thromboembolism in high-risk patients with non-valvular atrial fibrillation. Ann Intern Med 1998; 128:639–47.

148. Messe S, Silverman I, Kizer J, et al. Practice parameter: recurrent stroke with patent foramen ovale and atrial septal aneurysm. Report of the Quality Standards Subcommittee of the American Academy of Neurology. Neurology 2004;62:1042–50.

149. Kerut EK, Norfleet WT, Plotnick GD, Giles TD. Patent foramen ovale: a review of associated conditions and the impact of physiological size. J Am Coll Cardiol 2001;38:613–623.

150. Mattioli AV, Aquilina M, Oldani A, et al. Atrial septal aneurysm as a cardioembolic source in adult patients with stroke and normal carotid arteries. A multicentre study. Eur Heart J 2001;22:261–8.

151. Mas JL, Arquizan C, Lamy C, et al. Recurrent cerebrovascular events associated with patent foramen ovale, atrial septal aneurysm, or both. N Engl J Med 2001;345:1740–6.

152. De Castro S, Cartoni D, Fiorelli M, et al. Patent foramen ovale and its embolic implications. Am J Cardiol 2000;86:51G–52G.

153. Kizer JR, Devereux RB. Patent foramen ovale in young adults with unexplained stroke. N Engl J Med 2005;353:2361–72.

154. Hart RG, Kanter MC. Hematologic disorders and ischemic stroke. A selective review. Stroke 1990;21: 1111–21.

155. Munts AG, van Genderen PJ, Dippel DW, et al. Coagulation disorders in young adults with acute cerebral ischaemia. J Neurol 1998;245:21–5.

156. Hankey GJ, Eikelboom JW, van Bockxmeer FM, et al. Inherited thrombophilia in ischemic stroke and its pathogenic subtypes. Stroke 2001;32:1793–9.

157. Coull BM, Clark WM. Abnormalities of hemostasis in ischemic stroke. Med Clin North Am 1993;77:77–94.

158. Barinagarrementeria F, Cantu-Brito C, De La Pena A, Izaguirre R. Prothrombotic states in young people with idiopathic stroke. A prospective study. Stroke 1994;25:287–90.

159. APASS Investigators. Antiphospholipid antibodies and subsequent thrombo-occlusive events in patients with ischemic stroke. JAMA 2004;291:576–84.

160. Ferro D, Quintarelli C, Rasura M, et al. Lupus anticoagulant and the fibrinolytic system in young patients with stroke. Stroke 1993;24:368–70.

161. Chan WS, Ray J, Wai EK, et al. Risk of stroke in women exposed to low-dose oral contraceptives. A critical evaluation of the evidence. Arch Intern Med 2004;164:741–7.

162. Schienle HW, Seitz R, Rohner I, et al. Coagulation factors and markers of activation of coagulation in homocystinuria (HOCY): a study in two siblings. Blood Coagul Fibrinolysis 1994;5:873–8.

163. The VITATOPS (Vitamins to Prevent Stroke) Trial: rationale and design of an international, large, simple, randomised trial of homocysteine-lowering multivitamin therapy in patients with recent transient ischaemic attack or stroke. Cerebrovasc Dis 2002;13:120–6.

164. Brey RL, Coull BM. Cerebral venous thrombosis. Role of activated protein C resistance and factor V gene mutation. Stroke 1996;27:1719–20.

165. Ridker PM, Miletich JP, Stampfer MJ, et al. Factor V Leiden and risks of recurrent idiopathic venous thromboembolism. Circulation 1995;92: 2800–2.

166. Szolnoki Z, Somogyvari F, Kondacs A, et al. Evaluation of the roles of the Leiden V mutation and ACE I/D polymorphism in subtypes of ischaemic stroke. J Neurol 2001;248:756–61.

167. Zunker P, Hohenstein C, Plendl HJ, et al. Activated protein C resistance and acute ischaemic stroke: relation to stroke causation and age. J Neurol 2001; 248:701–4.

6

Thrombolytic/antithrombotic clinical trials in cardiology: an overview

Daniel Jenni and Jürg-Hans Beer

Thrombolytic trials in acute myocardial infarction

Streptokinase versus placebo

In the late 1960s and the 1970s, a number of controlled studies showed a benefit in myocardial infarction (MI) of a long-term infusion (over 24 h) of the fibrinolytic agent streptokinase applied in the first 24–72 h after the onset of infarction,[1,4] although other studies showed no significance.[2,3] The first comparison of an earlier lysis (3 h after onset) with (by that time) the usual later start of lysis showed no negative effect on 1 year mortality.[1] The European Cooperative Study Group, the first prospective randomized study, proved a mortality benefit after 6 months in patients treated with a 24 h streptokinase infusion starting at latest 12 h after onset of symptoms (absolute risk reduction (ARR) 15%).[5] As early as 1980, a Russian group found a greater benefit of streptokinase therapy in patients with onset of MI only 3–6 h before, with better outcome in younger patients (<65 years) and regardless of the time of infusion.[6]

At this time, a number of different trials were initiated investigating short-term application of streptokinase (1–1.5 MU over 1 h) followed by long-term infusion of heparin (72 h–7 days).[9–11] While these studies were under way, some groups tried to apply intracoronary streptokinase, but the results were not encouraging.[7,8] In 1986, the results of two smaller studies by Schreiber et al[10] and Bassand et al[11]

showed an improvement in left ventricular function after therapy with streptokinase, especially in patients with anterior wall infarction.[11]

In 1986 and 1987, the GISSI (Gruppo Italiano per lo Studio della Streptochinasi nell'Infarto miocardico) study, the first large randomized study comparing streptokinase and placebo, was able to prove a significant benefit of streptokinase (1.5 MU/1 h) given up to 6 h after onset of symptoms with regard to a reduced mortality after 21 days (ARR 2.3%)[12] and after 1 year (ARR 1.8%).[13] These results were even better for patients treated within 3 h after the beginning of the infarction.

The results of the pilot study ISIS, published in 1987,[14] showed a positive trend for reduction of reinfarction and mortality for patients treated with short-term intravenous streptokinase lysis (1.5 MU/1 h) followed by heparin (1000 IE/h over 48 h) and also a positive trend in reduction of reinfarction by aspirin. Also in 1987, White et al[15] showed in over 200 patients a significant reduction in early mortality after short-term application of streptokinase in the first 4 h after onset of symptoms, regardless of the location of the infarction. ISIS-2, a randomized double-blind placebo-controlled study with over 17 000 patients, showed a significant reduction in vascular mortality after MI with streptokinase alone (ARR 2.8%), aspirin alone (ARR 2.4%), and a combination of streptokinase and aspirin (ARR 5.2%).[16]

In 1986 and 1987, the ISAM (Intravenous Streptokinase in Acute Myocardial Infarction) Study Group could not prove a mortality benefit in their study with 1741 patients treated with streptokinase, but they did show a better left ventricular ejection fraction in those with anterior wall infarction treated with streptokinase compared with placebo.[17]

Urokinase versus placebo

Urokinase, another fibrinolytic agent, was also evaluated for use in MI. Urokinase usually does not induce antibodies and was thought to be particularly useful in patients with antibodies to streptokinase. In the mid 1970s, there were two small studies conducted with intravenous urokinase, which showed contradictory results.[18,19] There was only one larger randomized open-label study with urokinase versus placebo, which did not show significant results in 2201 patients (USIM, Urochinasi per via Sistemica nell'Infarto Miocardio).[20] The overall mortality was similar in the two groups. Due to these results and because of the better results of the alteplase trials, further use of urokinase was no longer promoted.

Alteplase (rtPA, tPA) versus placebo or streptokinase

Soon after the success of streptokinase, other agents for thrombolysis were evaluated in the same setting. The reasons for this search for other agents was primarily the side-effects of streptokinase (allergic reactions leading to hypotension), the production of antibodies against streptokinase after the first use (which prohibited repeated use in the same patient), and the fibrin-specificity.

One of these new agents was the recombinant tissue-type plasminogen activator (rtPA), also called alteplase. The advantage of rtPA is its property of binding to fibrin and also its activation through fibrin. This leads to fibrin-bound plasmin, which is protected from antiplasmin and is more effective. Usually, alteplase is given in a front-loaded manner (bolus plus infusion over 60 min). In 1987, the TIMI 1 (Thrombolysis in Myocardial Infarction) Study Group published its results of clinical and angiographic success of alteplase versus streptokinase in 290 patients.[21] It was shown that alteplase led to a more rapid reperfusion, but there was no difference in mortality and left ventricular function between the two groups. In 1988, ASAET (Anglo-Scandinavian

Study of Early Thrombolysis) showed a significant benefit of alteplase over placebo in acute MI (AMI) with regard to mortality after 1 month (ARR 2.6%)[22] and 6 months (ARR 2.7%),[23] but no difference in readmissions or development of heart failure. The TAMI 6 (Thrombolysis and Angioplasty in Myocardial Infarction study, however, showed no clinical benefit of thrombolysis in infarctions up to 24 h after onset, although the vessel patency was improved.[24]

There were further comparisons between alteplase and streptokinase. In 1990, GISSI presented results on 12 490 patients (GISSI 2) with AMI who were randomized to streptokinase or alteplase (either with or without heparin).[25] Together with these results, an international study group of the GISSI 2 trial published results from 20 891 patients.[26] There were no differences in the composite endpoint (death or severe left ventricular damage) after 15 days, after 1 month, and after 6 months between the three groups.[25–27] In KAMIT (Kentucky Acute Myocardial Infarction Trial), published in 1991, 216 patients were randomized either to alteplase or to streptokinase with half-dose alteplase.[28] The combined group had a greater patency at 90 minutes and a greater myocardial salvage after 7 days, but there was no effect on in-hospital mortality. In 1993, two studies showed contradictory results. In GUSTO I (Global Use of Strategies to Open Occluded Coronary Arteries) 41 021 patients were randomized to different regimes of alteplase, streptokinase, or the combination.[29] There was an absolute risk reduction of 0.9% for death and disabling stroke after 30 days in the group receiving alteplase with intravenous heparin. In ISIS 3 (Third International Study of Infarct Survival), 41 299 patients were randomized to alteplase, streptokinase, or anistreplase.[30] The differences were small and not significant – either for preventing recurrent infarction or for occurrence of stroke in the acute phase. The 35-day mortality was comparable and the 6-month survival was similar for all three groups.

Anistreplase (APSAC: anisoylated plasminogen–streptokinase activator complex)

The advantage of anistreplase (a modification of streptokinase) over other fibrinolytic agents such as streptokinase and alteplase lies in the fact that it is administered as a single bolus injection without the need for an infusion, due to its longer half-life, which was thought to result in better patency rates of the target vessel. The first trial of anistreplase versus placebo in AMI (AIMS, Anistreplase Intervention Mortality Study) was published in 1988.[31] The trial was terminated for ethical reasons after the inclusion of 1004 patients, because of an ARR of 6% for death after 30 days in the group receiving anistreplase. The ARR for death after 1 year was 7% in favor of the intervention group.[32]

The TEAM 2(second Trial of Eminase (anistreplase) in Acute Myocardial infarction) study[33] compared anistreplase with streptokinase in 370 patients with AMI and found no significant reduction in in-hospital mortality (ARR 1.1%). There have been a number of studies comparing anistreplase with alteplase. One of these was the already-mentioned ISIS-3.[30] The others were ENTIM (Etudes des Nouveaux Thrombolytiques dans l'Infarctus du Myocarde),[34] TEAM 3,[35] TAPS (rt-PA–APSAC Patency Study),[36] DUCCS 2 (second Duke University Clinical Cardiology Study)[37] and TIMI 4.[38] ENTIM showed no difference in mortality, infarct size, or left ventricular function after 3 weeks in 183 patients. In TEAM 3, 325 patients were randomized, and the only significant difference was a better left ventricular function in the alteplase group, although the nonsignificant ARR of 1.7% for mortality was in favor of anistreplase. A different result was found in TAPS (421 patients), where anistreplase led to a significant higher in-hospital mortality (plus 5.7% compared with alteplase), although reocclusion rates after 21 days were similar. DUCCS 2 also showed better results for alteplase in 162 patients – mainly due to more bleeding complications and a later electrocardiographic (ECG) normalization in the anistreplase group. In TIMI 4, alteplase again showed a trend to superiority in 382 patients regarding the combined endpoint of death, severe heart failure, a left ventricular function of less than 40%, reinfarction, reocclusion, lower TIMI flow grade, major hemorrhage, and severe anaphylaxis (ARR 7.7%).

Reteplase (rPA)

Reteplase is another reengineered fibrinolytic agent, which can be given in a double-bolus manner (10 U/kg body weight, 30 min apart), resulting in an easier and probably faster application. The first comparison of reteplase was performed against streptokinase in INJECT (International Joint Efficacy Comparison of Thrombolytics).[39] In 6010 randomized patients, no significant difference was found in death after 35 days or after 6 months (with a tendency in favor of reteplase, ARR 1.0%). Hypotension and anaphylactic reactions were significantly less in the reteplase group.

The other studies with reteplase were all performed against alteplase. In RAPID (Recombinant plasminogen activator Angiographic Phase II International Dose-finding study)[40] 606 patients were included, and double-bolus reteplase showed significantly better TIMI flow grade and late patency compared with standard-dose alteplase. The ARR for reocclusion was 4.9% and that for 30-day mortality was 2% in favor of reteplase (both results were not significant). The following study RAPID II[41] showed similar results in 324 patients, although the ARR for the 35-day mortality was now 4.3% in favor of reteplase ($p = 0.11$). After these encouraging results, the large GUSTO III study[42] with 15059 randomized patients, was eagerly awaited, but there were no significant differences between the two regimens with regard to the 30-day mortality and the occurrence of stroke.

Tenecteplase (TNK-tPA)

Tenecteplase is a variant of alteplase with a high fibrin specificity and resistance to plasminogen activator inhibitor 1 (PAI-1). The main advantage of tenecteplase compared with alteplase is that it is given in a single-bolus administration, versus bolus and infusion over 60 min for alteplase, because of a reduction in the systemic clearance of the agent. In 1997, the TIMI-10A study, a dose-finding study for tenecteplase,[43] showed encouraging results in primary patency rate in 113 patients.

A comparison between tenecteplase and alteplase was performed in the TIMI 10B trial,[44] which showed similar angiographic success for both drugs in AMI in 886 patients. The dose finding was also tested in the ASSENT-1 (Assessment of the Safety and Efficacy of a New Thrombolytic) study with 3235 patients enrolled,[45] where similar results to the TIMI 10A study emerged, with low incidences of death, nonfatal stroke, and severe bleeding. The ASSENT-2 study, published in 1999, compared single-dose tenecteplase with the standard regimen of alteplase in 16949 patients with AMI, and could not find any difference in 30-day mortality. The study was powered to prove an equal success rate, which was clearly achieved.[46] In addition, tenecteplase also showed a lower incidence of major bleeds (ARR 1.3%; $p = 0.0003$).

Saruplase (prourokinase)

Saruplase is a recombinant urokinase-type plasminogen activator, which is also administered in a front-loaded manner (bolus and infusion over 60 min). In 1989, the PRIMI (PRo-urokinase In Myocardial Infarction trial) Study Group published results on 401 patients who were compared between saruplase and streptokinase in AMI.[47] Coronary patency rates after 24 h were similar in both groups; bleeding complications were less in the saruplase group. In 1998, the COMPASS (COMparison trial of Saruplase and Streptokinase) Investigators compared 3089 patients with AMI between saruplase and streptokinase.[48] There were no significant differences in mortality after 30 days and after 1 year (ARR for saruplase 1% and 1.4%, respectively). Saruplase was associated with more hemorrhagic and less ischemic stroke.

Saruplase was also evaluated against urokinase (SUTAMI[49]) and alteplase (SESAM[50]). SUTAMI (Saruplase and Urokinase in the Treatment of Acute Myocardial Infarction) was designed only to compare the course of fibrinogen, thrombin–antithrombin III complex, and prothrombin fragments 1 and 2, and showed similar results for both drugs. In the SESAM (Study in Europe with Saruplase and Alteplase in Myocardial infarction) study, alteplase and saruplase were compared in 473 patients regarding the time to patency and the angiographic success. Both agents showed similar results regarding early patency, reocclusion rate, and safety profile.

Lanetoplase (nPA)

Lanetoplase, which is derived from alteplase, can also be given in a single-bolus manner, which provides faster and easier application compared with front-loaded regimens such as alteplase. The first large study with lanetoplase, published in 1998, was InTIME (Intravenous nPA for Treatment of Infarcting Myocardium Early),[51] an angiographically

documented dose-finding study in which single-dose lanetoplase in different regimens was compared with alteplase. In 602 patients, it was shown that lanetoplase at the highest dose (120 kU/kg) had a higher patency rate after 90 min than alteplase in the usual front-loaded application (bolus and 60 min infusion). Safety was comparable. Thereafter, InTIME II was initiated and powered to prove at least equality between lanetoplase and alteplase,[52] including 15 078 patients with AMI. No difference could be found in the endpoints of mortality after 30 days and after 6 months, and stroke, reinfarction, and percutaneous coronary intervention (PCI) after 30 days.

Overall statement

Currently, thrombolysis is still the standard of care in ST-elevation AMI (STEMI) (after the exclusion of patients with contraindications) if angioplasty is not available within 90 min and if the patient is not aged 75 years or older. Given the comparable study results for major cardiac events and the complications of most of the newer agents, together with the lack of meta-analyses because of differences in study protocols, recommendations are made on the basis of the simplicity of application and the costs of the different agents. Single-bolus injections are easier to apply in acute situations and can shorten the door-to-treatment time. Therefore, tenecteplase and lanetoplase (both rather expensive agents) should be used in daily routine; reteplase has the problem of a double-bolus injection, which may potentially lead to mistakes in use. Cerebral bleeding occurs in about 0.7% of patients with thrombolysis, with a clear increase from the age of 70 years and an excess rate in patients aged 75 years or older.

Antithrombotic trials

Intravenous/subcutaneous therapy

Unstable angina/acute myocardial infarction

Heparin. Although it had never really been tested, intravenous heparin therapy was from the middle of the 1980s the standard in unstable angina (UA) and AMI. The anticoagulant dose was usually adjusted for 1.5 times the baseline measurement of activated partial thromboplastin time (aPTT). As early as 1976, small studies showed not only a benefit in preventing deep venous thrombosis and pulmonary embolism but also a reduction of the ECG changes in AMI.[53] In 1982, Gritsiuk et al[54] showed a benefit of heparin versus glucose, insulin, and potassium in 121 patients with AMI with regard to ejection fraction and death. Only in 1988 were trial results published, by Theroux et al,[55] comparing aspirin 325 mg with therapeutic heparin and the combination of both in 479 patients with UA.[55] Heparin, aspirin, and the combination all significantly reduced the incidence of MI during hospitalization (up to 9 days) compared with placebo (ARR 11.2%, 9%, and 10.4%, respectively); there were no deaths in the treatment groups, compared with 1.7% in the placebo group (p=ns). The combination of aspirin and heparin led to a higher rate of serious bleeding compared with heparin alone (3.3% vs 1.7%). Heparin alone was also associated with a decrease in the occurrence of refractory angina during hospitalization. In 1993, the next study by the same group with 484 patients compared aspirin 325 mg with a therapeutic heparin dose for an average of 5 days, and showed an ARR of 2.9% for the prevention of the development of MI in the heparin group during hospitalization.[56]

Low-molecular-weight heparins (LMWH). LMWH, already established in the therapy of deep vein thrombosis, were the next agents thought to be at least as effective as unfractionated heparin in UA and AMI, and were certainly easier in terms of management (no need for monitoring, more reliable dose–response and bioavailability, and subcutaneous administration) with fewer side-effects (fewer heparin-induced thrombosis (HIT) II complication events).

In 1996, the FRISC (Fragmin during Instability in Coronary Artery Disease) study compared dalteparin (given twice daily for 6 days and then once daily up to 35–45 days) versus placebo in 1506 patients with UA.[57] Early mortality and early new MI (up to 6 days) were lower in the dalteparin group (ARR 3%), and after 40 days the positive effects persisted. After 4–5 months, however, there were no significant differences in rates of death, new MI, or revascularization. Side-effects were rare.

In 1997, dalteparin was compared with intravenous heparin in 1482 patients with UA or non-Q-wave infarction, and proved to be similar to unfractionated heparin in the composite clinical endpoint of death, MI, or recurrent angina in the first 6 days as well as from day 6 to 45 and in revascularization procedures until day 45 (FRIC: Fragmin in Unstable Coronary Artery Disease).[58] Also in 1997, the ESSENCE (Efficacy and Safety of Subcutaneous Enoxaparin in Non-Q-wave Coronary Events) trial was published, in which 3171 patients with UA or non-Q-wave infarction were randomized to enoxaparin or intravenous heparin for a minimum of 48 h up to 8 days.[59] At 14 days and at 30 days, the composite endpoint of death, MI, or recurrent angina was significantly lower for the enoxaparin group (ARR 3.2% vs 3.5%). The 1-year results showed a persistently positive effect, with about the same risk reduction for the composite endpoint (ARR 3.7%; p=0.022) and with less need for diagnostic catheterization (ARR 3.6%) and coronary revascularization (ARR 5.3%) in the enoxaparin group.[60]

The FRAX.I.S (Fraxiparine in Ischemic Syndrome) study evaluated nadroparin against unfractionated heparin in 3468 patients with two different regimens. One group received nadroparin subcutaneously twice daily for 6 days and the other group for 14 days. With respect to the primary endpoint (cardiac death, MI, refractory angina, or reoccurrence of UA at day 14), there were no significant differences between the three groups. However, the major bleeding rate was significantly elevated in the nadroparin 14-day group (absolute risk elevation 1.9% against unfractionated heparin; p=0.0035).[61]

The ACUTE (Antithrombotic Combination Using Tirofiban and Enoxaparin) study compared enoxaparin with unfractioned heparin in 525 patients with non-ST-elevation coronary syndromes who were also receiving tirofiban.[62] The total bleeding rate was slightly higher in the unfractioned heparin group (4.8% vs 3.5%), but the composite endpoint of death or MI occurred with similar frequency. Enoxaparin was better in reducing the need for revascularization due to refractory ischemia (ARR 3.7%) and in reducing rehospitalization due to unstable angina (ARR 5.5%).

A similar study with patients receiving eptifibatide comparing enoxaparin and unfractionated heparin, the INTERACT (INTegrilin and Enoxaparin Randomized assessment of Acute Coronary Treatment) study, was published early in 2003.[63]

In 746 patients with non-ST-elevation coronary syndromes, the composite endpoint of death or MI after 30 days was decreased (ARR 4%) in the enoxaparin group.

After its success in UA, enoxaparin was tested in 2000 in a pilot study in patients with STEMI in 20 patients, and was shown to produce stable therapeutic anti-factor Xa-levels during lysis with alteplase.[64] In the same year, a subgroup meta-analysis of ESSENCE and TIMI 11B in patients with STEMI showed a significant reduction in the composite endpoint (death, myocardial infarction, or emergency revascularization) in favor of enoxaparin after 43 days.[65] In 2001, the HART II (Heparin and Aspirin Reperfusion Therapy) trial in 400 patients controlled angiographically after lysis with alteplase combined with either enoxaparin or unfractionated heparin showed similar results for both groups with regard to restored TIMI grade 2 or 3 flow.[66] In the ENTIRE (ENoxaparin and Tenecteplase with or without gp IIb/IIIa Inhibitor as Reperfusion strategy in the STEMI trial) – TIMI 23 trial, enoxaparin proved once again to be as effective as unfractionated heparin in patients with lysis, either with full-dose tenecteplase or half-dose tenecteplase plus abciximab.[67] Enoxaparin reduced death and recurrent MI after 30 days (ARR 11.5%) in combination with full-dose tenecteplase compared with unfractioned heparin.

Further evidence for the superiority of enoxaparin in STEMI came in 2002 from Baird et al,[68] who showed in 300 patients undergoing lysis of a STEMI that enoxaparin reduced the triple endpoint of death, nonfatal MI or readmission with UA by 10% after 90 days.[68] There was no difference in major haemorrhage. The AMI-SK study[69] showed a similar benefit in 496 patients with AMI who had a lysis with streptokinase: the ARR for enoxaparin for the composite endpoint of death, reinfarction, or recurrent angina at 30 days was 8% compared with unfractionated heparin.

Finally, the ASSENT-3 study, published in 2001, compared three different regimens in 6095 patients: full-dose tenecteplase and enoxaparin, half-dose tenecteplase and abciximab, and full-dose tenecteplase and unfractioned heparin.[70] With regard to the primary endpoint (30-day mortality, in-hospital reinfarction, and in-hospital refractory ischemia), the enoxaparin and abciximab groups were significantly better (ARR 4% and 4.3%, respectively). The same was true when serious bleeds and intracranial haemorrhage were taken into account in a composite endpoint, with an ARR of 3.3% for the enoxaparin group and 2.8% for the abciximab group. The therapeutic effects of the enoxaparin and abciximab groups were similar.

There is still debate whether the effectiveness of LMWH differs between products. This discussion remains speculative since there are no head-to-head comparisons available between LMWH. It has been proposed that the ratio of antithrombin to anti-factor Xa effects may be the key difference. The reasons why LMWH seems to do better than unfractionated heparin may include the handling, dosing, and control of the unfractionated heparin.

The present standard of care in acute coronary syndromes is the use of LMWH, with enoxaparin, dalteparin, and nadroparin being the best studied agents and showing the best results compared with unfractionated heparin. In summary, the current recommendation is to use LMWH for at least 6 days at therapeutic dosage for conservative management of acute coronary syndromes.

Hirudin. The promise of hirudin compared with heparin came from a more predictable dose–response, easier monitoring, direct and high-affinity inhibition of thrombin (including clot-bound thrombin), and the absence of heparin-induced thrombopenia. The TIMI 5 study, published in 1994, showed in 246 patients with AMI and lysis with alteplase an encouraging advantage of hirudin over unfractionated heparin in the composite endpoint of in-hospital death or reinfarction, with an ARR of 9.9%.[71] Major hemorrhages were also significantly fewer in the hirudin group (ARR 3.5%). The TIMI 9B study followed TIMI 5, with more patients being randomized. In the study population of 3002 patients, no differences in predefined primary and composite endpoints could be shown. In addition, subgroup analysis could not find a subgroup with an advantage for hirudin therapy.[72]

With regard to UA, a first study (GUSTO IIa) comparing hirudin with unfractionated heparin had been interrupted after 2564 patients due to a higher rate of hemorrhagic strokes in the hirudin group.[73] Because a dosage problem was believed to be responsible, the study was relaunched (as GUSTO IIb) with a lower dose of hirudin, and published in 1996: 12 142 patients with UA or non-Q-wave infarction were randomized to either heparin or hirudin. Hirudin reduced slightly the incidence of non-fatal MI after 30 days, but the composite endpoint of death, reinfarction, or nonfatal infarction showed only a trend in favor of hirudin (ARR 0.9%).

Another study performed in 1205 patients with AMI and lysis with streptokinase showed no effect of subcutaneous lepirudin (recombinant hirudin) compared with subcutaneous heparin in restoring TIMI grade 3 flow in the infarction-related vessel and no effect on the composite clinical endpoint (death, nonfatal stroke, nonfatal reinfarction, rescue PCI, or refractory angina) or mortality after 1 year (HIT-4).[75] At present, hirudin is approved by the US Food and Drug Administration for use in patients after PCI.

Glycoprotein (GP)IIb/IIIa inhibitors. In 1997, two landmark studies proved the efficacy of this new group of antiplatelet drugs in preventing ischemic complications after PCI in elective and urgent revascularization procedures. EPILOG (Evaluation of PTCA to Improve Long-term Outcome with abciximab GPIIb/IIIa receptor blockade) compared abciximab and low-dose heparin versus placebo with standard heparin in 2792 patients undergoing elective or urgent revascularization.[76] The abciximab group showed an ARR of 6.5% for the composite endpoint of death, myocardial infarction, or urgent revascularization. In the same year, the CAPTURE (Chimeric 7E3 Antiplatelet Therapy in Unstable angina REfractory to standard treatment) trial showed a periprocedural benefit of abciximab in 1265 patients with UA undergoing angioplasty,[77] with fewer events (death, myocardial infarction, or repeated intervention) after 30 days (ARR 4.6%) but similarity after 6 months.

In 2001, the ADMIRAL (Abciximab before Direct angioplasty and stenting in Myocardial Infarction Regarding Acute and Long-term follow-up) study compared abciximab versus placebo before angioplasty and stenting in 300 patients with AMI.[78] Abciximab led to better immediate and late (6 months) angiographic success and to a reduction of the composite endpoint death, reinfarction, and urgent revascularization after 30 days (ARR 8.6%) and after 6 months (8.5%). When GPIIb/IIIa inhibitors were studied in revascularization procedures, they were also thought to be potentially beneficial in the management of UA and non-Q-wave infarction.

Four studies were reported in 1998 that compared different GPIIb/IIIa inhibitors either with placebo or with heparin. The PURSUIT (Platelet glycoprotein IIb/IIIa in Unstable angina: Receptor Suppression Using Integrilin Therapy) investigators looked at 10948 patients with acute coronary syndromes who received either eptifibatide or placebo on top of intravenous heparin and aspirin.[79] The frequency of the composite endpoint (death or nonfatal MI) was reduced in the eptifibatide group after 7 and 30 days (ARR 1.5% for both).

In the PRISM (Platelet Receptor inhibition in Ischemic Syndrome Management) study, 3232 patients with UA were randomized to either tirofiban or intravenous heparin.[80] At 48 hours, significantly fewer patients in the tirofiban group reached the composite endpoint of death, MI or refractory ischemia (ARR 1.8%); after 30 days, the difference was no longer significant but showed a trend in favor of tirofiban (ARR 1.3%). Mortality after 30 days was significantly reduced in the tirofiban group (ARR 1.3%).

PRISM-PLUS looked at 1915 patients with UA/non-Q-wave infarction and randomized them to intravenous heparin, tirofiban, or both.[81] Tirofiban alone had an excess mortality at 7 days (plus 3.5%) compared with heparin alone, but the combination significantly reduced the short- and long-term composite endpoint (see PRISM) at 6 days, 30 days, and 6 months (ARR 5%, 4.8%, and 4.4%, respectively).

Finally in 1998, the PARAGON (Platelet IIb/IIIa Antagonism for the Reduction of Acute coronary syndrome events in the Global Organization Network) investigators published results from 2282 patients with UA/non-Q-wave infarction who were randomized to different regimens of lamifiban with and without heparin or to heparin alone.[82] The composite primary endpoint of death or non-fatal MI was not significantly different after 30 days, but turned out to be significantly different for the lower dose of lamifiban after 6 months (ARR 4.2%). In a subsequent study, PARAGON B, 1160 patients with non-ST-elevation acute coronary syndromes were randomized to lamifiban or placebo in addition to heparin or LMWH.[83] In the subgroup of patients who were troponin T-positive at study entry, there was a clear reduction of the primary endpoint (death, MI, or recurrent ischemia) in the lamifiban group at 30 days (ARR 8.4%).

The large GUSTO IV-ACS study was published in 2001, with 7800 patients with non ST-elevation acute coronary syndromes not undergoing early revascularization being randomized to different regimens of abciximab or placebo.[84] Concomitant therapy was also studied in a subgroup (heparin versus dalteparin). At 30 days, there were no differences in the primary endpoint (death or MI) and there was no subgroup showing a benefit of the intervention strategy. The authors therefore concluded that abciximab was not beneficial in the studied population who were not undergoing early angiography. The results after 1 year were published in 2003, and again showed no benefit in mortality.[85] Patients with low/negative cardiac troponin and those with elevated C-reactive protein (CRP) even had an excess mortality when treated for 48h with abciximab (absolute risk increase 2.7% ($p=0.02$) vs 4.2% ($p=0.04$)).

For patients with STEMI, the first results with GPIIb/IIIa inhibitors were published in 1997. The IMPACT-AMI study was an angiographic dose-finding study for integrilin in 180 patients with STEMI who received alteplase for lysis.[86] It could be shown that integrilin led to a better reperfusion after 90 min, but there was no clinical difference in outcome. PARADIGM (Platelet Aggregation Receptor Antagonist Dose Investigation and Reperfusion Gain in Myocardial Infarction) studied lamifiban in the same setting in 353 patients and could not show any benefit in TIMI grade 3 flow rate, death, reinfarction, or refractory ischemia.[87]

In 2000, after an initial dose-finding study in 304 patients, the SPEED (Strategies for Patency Enhancement in the Emergency Department) investigators randomized 224 patients with STEMI to full-dose reteplase or to abciximab and half-dose reteplase.[88] Overall, there was no significant difference in TIMI flow grade in the angiographic control at 60–90 min after therapy between the two groups, but a subgroup of the abciximab group with 60 U/kg bolus of heparin showed a better TIMI grade 3 flow. Major bleeding showed a trend to occur more frequently in the combined group. Another angiographic study, TIMI 14, published in 1999, was also a dose-finding study in 888 patients comparing different combinations of alteplase/streptokinase and abciximab

with either substance alone.[89] Ninety minutes after initiation of therapy, the TIMI grade 3 flow rate was significantly higher in the half-dose alteplase/ abciximab group than in conventional lysis (77% vs 62%).

The largest trial investigating the effect of abciximab and reduced dose alteplase versus alteplase alone was GUSTO V, which was published in 2001.[90] In this trial, 16 588 patients with AMI were randomized to either of the two groups. The endpoint of death or reinfarction after 7 days was reduced in the combination group (ARR 1.4%), and with an additional endpoint (urgent revascularization) the difference was even larger (ARR 4.6%). These advantages were somewhat outweighed by an augmentation of nonserious and serious bleeds. In patients older than 75 years, the rate of intracranial bleeding was doubled. A 1-year follow-up of GUSTO V in 2002 showed no significant difference in terms of mortality between the two groups.[91] As with LMWH, there are no head-to-head comparisons of different GPIIb/IIIa inhibitors in AMI and acute coronary syndromes without coronary intervention.

In summary, at present, GPIIb/IIIa inhibitors are not used routinely in patients undergoing thrombolysis in AMI. Tirofiban and integrelin are used in acute coronary syndromes not immediately undergoing revascularization. Abciximab is used preferably in patients undergoing PCI based on currently available data. For reasons of cost and because outcomes do not seem to hold longer than 1 year, tirofiban may be used for this indication as well.

Oral antiplatelet therapy

Secondary prevention

In the early 1970s, smaller randomized studies were conducted to demonstrate an effect of aspirin in secondary prevention after MI. A first overview of seven randomized prospective trials and two case–control studies showed no difference between aspirin and placebo but a favorable trend for the antithrombotic agent.[92]

In 1975, a prospective study evaluated the use of aspirin in 1 million people regardless of earlier coronary events, and showed no difference in coronary death between people who frequently took aspirin and those who did not.[93] Thereafter, several studies including up to 1600 patients per study demonstrated a significant reduction or a trend of risk reduction of coronary heart disease (CHD) and of recurrent MI.[94–96]

In 1980, three controversial studies were published that led to further confusion about the use of aspirin in CHD.[97–99] The Aspirin in Myocardial Infarction Study (AMIS) evaluated 4524 persons after at least one MI in a randomized, double-blinded, placebo-controlled manner, and showed a total mortality rate of 10.8% in the aspirin group versus 9.7% in the placebo group and no difference in the combination endpoint of coronary mortality and nonfatal MI (14.1% for aspirin and 14.8% for placebo).[97] In the same year, the Persantine [dipyridamole] – Aspirin Reinfarction Study (PARIS) randomized 2026 patients after MI to three different groups, and found a strong trend towards lower total mortality (relative risk reduction (RRR) 18%), lower coronary mortality (RRR 21%), and less nonfatal myocardial infarction (RRR 24%) in the aspirin group.[98] These results were statistically significant only if patients were analyzed who started taking aspirin in the first 6 months after the MI.

Further evidence for a beneficial effect of aspirin came from the German–Austrian Aspirin Trial with 946 patients who were randomly allocated to 1.5 g aspirin, phenprocoumon, or placebo after an MI.[99] Coronary death was significantly reduced in the aspirin group compared with placebo (ARR 3.1%) and also compared with phenprocoumon (ARR 4%). Furthermore, coronary events were reduced in the same manner, with an ARR of 4.4% in favor of aspirin compared with placebo.

In 1986, the PARIS II trial was published, in which 3128 patients were randomized in a group with dipyridamole and aspirin versus placebo after MI.[100] A significance in favor of the treatment group was shown for coronary events (nonfatal MI or cardiac death) with a risk reduction of 30% after 1 year and of 24% at the end of the study. Thereafter, the use of aspirin in CHD was strongly supported in every review. Dipyridamole alone and in combination with aspirin is not recommended because of the negative results in the PARIS study.

In 1992, the Swedish Angina Pectoris Aspirin Trial (SAPAT) randomly assigned 2035 patients with stable angina in a double-blinded manner either to aspirin (75 mg) or to placebo.[101] All patients received sotalol for control of symptoms. After a follow-up duration of 50 months, the aspirin group showed a significant reduction of 34% (81 vs 124 patients; ARR 4.2%) in the primary outcome, defined as MI or sudden death.

In 1985, cardiologists investigated another antiplatelet substance for secondary prevention. The thienopyridine ticlopidine, already proven to be effective in cerebrovascular disease, showed an effect in preventing aortocoronary bypass graft occlusion. In the study by Rothlin et al,[102] the patency rate of bypass vessels per patient was similar in the group receiving ticlopidine to that in the group receiving acenocoumarol, which was the standard medication at that time. These results were confirmed by another study, by Limet et al,[103] who compared ticlopidine against placebo in 173 patients undergoing coronary artery bypass grafting (475 grafts). Because of the side-effects of ticlopidine, its use in long-term secondary prevention remained controversial, although Ishikawa et al[104] demonstrated an effect in preventing coronary events after a first MI.

Meanwhile another thienopyridine, clopidogrel, emerged as a valuable alternative without the hematological side-effects of ticlopidine. In 1996, the CAPRIE (Clopidogrel versus Aspirin in Patients at Risk of Ischaemic Events) study compared 75 mg clopidogrel with 325 mg aspirin in 19185 patients with previous signs of atherosclerotic disease (MI, ischemic stroke, or peripheral arterial disease).[105] With a mean follow-up of 1.91 years, clopidogrel showed a significant RRR of 8.7% for the combined endpoint of ischemic stroke, MI, or vascular death. The ARR, however, was only 0.51% compared with ASA. The absolute risk per year was 5.83% for the combined endpoint in the aspirin group, which is rather low for such a high-risk population. The small ARR resulted in a number to treat to prevent 1 event in 1 year (NNT) of 196 patients, which led to much discussion about the cost–benefit of clopidogrel use. With the actual prices for the two drugs the costs per patient per year are 1117 Swiss Francs and the costs per event saved 218 984 Swiss Francs.

A collaborative meta-analysis published in 2002 examined all randomized antiplatelet trials available before September 1997 in patients at high risk of occlusive vascular events.[106] The results showed an ARR of 3.6% for having a serious vascular event for any platelet therapy after previous MI, an ARR of 3.8%

after a cerebrovascular event, and an ARR of 2.2% for other high-risk patients. Aspirin was the most widely studied drug, with doses of 75–150 mg daily proving to be as least as effective as higher doses. Ticlopidine showed overall an RRR of 12% compared with ASA, which is quite similar to that of clopidogrel (RRR 10% compared with aspirin). Addition of dipyridamole to aspirin showed no effect at all.[106]

Currently under way is the CHARISMA (Clopidogrel for High Atherothrombotic Risk and Ischemic Stabilization, Management and Avoidance) study, which compares the combination of clopidogrel and aspirin with clopidogrel alone in atherosclerotic high-risk patients.

Unstable angina/acute myocardial infarction

In 1983, approximately 10 years after the first trials of the use of aspirin in secondary prevention of CHD, the first study on its use in UA showed a beneficial effect in the prevention of AMI and death. The Veterans Administration Cooperative Study included 1266 men with UA and randomized them to groups with either placebo or 324 mg aspirin daily for 12 weeks.[107] The aspirin group had a significant ARR of 5.1% for the combined endpoint of AMI or death compared with placebo, with a greater effect on the prevention of AMI. These results were confirmed by a Canadian multicenter trial in 1985, which showed a significant ARR of 8.4% for aspirin (1000 mg daily) in the combined endpoint of death or MI versus placebo or sulfinpyrazone.[108]

The thienopyridines have also been tested in the secondary prevention of UA. In 1990, Balsano et al[109] studied 652 patients with UA who were randomly assigned to conventional therapy (β-blockers, nitrates, and calcium antagonists) with or without ticlopidine 250 mg twice daily. They found a significant ARR of 6.3% for ticlopidine for the combined endpoint of vascular death or nonfatal MI compared with placebo. The ARR for any MI was 5.8%. Even better results were obtained from a subgroup analysis of patients with transient ischemic ECG changes.[110]

In 2001, data were published from the CURE (Clopidogrel in Unstable angina to prevent Recurrent ischemic Events) study, in which clopidogrel was tested in addition to aspirin in patients with acute coronary syndromes without ST elevation.[111]

This study randomized 12 562 patients into two treatment groups, either aspirin alone or aspirin and clopidogrel with a loading dose of 300 mg and a maintenance dose of 75 mg daily for 3–12 months. The composite endpoint of cardiovascular death, nonfatal MI, or stroke was reduced, with an ARR of 2.1% in the clopidogrel group. This number remained quite stable when refractory ischemia was added to the primary endpoint (ARR 2.3%). The results were compromised somewhat by an increase of the major bleed rate by 1.0% (absolute risk). Because of numerous doubts about the benefit of clopidogrel over time and in subgroups of patients, two further analyses of the same study have been published. These demonstrated a significant positive effect for clopidogrel in different risk groups stratified according to the TIMI risk score.[112] The most positive effects were obtained in the highest-risk group (ARR 4.8%); significant effects of clopidogrel on the primary endpoint were found after 30 days (ARR 1.1%) and beyond 30 days (ARR 1.1%).[113] The effect started as early as 24 h after the beginning of therapy.

After success with the intravenous application of GPIIb/IIIa inhibitors in patients undergoing coronary interventions, a number of oral GPIIb/IIIa inhibitors have been developed, but all three studies that looked at the effect of these agents in UA – SYMPHONY (Sibrafiban versus aspirin to Yield Maximum Protection from ischemic Heart events post-acute coronary syndromes) for sibrafiban[114] and OPUS (Orofiban in Patients with Unstable Coronary Syndromes) – TIMI-16 for orbofiban[115] or after stent implantation during PCI (EXCITE, Evaluation of oral Xemilofibran In controlling Thrombotic Events[116]) showed no effect[114,116] or a negative effect[115] on cardiovascular events and death.

After percutaneous coronary intervention

Because of a high rate of early stent thrombosis after PCI, the initial recommendations were to establish anticoagulation therapy with initial heparin followed by oral anticoagulation. In 1995, Van Belle et al[117] reported a small series of 45 patients who were treated with ASA 200 mg/day, ticlopidine 500 mg/day and periprocedural heparin. There was no early stent thrombosis in any of the patients. The study by Schomig et al[118] a year later confirmed this early result.

They randomized 517 patients either to aspirin and ticlopidine or to aspirin, intravenous heparin, and phenprocoumon. The group with ticlopidine showed a significant ARR of 11.1% for the primary non-cardiac endpoint (death from noncardiac causes, cerebrovascular events, severe hemorrhage, or peripheral vascular events) and an ARR of 4.6% for the primary cardiac endpoint (cardiac death, MI, repeated angioplasty, or aortocoronary bypass surgery). Occlusion of the stented vessel occurred in 0.8% of the ticlopidin group and in 5.4% of the phenprocumon group.[118]

Clopidogrel has been compared with ticlopidine for the prevention of stent thrombosis. Three studies with about 3200 patients by Moussa et al,[119] Müller et al,[120] and Bertrand et al[121] (CLASSICS) all found a comparable effect in preventing stent thrombosis with less noncardiac side-effects. Moreover, the PCI-CURE study investigated the effect of clopidogrel pretreatment (a median of 6 days) and long-term therapy (median 9 months) with clopidogrel in patients with UA undergoing PCI, and found a significant ARR of 1.9% for primary endpoint events (cardiovascular death, MI, and urgent target-vessel revascularization) in favor of the clopidogrel group.[122] The CREDO (Clopidogrel for Reduction of Events During Observation) study was similarly designed, and analyzed the effect of clopidogrel in patients undergoing elective PCI.[123] The significant ARR for clopidogrel for the same primary endpoint as in PCI-CURE was 3%, but there was also a trend towards more major bleeding in this group (an absolute increase of 2.1%). In March 2003, however, a further follow-up over a median 28 months of the study by Müller et al[120] showed a higher risk of cardiac death and nonfatal MI of 5.8% in the group treated with clopidogrel for 30 days (40 patient events) compared with ticlopidine.[124] This raises some concern about the widespread use of clopidogrel, and further studies should bring more clarity.

At present, there is a class 1 indication for the use of aspirin in either chronic or acute CHD. In the case of aspirin intolerance, clopidogrel is the alternative. In patients with acute coronary syndromes not undergoing PCI, the use of clopidogrel is additional to aspirin in medium- and high-risk situations for up to 9 months.

References

1. Wegner H, Dadaliaris D, Engelmann L, et al. Comparison of short and protracted streptokinase therapy in acute myocardial infarction. Z Gesamte Inn Med 1975;30:186–9.

2. Aber CP, Bass NM, Berry CL, et al. Streptokinase in acute myocardial infarction: a controlled multicentre study in the United Kingdom. BMJ 1976;ii:1100–4.

3. Australian multicentre trial of streptokinase in acute myocardial infarction. Med J Aust 1977;1:553.

4. Benda L, Haider M, Ambrosch F. Results of the Austrian myocardial infarction study on the effects of streptokinase. Wien Klin Wochenschr 1977;89:779–83.

5. European Cooperative Study Group for Streptokinase Treatment in Acute Myocardial Infarction. Streptokinase in acute myocardial infarction. N Engl J Med 1979;301:797–802.

6. Liusov VA, Koniaev BV, Belousov IuB, et al. Effectiveness and the methods of using streptokinase in myocardial inarct and preinfarct stenocardia. Kardiologiia 1980;20:46–51.

7. De Feyter PJ, van Eenige MJ, de Jong JP, et al. Experience with intracoronary streptokinase in 36 patients with acute evolving myocardial infarction. Eur Heart J 1982;3:441–8.

8. Khaja F, Walton JA, Brymer JF, et al. Intracoronary fibrinolytic therapy in acute myocardial infarction. Report of a prospective randomized trial. N Engl J Med 1983;308:1305–11.

9. Hillis LD, Borer J, Braunwald E, et al. High dose intravenous streptokinase for acute myocardial infarction: preliminary results of a multicenter trial. J Am Coll Cardiol 1985;6:957–62.

10. Schreiber TL, Miller DH, Silvasi DA, et al. Randomized double-blind trial of intravenous streptokinase in acute myocardial infarction. Am J Cardiol 1986;58:47–52.

11. Bassand JP, Faivre R, Becque O, et al. Intravenous streptokinase versus heparin in recent acute myocardial infarction. Randomized multicenter study in the Franche-Comte. Arch Mal Coeur Vaiss 1986;79:421–8.

12. Gruppo Italiano per lo Studio della Streptochinasi nell'Infarto miocardico (GISSI). Effectiveness of intravenous thrombolytic treatment in acute myocardial infarction. Lancet 1986;i:397–401.

13. Gruppo Italiano per lo Studio della Streptochinasi nell'Infarto miocardico (GISSI). Long-term effects of intravenous thrombolysis in acute myocardial infarction: final report of the GISSI study. Lancet 1987;ii:871–4.

14. The ISIS Collaborative Group. Randomized factorial trial of high-dose intravenous streptokinase, of oral aspirin and of intravenous heparin in acute myocardial infarction. ISIS (International Studies of Infarct Survival) pilot study. Eur Heart J 1987;8:634–42.

15. White HD, Norris RM, Brown MA, et al. Effect of intravenous streptokinase on left ventricular function and early survival after acute myocardial infarction. N Engl J Med 1987;317:850–5.

16. The ISIS Collaborative Group. Randomized trial of intravenous streptokinase, oral aspirin, both, or neither among 17 187 cases of suspected acute myocardial infarction: ISIS-2. Lancet 1988;ii:349–60.

17. The ISAM Study Group. A prospective trial of Intravenous Streptokinase in Acute Myocardial Infarction (ISAM). Mortality, morbidity and infarct size at 21 days. N Engl J Med 1986;314:1465–71.

18. Brochier M, Raynaud R, Planiol T, et al. Treatment by urokinase of myocardial infarction and threatened infarction. Randomised study of 120 cases. Arch Mal Coeur Vaiss 1975;68:563–9.

19. The European Collaborative Group. Controlled trial of urokinase in myocardial infarction. A European Collaborative Study. Lancet 1975;ii:624–6.

20. Rossi P, Bolognese L. Comparison of intravenous urokinase plus heparin versus heparin alone in acute myocardial infarction. Am J Cardiol 1991;68:585–92.

21. Chesebro JH, Knatterud G, Roberts R, et al. Thrombolysis in Myocardial Infarction (TIMI) Trial, phase I: a comparison between intravenous tissue plasminogen activator and intravenous streptokinase. Clinical findings through hospital discharge. Circulation 1987;76:142–54.

22. Wilcox RG, von der Lippe G, Olsson CG, et al. Trial of tissue plasminogen activator for mortality reduction in acute myocardial infarction. Anglo-Scandinavian Study of Early Thrombolysis (ASAET). Lancet 1988; ii:525–30.

23. Wilcox RG, von der Lippe G, Olsson CG, et al. Effects of alteplase in acute myocardial infarction: 6 month results from the ASAET study. Lancet 1990;335: 1175–8.

24. Califf RM, Vandormael M, Grines CL, et al. A randomized trial of late perfusion therapy for acute myocardial infarction. Circulation 1997;85:2090–9.

25. Gruppo Italiano per lo Studio della Sopravvivenza nell'Infarto miocardico (GISSI). GISSI-2: a factorial randomized trial of alteplase vs streptokinase and heparin vs no heparin among 12 490 patients with acute myocardial infarction. Lancet 1990;336:65–71.

26. The International Study Group. In-hospital mortality and clinical course of 20 891 patients with suspected acute myocardial infarction randomized between alteplase and streptokinase with or without heparin. Lancet 1990;336:71–5.

27. GISSI-2 and International Study Group. Six-month survival in 20 891 patients with acute myocardial infarction randomized between alteplase and streptokinase with or without heparin. Eur Heart J 1992; 13:1692–7.

28. Grines CL, Nissen SE, Booth DC, et al. A prospective, randomized trial comparing combination half-dose tissue-type plasminogen activator and streptokinase with full-dose tissue-type plasminogen activator. Circulation 1991;84:540–9.

29. The GUSTO Investigators. An international randomized trial comparing four thrombolytic strategies for acute myocardial infarction. N Engl J Med 1993; 329:673–82.

30. The ISIS-3 (Third International Study of Infarct Survival) Collaborative Group. ISIS-3: a randomized comparison of streptokinase vs tissue plasminogen activator vs anistreplase and of aspirin plus heparin vs aspirin alone among 41 299 cases of suspected acute myocardial infarction. Lancet 1992;339:753–70.

31. The AIMS Group. Effect of intravenous APSAC on mortality after acute myocardial infarction: preliminary report of a placebo-controlled trial. Lancet 1988;i:545–9.

32. The AIMS Group. Long-term effects of intravenous anistreplase in acute myocardial infarction: final report of the AIMS Study. Lancet 1990;335:427–31.

33. Anderson JL, Sorensen SG, Moreno FL, et al. Multicenter patency trial of intravenous anistreplase compared with streptokinase in acute myocardial infarction. Circulation 1991;83:126–40.

34. Lusson J-R, Anguenot T, Wolf J-E, et al. Comparative effects of APSAC and rt-PA on infarct size and left ventricular function in acute myocardial infarction. A multicentre randomized study. Circulation 1991; 84:1107–17.

35. Anderson JL, Becker LC, Sorensen SG, et al. Anistreplase versus alteplase in acute myocardial infarction: comparative effects on left ventricular

function, morbidity and 1-day coronary artery patency. J Am Coll Cardiol 1992;20:753–66.

36. Neuhaus K-L, von Essen R, Tebbe U, et al. Improved thrombolysis in acute myocardial infarction with front-loaded administration of alteplase: results of the rt-PA-APSAC patency study. J Am Coll Cardiol 1992;19:885–91.

37. O'Connor CM, Meese R, McNulty S, et al. A randomized factorial trial of reperfusion strategies and aspirin dosing in acute myocardial infarction. Am J Cardiol 1996;77:791–7.

38. Cannon CP, McCabe CH, Diver DJ, et al. Comparison of front-loaded recombinant tissue-type plasminogen activator, anistreplase and combination thrombolytic therapy for acute myocardial infarction: results of the Thrombolysis in Myocardial Infarction (TIMI) 4 trial. J Am Coll Cardiol 1994;24:1602–10.

39. International Joint Efficacy Comparison of Thrombolytics. Randomized, double-blind comparison of reteplase double-bolus administration with strepto kinase in acute myocardial infarction (INJECT): trial to investigate equivalence. Lancet 1995;346:329–36.

40. Smalling RW, Bode C, Kalbfleisch J, et al. More rapid, complete and stable coronary thrombolysis with bolus administration of reteplase compared with alteplase infusion in acute myocardial infarction. Circulation 1995;91:2725–32.

41. Bode C, Smalling RW, Berg G, et al. Randomized comparison of coronary thrombolysis achieved with double bolus reteplase (recombinant plasminogen activator) and front loaded, accelerated alteplase (recombinant tissue plasminogen activator) in patients with acute myocardial infarction. Circulation 1996;94:891–8.

42. The Global Use of Strategies to Open Occluded Coronary Arteries (GUSTO) III Investigators. A comparison of reteplase with alteplase for acute myocardial infarction. N Engl J Med 1997;337:1118–23.

43. Cannon CP, McCabe CH, Gibson M, et al. TNK-tissue plasminogen activator in acute myocardial infarction of the Thrombolysis In Myocardial Infarction (TIMI) 10A dose ranging trial. Circulation 1997;95:351–6.

44. Cannon CP, Gibson CM, McCabe CH, et al. TNK-tissue plasminogen activator compared with front loaded alteplase in acute myocardial infarction. Results of the TIMI 10B trial. Circulation 1998;98: 2805–14.

45. Van de Werf F, Cannon CP, Luyten A, et al. Safety assessment of single-bolus administration of TNK tissue-plasminogen activator in acute myocardial infarction: the ASSENT-1 trial. Am Heart J 1999; 137:786–91.

46. Assessment of the Safety and Efficacy of a New Thrombolytic (ASSENT-2) Investigators. Single-bolus tenecteplase compared with front-loaded alteplase in acute myocardial infarction: The ASSENT-2 double-blind randomized trial. Lancet 1999;354:716–22.

47. PRIMI Trial Study Group. Randomized double-blind trial of recombinant pro-urokinase against streptokinase in acute myocardial infarction. Lancet 1989; i:863–8.

48. Tebbie U, Michels R, Adgey J, et al. Randomized, double-blind study comparing saruplase with streptokinase therapy in acute myocardial infarction: the COMPASA equivalence trial. J Am Coll Cardiol 1998;31:487–93.

49. Hoffmann JJ, Michels HR, Windeler J, Günzler WA. Plasma markers of thrombin activity during coronary thrombolytic therapy with saruplase or urokinase: no prediction of reinfarction. Fibrinolysis 1993;7:330–4.

50. Bär FW, Meyer J, Vermeer F, et al. Comparison of saruplase and alteplase in acute myocardial infarction. Am J Cardiol 1997;79:727–32.

51. den Heijer P, Vermeer F, Ambrosioni E, et al. Evaluation of a weight-adjusted single-bolus plasminogen activator in patients with myocardial infarction. A double-blind, randomized angiographic trial of lanctoplase versus alteplase. Circulation 1998;98:2217–25.

52. The InTIME-II Investigators. Intravenous nPA for the treatment of infarcting myocardium early. InTIME-II, a double-blind comparison of single-bolus lanetolase vs accelerated alteplase for the treatment of patients with acute myocardial infarction. Eur Heart J 2000; 2005–13.

53. Saliba MJ Jr, Kuzman WJ, Marsh DG, Lasry JE. Effect of heparin in anticoagulant doses on the electrocardiogram and cardiac enzymes in patients with acute myocardial infarction. A clinical pilot study. Am J Cardiol 1976;37:605–7.

54. Gritsiuk AI, Netiazhenko VZ, Amosova EN, et al. Effectiveness of heparin in patients with acute myocardial infarction. Kardiologiia 1982;22:31–7.

55. Theroux P, Ouimet H, McCans J, et al. Aspirin, heparin, or both to treat acute unstable angina. N Engl J Med 1988;319:1105–11.

56. Theroux P, Waters D, Qiu S, et al. Aspirin versus heparin to prevent myocardial infarction during the acute phase of unstable angina. Circulation 1993;88: 2045–48.

57. Fragmin During Instability in Coronary Artery Disease (FRISC) Study Group. Low-molecular-weight heparin during instability in coronary artery disease. Lancet 1996;347:561–8.

58. Klein W, Buchwald A, Hillis SE, et al. Comparison of low-molecular weight heparin with unfractioned

heparin acutely and with placebo for 6 weeks in the management of unstable coronary artery disease. Fragmin In Unstable Coronary Artery Disease Study (FRIC). Circulation 1997;96:61–8.

59. Cohen M, Demers C, Gurfinkel EP, et al. A comparison of low-molecular-weight heparin with unfractionated heparin for unstable coronary artery disease. N Engl J Med 1997;337:447–52.

60. Goodman SG, Cohen M, Bigonzi F, et al. Randomized trial of low-molecular-weight heparin (enoxaparin) vs unfractionated heparin for unstable coronary artery disease. 1-year results of the ESSENCE study. J Am Coll Cardiol 2000;36:693–8.

61. The FRAX.I.S Study Group. Comparison of two treatment durations (6 days and 14 days) of low molecular weight heparin with a 6-day treatment of unfractionated heparin in the initial management of unstable angina or non-Q wave myocardial infarction: FRAX.I.S (FRAXiparine in Ischemic Syndrome). Eur Heart J 1999;20:1553–62.

62. Cohen M, Theroux P, Borzak S, et al. Randomized double-blind safety study of enoxaparin versus unfractionated heparin in patients with non-ST-segment elevated acute coronary syndromes treated with tirofiban and aspirin. The ACUTE II study. The Antithrombotic Combination Using Tirofiban and Enoxaparin. Am Heart J 2002;144:470–7.

63. Goodman SG, Fitchett D, Armstrong PW, et al. Randomized evaluation of the safety and efficacy of enoxaparin versus unfractionated heparin in high-risk patients with non-ST-segment elevation acute coronary syndromes receiving the glycoprotein IIb/IIIa inhibitor eptifibatide. Circulation 2003;107:238–44.

64. Ross AM, Coyne K, Hammond M, Lundergan CF. Low-molecular-weight heparins in acute myocardial infarction, rationale and results of a pilot study. Clin Cardiol 2000;23:483–5.

65. Cohen M, Antman EM, Gurfinkel E, et al. Impact of enoxaparin low-molecular-weight heparin in patients with acute Q-wave myocardial infarction. Am J Cardiol 2000;86:553–6.

66. Ross AM, Molhoek P, Lundergan C, et al. Randomized comparison of enoxaparin, a low-molecular-weight heparin, with unfractionated heparin adjunctive to recombinant tissue plasminogen activator thrombolysis and aspirin: second trial of Heparin and Aspirin Reperfusion Therapy (HART II). Circulation 2001; 104:648–52.

67. Antman EM, Louwerenburg HW, Baars HF, et al. Enoxaparin as adjunctive antithrombin therapy for ST-elevated myocardial infarction: results of the ENTIRE–Thrombolysis in Myocardial Infarction (TIMI) 23 trial. Circulation 2002;105:1642–9.

68. Baird SH, Menown IB, Mcbride SJ, et al. Randomized comparison of enoxaparin with unfractionated heparin following fibrinolytic therapy for acute myocardial infarction. Eur Heart J 2002;23:627–32.

69. Simoons M, Krzeminska-Pakula M, Alonso A, et al. Improved reperfusion and clinical outcome with enoxaparin adjunct to streptokinase thrombolysis in acute myocardial infarction. The AMI-SK study. Eur Heart J 2002;23:1282–90.

70. The Assessment of the Safety and Efficacy of a New Thrombolytic Regimen (ASSENT)-3 Investigators. Efficacy and safety of tenecteplase in combination with enoxaprin, abciximab, or unfractionated heparin: the ASSENT-3 randomised trial in acute myocardial infarction. Lancet 2001;358:605–13.

71. Cannon CP, McCabe CH, Henry TD, et al. A pilot trial of recombinant desulfatohirudin compared with heparin in conjunction with tissue-type plasminogen activator and aspirin for acute myocardial infarction: results of the Thrombolysis in Myocardial Infarction (TIMI) 5 trial. J Am Coll Cardiol 1994;23:993–1003.

72. Antman EM. Hirudin in acute myocardial infarction. Thrombolysis and Thrombin Inhibition in Myocardial Infarction (TIMI) 9B trial. Circulation 1996;94:911–21.

73. The Global Use of Strategies to Open Occluded Coronary Arteries (GUSTO) IIa Investigators. Randomized trial of intravenous heparin versus recombinant hirudin for acute coronary syndromes. Circulation 1994;90:1631–7.

74. The Global Use of Strategies to Open Occluded Coronary Arteries (GUSTO) IIb Investigators. A comparison of recombinant hirudin with heparin for the treatment of acute coronary syndromes. N Engl J Med 1996;335:775–82.

75. Neuhaus K-L, Molhoek GP, Zeymer U, et al. Recombinant hirudin (lepirudin) for the improvement of thrombolysis with streptokinase in patients with acute myocardial infarction. Results of the HIT-4 trial. J Am Coll Cardiol 1999;34:966–73.

76. The EPILOG Investigators. Platelet glycoprotein IIb/IIIa receptor blockade and low-dose heparin during percutaneous coronary revascularization. N Engl J Med 1997;336:1689–96.

77. The CAPTURE Investigators. Randomised, placebo-controlled trial of abciximab before and during coronary intervention in refractory unstable angina: the CAPTURE study. Lancet 1997;349:1429–35.

78. Montalescot G, Barragan P, Wittenberg O, et al. Platelet glycoprotein IIb/IIIa inhibition with coronary stenting for acute myocardial infarction. N Engl J Med 2001:1895–903.

79. The PURSUIT Trial Investigators. Inhibition of platelet glycoprotein IIb/IIIa with epitifibatide in

patients with acute coronary syndromes. N Engl J Med 1998;339:436–43.

80. The PRISM Investigators. A comparison of aspirin plus tirofiban with aspirin plus heparin for unstable angina. N Engl J Med 1998;378:1498–1505.

81. PRISM-PLUS Investigators. Inhibition of the platelet glycoprotein IIb/IIIa receptor with tirofiban in unstable angina and non-Q-wave myocardial infarction. N Engl J Med 1998;338:1488–97.

82. The PARAGON Investigators. International, randomized, controlled trial of lamifiban (a platelet glycoprotein IIb/IIIa inhibitor), heparin, or both in unstable angina. Circulation 1998;97:2386–95.

83. Newby LK, Ohman EM, Christenson RH, et al. Benefit of glycoprotein IIb/IIIa inhibition in patients with acute coronary syndromes and troponin T-positive status. Circulation 2001;2891–6.

84. The GUSTO-IV-ACS Investigators. Effect of glycoprotein IIb/IIIa receptor blocker abciximab on outcome in patients with acute coronary syndromes without early coronary revascularisation: the GUSTO-IV-ACS randomised trial. Lancet 2002;357:1915–24.

85. Ottervanger JP, Armstrong P, Barnathan ES, et al. Long-term results after the glycoprotein IIb/IIIa inhibitor abciximab in unstable angina: one-year survival in the GUSTO-IV-ACS (Global Use of Strategies To Open Occluded Coronary Arteries IV–Acute Coronary Syndrome) trial. Circulation 2003;107:437–42.

86. Ohman EM, Kleiman NS, Gacioch G, et al. Combined accelerated tissue-plasminogen activator and platelet glycoprotein IIb/IIIa integrin receptor blockade with integrilin in acute myocardial infarction. Results of a randomized, placebo-controlled, dose ranging trial. Circulation 1997;95:846–54.

87. The PARADIGM Investigators. Combining thrombolysis with the platelet glycoprotein IIb/IIa inhibitor lamifiban: results of the Platelet Aggregation Receptor Antagonist Dose Investigation and Reperfusion Gain in Myocardial Infarction (PARADIGM) trial. J Am Coll Cardiol 1998;32:2003–10.

88. The SPEED Group. Trial of abciximab with and without low-dose reteplase for acute myocardial infarction. Circulation 2000;101:2788–94.

89. Antman EM, Giugliano RP, Gibson M, et al. Abciximab facilitates the rate and extent of thrombolysis. Results of the Thrombolysis In Myocardial Infarction (TIMI) 14 trial. Circulation 1999;99:2720–32.

90. The GUSTO-V Investigators. Reperfusion therapy for acute myocardial infarction with fibrinolytic therapy or combination reduced fibrinolytic therapy and platelet glycoprotein IIb/IIIa inhibition: the GUSTO-V randomised trial. Lancet 2001;357: 1905–14.

91. Lincoff AM, Califf RM, Van de Werf F, et al. Mortality at 1 year with combination platelets glycoprotein IIb/IIIa inhibition and reduced-dose fibrinolytic therapy vs conventional fibrinolytic therapy for acute myocardial infarction: GUSTO-V randomized trial. JAMA 2002;288:2130–5.

92. Klimt CR, Doub PH, Doub NH. Clinical trials in thrombosis: secondary prevention of myocardial infarction. Thromb Haemost 1976;35:49–56.

93. Hammond EC, Garfinkel L. Aspirin and coronary heart disease: findings of a prospective study. BMJ 1975;ii:269–71.

94. Czaplicki S, Gietka J, Sulek K. The frequency of coronary heart disease and myocardial infarction in rheumatoid arthritis patients. Cor Vasa 1978;20: 249–54.

95. Vogel G, Fischer C, Huyke R. Prevention of reinfarction with acetylsalicylic acid. Folia Haematol Int Mag Klein Morphol Blutforsch 1979;106:797–803.

96. Elwood PC, Sweetnam PM. Aspirin and secondary mortality after myocardial infarction. Lancet 1979;ii: 1313–15.

97. The AMIS Investigators. A randomized, controlled trial of aspirin in persons recovered from myocardial infarction. JAMA 1980;243:661–9.

98. The PARIS Investigators. Persantine and aspirin in coronary heart disease. The Persantine–Aspirin Reinfarction Study Research Group. Circulation 1980;62:449–61.

99. Breddin K, Loew D, Lechner K, et al. The German Austrian Aspirin Trial: a comparison of acetylsalicylic acid, placebo and phenprocoumon in secondary prevention of myocardial infarction. Circulation 1980;62:V63–72.

100. Klimt CR, Knatterud GL, Stamler J, Meier P. Persantine–Aspirin Reinfarction Study. Part II. Secondary coronary prevention with persantine and aspirin. J Am Coll Cardiol 1986;7:251–69.

101. Juul-Moller S, Edvardsson N, Jahnmatz B, et al. Double-blind trial of aspirin in primary prevention of myocardial infarction in patients with stable chronic angina pectoris. The Swedish Angina Pectoris Aspirin Trial (SAPAT) Group. Lancet 1992;340:1421–5.

102. Rothlin ME, Pfluger N, Speiser K, et al. Platelet inhibitors versus anticoagulants for prevention of aorta-coronary bypass graft occlusion. Eur Heart J 1985;6:168–75.

103. Limet R, David JL, Magotteaux P, et al. Prevention of aorta–coronary bypass graft occlusion. Beneficial effect of ticlopidine on early and late patency rates of venous coronary bypass grafts: a double-blind study. J Thorac Cardiovasc Surg 1987;94:773–83.

104. Ishikawa K, Kanamasa K, Hama J, et al. Aspirin plus either dipyridamole or ticlopidine is effective in preventing recurrent myocardial infarction. Secondary Prevention Group. Jpn Circ J 1997;61:38–45.

105. The CAPRIE Steering Committee. A randomised, blinded, trial of Clopidogrel versus Aspirin in Patients at Risk of Ischaemic Events (CAPRIE). Lancet 1996;348:1329–39.

106. The Antithrombotic Trialists' Collaboration. Collaborative meta-analysis of randomised trials of antiplatelet therapy for prevention of death, myocardial infarction, and stroke in high risk patients. BMJ 2002;324:71–86.

107. Lewis HD Jr, Davis JW, Archibald DG, et al. Protective effects of aspirin against acute myocardial infarction and death in men with unstable angina. Results of a Veterans Administration Cooperative Study. N Engl J Med 1983;309:396–403.

108. Cairns JA, Gent M, Singer J, et al. Aspirin, sulfinpyrazone, or both in unstable angina. Results of a Canadian multicenter trial. N Engl J Med 1985;313:1369–75.

109. Balsano F, Rizzon P, Violi F, et al. Antiplatelet treatment with ticlopidine in unstable angina. A controlled multicenter clinical trial. The Studio della Ticlopidina nell'Angina Instabile Group. Circulation 1990;82:17–26.

110. Scrutinio D, Lagioia R, Rizzon P. Ticlopidine tratment for patients with unstable angina at rest. A further analysis of the study of ticlopidine in unstable angina. Eur Heart J 1991;12(Suppl G):27–9.

111. Yusuf S, Zhao F, Metha SR, et al. Effects of clopidogrel in addition to aspirin in patients with acute coronary syndromes without ST-segment elevation. N Engl J Med 2001;345:494–502.

112. Budaj A, Yusuf S, Metha SR, et al. Benefit of clopidogrel in patients with acute coronary syndromes without ST-segment elevation in various risk groups. Circulation 2002;106:1622–6.

113. Yusuf S, Metha SR, Zhao F, et al. Early and late effects of clopidogrel in patients with acute coronary syndromes. Circulation 2003;25:966–72.

114. The SYMPHONY Investigators. Comparison of sibrafiban with aspirin for prevention of cardiovascular events after acute coronary syndromes: a randomised trial. Lancet 2000;355:337–45.

115. Cannon CP, McCabe CH, Wilcox RG, et al. Oral Glycoprotein IIb/IIIa Inhibition with Orofiban in Patients with Unstable Coronary Syndromes (OPUS-TIMI-16) trial. Circulation 2000;102:149–156.

116. O'Neill WW, Serruys P, Knudtson M, et al. Long-term treatment with a platelet glycoprotein receptor antagonist after percutaneous coronary revascularization. N Engl J Med 2000;342:1316–24.

117. Van Belle E, McFadden EP, Lablanche JM, et al. Two-pronged antiplatelet therapy with aspirin and ticlopidine without systemic anticoagulation. An alternative therapeutic strategy after bailout stent implantation. Coron Artery Dis 1995;6:341–5.

118. Schomig A, Neumann FJ, Kastrati A, et al. A randomized comparison of antiplatelet and anticoagulant therapy after the placement of coronary-artery stents. N Engl J Med 1996;334:1084–9.

119. Moussa I, Oetgen M, Roubin G, et al. Effectiveness of clopidogrel and aspirin versus ticlopidine and aspirin in preventing stent thrombosis after coronary stent implantation. Circulation 1999;99:2364–6.

120. Müller C, Büttner HJ, Petersen J, Roskamm H. A randomized comparison of clopidogrel and aspirin versus ticlopidine and aspirin after the placement of coronary-artery stents. Circulation 2000;101:590–3.

121. Bertrand ME, Rupprecht HJ, Urban P, et al. Double-blind study of the safety of clopidogrel with and without a loading dose in combination with aspirin compared with toclopidine in combination with aspirin after coronary stenting. The Clopidogrel Aspirin Stent International Cooperative Study (CLASSICS). Circulation 2000;102:624–9.

122. Metha SR, Yusuf S, Peters RJ, et al. Effects of pretreatment with clopidogrel and aspirin followed by long-term therapy in patients undergoing percutaneous coronary intervention: the PCI-CURE study. Lancet 2001;358:527–33.

123. Steinhubl SR, Berger PB, Mann JT 3rd, et al. Early and sustained dual oral antiplatelet therapy following percutaneous coronary intervention: a randomized controlled trial. JAMA 2002;288:2411–20.

124. Müller C, Roskamm H, Neumann FJ, et al. A randomized comparison of clopidogrel and aspirin versus ticlopidin and aspirin after the placement of coronary artery stents. J Am Coll Cardiol 2003;41:969–73.

7

Study design for thrombolytic and antithrombotic treatment trials in acute stroke: mistakes and lessons

Kennedy R Lees and Graeme J Hankey

Introduction

Stroke clinicians need to know which treatments for acute stroke are effective and what their risks are. It is not good enough to base such assessments on theory alone; a treatment suggested by theory must be thoroughly tested in clinical practice. Appropriate evaluation (Table 7.1) usually requires enormous efforts and resources, but this is severalfold less than the costs of misplaced enthusiasm that leads to the introduction of, and perseverence with, ineffective or dangerous treatments.

It is rare for treatments for stroke to have a dramatically favorable effect. If ever they do, the effect should be obvious without randomized trials. In these circumstances, the treatment is widely accepted as being effective and is adopted into clinical practice. However, in reality, there remains considerable variation in the treatment of stroke among different clinicians, centers, and countries. One of the main reasons for such variation in practice is the uncertainty that exists about the safety and effectiveness of various treatments for stroke; this in turn reflects the lack of reliable evidence about the relative safety and effectiveness of these treatments, which are likely to have modest effects at best in the types and subtypes of stroke patients that we can currently recognize and study. Such modest treatment effects, if they truly exist, are important to recognize because they can be

clinically worthwhile for the patient, and also for public health if they are safe, inexpensive and widely applicable. However, they can be easily overestimated, or underestimated and even missed, in studies by equally modest errors, such as systematic error (bias) and random error (Table 7.2). Reliable and accurate identification of modest, but important, treatment effects therefore requires simultaneous minimization of systematic errors and random errors (Table 7.3), in addition to careful attention to other aspects of the study design.

In the last decade, more than a dozen clinical trials of thrombolytic or antithrombotic treatment in acute stroke have been published, but few have been clearly positive. There are several possible reasons for the many so-called 'negative' trials; we may have:

- misunderstood the etiology and pathogenesis of ischemic stroke
- developed inappropriate drugs for stroke
- misunderstood the pharmacology of these drugs and how they interact with each other
- developed invalid animal models of ischemic stroke for testing drugs
- tested the treatments by inappropriate study designs and failed to mimimize random error

In this chapter, we shall confine ourselves to discussing the strengths and weaknesses of various

Table 7.1   Key elements in the design of a clinical trial of a treatment for stroke treatment or prevention

Hypothesis and aim
- Are the study hypothesis and aim clearly stated?
- Did the study hypothesis prespecify any proposed subgroup analyses (a priori)?

Design
- What is the study design?
- Is it a randomized trial?
- Is the method of randomization described?

Patients
- Were the patients selected according to appropriate diagnostic criteria?

Follow-up
- Were all patients followed up prospectively at prespecified, regular intervals?
- Was patient follow-up complete?

Outcome measures
- Is the primary measure of outcome:
  - Relevant to the patient (e.g. death, functional dependency, serious vascular event)?
  - Relevant to the intervention (i.e. potentially modifiable)?
  - Valid (measures what it is supposed to measure)?
  - Reliable (reproducible)?
  - Simple?
  - Communicable?
- Avoid surrogate outcomes in phase III studies:
  - Surrogate outcomes may reflect only one part of the disease process, and their treatment may not produce worthwhile improvements in survival and functional outcome
  - Treating surrogate outcomes may be hazardous

Outcome evaluation
- Were the outcome events recorded in such a way as to reduce the risk of bias (i.e. blind to the assigned treatment)?

Statistical analysis
- Is the primary analysis by intention-to-treat (i.e. is the final analysis based on the groups to which all randomized patients were originally allocated)?
- Are there subgroup analyses?
- When are additional ('on-treatment') analyses appropriate?

Table 7.2   Common epidemiological sources of error in studies of interventions for stroke

Systematic errors (biases) in the assessment of treatment
- Selection bias (systematic pretreatment differences in comparison groups)
- Performance bias (systematic differences in the care provided apart from the intervention being evaluated)
- Attrition bias (systematic differences in withdrawals from the trials)
- Recording/detection bias (systematic differences in outcome assessment)

Random errors in the assessment of treatment effects
- These relate to the impact of the play of chance on comparisons of the outcome between those exposed and not exposed to the treatment of interest
- They are determined by the number of relevant outcome events in the study
- The potential error can be quantified by means of a confidence interval, which indicates the range of effects statistically compatible with the observed result
- They can prevent real effects of treatment being detected or their size being estimated reliably

Table 7.3   Some strategies to reliably identify or exclude modest treatment effects

Minimization of systematic error

- Proper randomization
- Analysis by allocated treatment (including all randomized patients: intention-to-treat)
- Outcome evaluation blind to the allocated treatment
- Chief emphasis on overall results (without undue data-dependent emphasis on particular subgroups)
- Systematic review of all relevant studies (without undue data-dependent emphasis on particular studies)

Minimization of random error

- Large numbers of major outcomes (with streamlined study methods to facilitate recruitment)
- Systematic review of all relevant studies (yielding the largest possible number of major outcome events)

methodological issues in the design of acute stroke trials (Table 7.4), concentrating on areas where lessons have been learned or mistakes avoided, and where subsequent or future trials are able to benefit. By its nature, this exercise has negative aspects and should not be taken out of context as overly critical. At the outset, therefore, we wish to stress that the positive features of nearly all of the trials that we shall review greatly outweigh their problems. Indeed, the design flaws were frequently anticipated by the investigators or have been recognized during reporting. It is the nature of clinical research that a compromise is usually required between the scientifically ideal approach and the practicalities of conducting research in acutely ill patients, often with an inadequate budget and with competition for resources. Hindsight is powerful.

Objectives of the trial – importance of phase I/II trials in acute stroke

The primary objective(s) of the trial are crucial in determining its design. Rigorously designed phase III (pivotal efficacy) trials are required to evaluate the clinical benefit of potential therapies for acute stroke. However, prior to the design of these large-scale studies, smaller phase I (initial first human studies without therapeutic benefit, typically with healthy subjects and defining maximally tolerated doses) and phase II (dose range-finding studies exploring efficacy or surrogate endpoints in patients with the potential to benefit from treatment) trials are necessary to define both the safety profile of a given therapy and to establish

a dose range for efficacy. Late phase II studies usually address a hypothesis of biological activity of a drug (proof of concept), but are not usually sufficiently powered to determine conclusive efficacy.

Therefore, before a drug is of proven efficacy and safety, it is appropriate to undertake explanatory trials to ensure that the circumstances for its use are optimized before subjecting large numbers of patients to the treatment in a pragmatic trial. Some of the trials of intravenous streptokinase in acute ischaemic stroke (MAST-I (Multicenter Acute Stroke Trial – Italy)[1] and MAST-E (Europe)[2]) took a pragmatic approach before the safety and efficacy of streptokinase at the dose of 1.5 MU had been established. The Australian Streptokinase Trial also used the same dose, but adopted the reasonable a priori hypothesis that treatment would be safer and more effective if administered early.[3] The NINDS (National Institute of Neurological Disorders and Stroke) trial took this considerably further, and was the only trial of intravenous thrombolysis to produce a clearly positive result.[4] The PROACT-II (Prolyse in Acute Cerebral Thromboembolism) trial of intra-arterial thrombolysis was also an explanatory trial with a positive result.[5] It is irresponsible, and potentially hazardous (for the stroke community), to proceed directly to a pragmatic trial that does not carefully control patient selection, center selection, monitoring procedures, and data collection unless a treatment has been proven to be effective and safe, and accepted by the medical community. It is preferable to expand the indications for a drug gradually and under carefully controlled circumstances than to risk loss of a potentially effective treatment through unrestrained enthusiasm. Perhaps streptokinase may have had a place in stroke treatment if MAST-E and MAST-I had taken the approach of the Australian

Table 7.4 Specific areas in which the study design may have been suboptimal in recent acute stroke treatment trials and which should be considered for future trials

1. Objectives
- Pragmatic trial versus explanatory trial
- Importance of phase I/II trials

2. Patient selection
- Generalizability versus specificity of treatment effect
- Stroke etiology
- Stroke severity
- Time since stroke onset
- Brain imaging findings

3. Center selection
- Training
- Monitoring
- Feedback

4. Data collection
- Screening data (inclusion and exclusion criteria)
- Important etiological and prognostic characteristics of patients at baseline
- Demography (e.g. patient weight)
- Postrandomization CT scans (recording of hemorrhagic transformation)
- Safety data (e.g. blood pressure, aspirin use)

5. Treatment selection
- Drug
- Dose
- Duration of treatment

6. Treatment allocation
- Minimization of systematic bias (randomization)
- Minimization of outcome evaluation bias (blinding)

7. Concomitant treatment
- Antihypertensive drugs
- Antiplatelet drugs
- Heparin

8. Outcome selection
- Primary endpoint:
  - Relevant
  - Valid
  - Reliable
  - Sensitive to change
  - Communicable
- Secondary endpoints (e.g. infarct size)

9. Follow-up
- Prospective
- Sufficient time to realize major outcomes
- Completeness

10. Outcome evaluation
- Blinding
- Regularity and frequency

11. Sample size
- Clinically important difference (i.e. target)
- Power

12. Analysis
- Intention-to-treat
- 'On-treatment' (efficacy)
- Subgroup analyses

13. Collaboration
- Planning
- Conduct
- Post-trial analysis (data availability)

Streptokinase Trial or of NINDS. The coordinators of IST-III (International Stroke Trial), an ongoing placebo-controlled, randomized trial of intravenous recombinant tissue-type plasminogen activator (rtPA, alteplase) within 6 h of onset of ischemic stroke, will need to pay close attention to center selection, training of investigators, and screening logs if the potential risks are not to be realized. Provided that patients who are treated with open-label alteplase alongside trial patients within IST-III centers are recorded in similar detail and that only centers with a proven record of selecting patients who can be treated with a low rate of hemorrhagic complications are included, this trial may play a valuable role in extending the indications for alteplase. On the other hand, experience with ancrod has suggested that although it was safe and effective when used within 3 h of stroke onset, a European trial with a later time window failed to confirm benefit and ancrod is not currently in clinical development.[6] Notwithstanding these comments, a trial must be practical. One of the greatest criticisms of the NINDS trial is the short time to treatment that was required: 90 min in half of the patients. It was a testament to the investigators that they achieved this in over 300 patients, but it has proven very difficult for most centers to emulate this.

Patient selection

Generalizability versus specificity of treatment effect

Patient selection for trials represents a compromise between generalizability (e.g. including all types of patients with stroke) and the likelihood of achieving a positive result (e.g. including only specific types of patients with stroke who are most likely to respond favorably to the study treatment).

Stroke etiology

The causes of ischemic stroke are heterogeneous. About one-fifth of all cerebral infarcts are caused by in situ atherothrombosis (i.e. plaque erosion or fissure followed by platelet aggregation, and fibrin thrombus), another two-fifths are caused by atherothromboembolism, one-fifth by embolism from the heart of a variety of materials (e.g. fresh thrombus, organized thrombus, calcium, prosthetic valves, bacteria, or tumor), and one-fifth by other causes (e.g. arterial dissection, arteritis, or procoagulant states).[7] It is unrealistic to expect effective treatments for one cause to be as widely applicable and effective for all etiological subtypes of ischemic stroke. The *overall* effect of any treatment is likely to be *modest*, at best. This has been a problem in all the thrombolytic and antithrombotic stroke trials because of the lack of reliable and valid criteria for accurately classifying ischemic stroke acutely into etiological subtypes.

Stroke severity

Stroke severity is an important prognostic factor, which is relevant to patient selection and trial design. This is because most acute stroke trials rely on distinguishing between favorable and unfavorable outcomes, and recruitment of patients with an inevitably favorable or an inevitably unfavorable outcome simply dilutes the population who will contribute to assessment of the intervention (and thus may negate an important modest treatment effect in subgroup(s) of patients). For example, after 800 patients were randomized in the TAIST (Tinzaparin in Acute Ischaemic Stroke) trial, it became clear that the recruited patients had milder strokes than anticipated and that the risk of developing deep vein thrombosis (DVT) and associated complications was much lower than predicted.[7] The initial entry criterion, of a Scandinavian Stroke Scale Score of 53 or less, was modified to 40 or less in subsequent patients. This use of severity restriction is common to trials in all therapeutic areas, but has an additional relevance to antithrombotic trials in acute

stroke. The main risk from antithrombotic treatment is hemorrhagic transformation, and one of the prime influences on spontaneous hemorrhagic transformation is the initial stroke severity. Thus, there is a complex relationship between initial severity, risk of treatment, and potential benefit. MAST-E aimed to recruit moderately severe patients on the grounds that the potential dangers of streptokinase precluded treatment of patients with a naturally good prognosis.[8] In practice, this strategy produced a much higher incidence of hemorrhagic complications than treatment of allcomers,[1,4] and possibly contributed to the rapid realization that streptokinase was dangerous in acute stroke.[9] In contrast, the NINDS trial had a more open approach to severity (although this was carefully recorded) but a highly selective policy on the basis of time from stroke onset.

Time since stroke onset

Ischemia of the brain is followed by a time- and flow-dependent cascade of unique, complex chemical events: falling energy (ATP) production; overstimulation of neuronal glutamate receptors (excitotoxicity); excessive intraneuronal accumulation of sodium, chloride, and calcium ions; generation of free radicals; spreading damage; and mitochondrial injury. The time available to rescue ischemic, functionally impaired, but surviving brain tissue (the ischemic penumbra) may be up to 17 h in some patients, but is probably only a few hours in most. Consequently, the benefits of treatments that aim to rescue ischemic tissue are likely to be greater if given very early; 'time is brain'.

The decision by the NINDS trial investigators to stratify patients on the basis of time from stroke onset substantially enhanced the opportunity for demonstrating benefit and may have reduced the potential risk. Only two trials have used such an aggressive strategy for selection on the basis of time from stroke onset, and both of these trials in stroke have indicated a benefit.[4,6] The Australian Streptokinase Trial used an intermediate approach with a 4 h window.[3] In reporting the trial, the Australian investigators readily admitted that they expected efficacy to be restricted to patients who could be treated early, but in planning the trial they were constrained by potential difficulties in obtaining centers and recruiting patients if the upper limit of the time window were set at less than 4 h.

Time from stroke onset has also been relevant in trials of heparin and aspirin in acute ischemic stroke. Heparin and antiplatelet drugs are generally administered for periods of days or weeks. While there is a natural desire to start treatment as early as possible after stroke, before DVT or recurrent stroke has a chance to initiate, the first 24 h is probably the time of maximum risk of hemorrhagic transformation. It is possible that later initiation of treatment (e.g. delaying this until approximately 48 h) would have avoided exacerbating hemorrhagic transformation and may thus have rendered treatment safer.[7,10]

Brain imaging

The findings on brain imaging may also facilitate patient selection, as shown in ECASS (European Cooperative Acute Stroke Study).[11] On the basis of prior evidence,[12] an arbitrary limit of infarct size on the prerandomization computed tomography (CT) scan was constructed: patients with hypodensity affecting more than one-third of the middle cerebral artery territory or with mass effect affecting the hemisphere should be excluded. The success of this strategy was limited by issues of training and reproducibility (see below), but its potential value is confirmed by the contrast between the target population and the intention-to-treat population results from ECASS.[11]

For trials involving antithrombotic treatment such as aspirin and heparin, a pretreatment CT scan to exclude hemorrhage should be mandatory; even 'mild' treatments such as aspirin can increase the risk of hemorrhagic transformation. Even though no overall deleterious effect of aspirin was demonstrated in the IST, the safety of aspirin administration in patients who had not been scanned or who had intracerebral hemorrhage on their scan has not been proven; the trial was underpowered to examine this subgroup and it would have been unethical to continue treatment in patients known to have hemorrhage.[13]

Plain CT is not the only potential imaging investigation prior to antithrombotic treatment, however. The suggestion that large established infarcts will not benefit but have increased risk, the evidence that only a proportion of patients still have arterial occlusion when they are first assessed after acute stroke, and the positron-emission tomography (PET) data

demonstrating that not all patients have viable tissue still present all indicate that more advanced imaging methods may be worth considering for selection of patients for thrombolytic trials.[5,11,14,15] Trials such as the DIAS (Desmotoplase in Acute Stroke) trial are exploring the use of mismatch between magnetic resonance imaging (MRI) perfusion and diffusion lesion size to identify patients who may still have salvageable tissue.

Center selection

Training

It is straightforward to write a protocol with complex entry criteria for a trial and to produce detailed workbooks, procedural manuals, etc. to guide recruitment. Unfortunately, in the middle of the night in an emergency department faced with a patient who has neurological deficit and a limited time in which to complete assessments, let alone read the procedural manual, only two approaches together can save the trial. First, the main entry criteria need to be clear and easy to remember. Second, all of the investigators need to be thoroughly trained. This was the major lesson to be learned from ECASS I, where the entry criteria were clear and in retrospect well justified, but 10% of patients recruited to their trial had major protocol violations, especially on CT interpretation grounds. The ECASS investigators had anticipated the potential for problems and had distributed a booklet and example scans in advance of the trial. Even so, either because investigators had not been adequately trained or because not all investigators at each site who would be involved in the trial had received this training, a sufficient number of patients entered the trial inappropriately to convert a useful benefit into a nonsignificant trend.[11] The additional training provided for ECASS II, with the use of CD-ROM, feedback to the investigators, accreditation, etc. halved the rate of protocol violations.[14]

Monitoring and feedback

When issues about training arise and entry criteria are so important, there is a need for continuous monitoring of recruitment at each center and rapid feedback from the trial steering committee or sponsor to deal immediately with protocol violations. These quality control measures have been successfully used in other trials such as POST (Potassium Opener in Stroke Trial).[16]

Data collection

Inclusion and exclusion criteria for screening patients

Clearly defined inclusion and exclusion criteria assist patient selection, and a screening log of excluded patients helps to identify the type of patients who are not exposed to the study drug. The latter is particularly important in trials that base randomization on the 'uncertainty principle'. For example, the IST included only patients in whom the investigator was uncertain of the benefits of heparin and aspirin and, if he/she proceeded without a CT scan, in whom he/she was confident that hemorrhagic stroke was extremely unlikely.[13] This level of uncertainty or confidence in difficult clinical distinctions means that, despite the large numbers of patients in the trial and the consistency of effect across subgroups, there remains a small concern that patients who would clearly benefit from treatment such as heparin or would clearly be at risk from antithrombotic treatment cannot be identified. As a result, heparin is still widely used for DVT prevention and for treatment of certain categories of ischemic stroke.

Baseline data for important etiological and prognostic characteristics of randomized patients

The purpose of collecting baseline data is to be able to identify at the end of the trial which type of stroke patients were enrolled into the trial (and to whom the results can be generalized), and perhaps which type of patients responded favorably, unfavorably, or not at all to the study treatment.

Baseline data that could have been useful in trials of streptokinase include patient weight, to allow an accurate interpretation of the dose–response of

streptokinase. It is also important to collect routine prognostic and safety data such as blood pressure levels, aspirin use, etc. There may be obvious interactions between blood pressure treatment, aspirin use, and other antithrombotic treatment, and again post hoc analysis requires the data to consider the safety of interactions.

Because there is limited time for collecting baseline data in acute stroke trials, it is important that any such data are absolutely essential and time is used efficiently. Trials that disregard this issue and possibly those that require baseline diffusion and perfusion MRI scans, will recruit slowly. Nevertheless, trials without adequate baseline data can be difficult to interpret, particularly when safety issues such as hemorrhagic transformation are raised.

Treatment selection

Drug

If it is difficult to establish the efficacy and safety of a single drug, it is substantially more difficult to compare drugs of a similar class. Of the thrombolytic agents, streptokinase and tPA have been most widely used. Following the termination of MAST-E,[9] the other large streptokinase trials were also halted for safety reasons.[1,3] It is unclear from meta-analysis whether streptokinase is substantially worse than tPA, but the detailed trial reports reflect clinically worrying hypotension with streptokinase as well as prolonged effects on the coagulation system – both of which are probably deleterious in acute stroke. In retrospect, streptokinase was probably not the ideal choice of drug, because of the known risk of hypotension and association between hypotension and poorer outcome in stroke.[17,18]

Dose of drug

Quite apart from difficulty with choice of drug, thrombolytic trials have also suffered from a possible problem with choice of dose. Too high a dose was blamed by some for the disappointing results of the streptokinase trials, and there is certainly evidence that heavier patients suffered less than lighter patients from the fixed dose of streptokinase used in MAST-E.[19] The streptokinase trials were commenced without dose-ranging studies in stroke, yet it is now clear that safety and effectiveness have a different dose–response in stroke than for treatment of occlusion in other vessels.[20] Such studies were conducted with tPA, but were too small and involved only dose escalation rather than randomization among doses.[12,20] Similar criticisms can be levelled at heparin trials, except that the IST considered two dose levels of subcutaneous heparin and was at least based on common practice.[13] There are now excellent modern approaches to the conduct of randomized, double-blinded trials in which the optimal dose may not be known but a reasonable dose range to study has been established (for a review, see http://lib.stat.cmu.edu/bayesworkshop/Bayespp.html). This approach uses adaptive randomization among potentially active doses, online feedback of outcome to the randomization computer, and construction of a dose–response curve with Bayesian statistical methodology to assist with dose selection.

Duration of treatment

A further problem, particularly with the heparin trials, concerns duration of treatment. We have mentioned above the risks of commencing treatment during the period of maximal risk of hemorrhagic transformation. A long-acting thrombolytic drug given early after stroke will have effects that overlap with this period of increased risk, potentially offsetting benefit. Conversely, heparin treatment given for a period of only 7 or 10 days, even if commenced after the period of initial risk has elapsed, may have an inadequate effect if prevention of DVT and pulmonary embolism is the presumed mechanism of action. It would probably be necessary to continue treatment for as long as the patient is relatively immobile. Certainly, to administer treatment for 7 or 10 days to prevent thrombotic complications but to measure outcome 3 or 6 months later and include thrombotic events occurring between cessation of treatment and the follow-up period is a recipe for a negative trial.[7]

Treatment allocation

Minimization of systematic bias (randomization)

The reason for random allocation of treatment in clinical trials is to maximize the likelihood that each type of patient will have been allocated in similar proportions to the different treatment strategies being investigated. Nonrandomized methods (e.g. observational studies) may cause moderate or large biases.

It is crucial to ensure that the method of randomization is described. In other words, was the decision to enter each patient made irreversibly in ignorance of which trial treatment that each patient would be allocated? If not (e.g. if 'randomization' was based on an odd or even day of the week or date of birth), foreknowledge of the next treatment allocation could affect the decision to enter the patient, and those allocated one treatment might then differ systematically from those allocated another.

Minimization of observer bias (blinding)

The patient and attending clinicians should ideally be blind to the treatment allocation, particularly if any knowledge of treatment allocation could influence the final evaluation of outcome. See the section below on outcome evaluation.

Concomitant treatment

There is a substantial potential for concomitant treatment to influence outcome after stroke.

Neuroprotection

Only one small trial has studied the effectiveness and safety of thrombolysis combined with a neuroprotective agent. There have been no trials of the combination of thrombolysis, antiplatelet therapy, and one or more neuroprotective drugs that act on different parts of the cascade of ischemic neuronal injury. Neuroprotective drugs need access to the ischemic tissue before they can hope to work, and recanalized arteries need to remain recanalized and not rethrombose.

Antithrombotic and anthypertensive therapy

Thrombolytic agents dissolve red blood cell thrombus, but predispose to rethrombosis through platelet activation, release of bound thrombin, and activation of factors V and VIII by plasmin. It appears logical to add an antiplatelet agent to a thrombolytic agent in an attempt to maintain arterial recanalization and prevent rethrombosis. However, there is also the theoretical risk of an increase in hemorrhagic adverse events with the combination. Indeed, a significant interaction was detected between streptokinase and aspirin in MAST-I,[1] where a factorial design had been used. There is also the potential for an interaction between streptokinase and heparin, which was widely used in MAST-E.[2] While there may be insufficient evidence to guide treatment policies within trials on topics such as use of aspirin, heparin, or blood pressure reduction, at the very least it is essential to record concomitant treatment of a type that is anticipated to interact with the trial therapy. This was undertaken in MAST-E,[2] but the very simple approach taken to case report forms in some large pragmatic trials does not always allow detailed interpretation.

Outcome selection

Primary outcome event

Among the many trials of intravenous thrombolysis in acute stroke, the primary outcome was a functional measure of death and dependency at 3–6 months after stroke. Only one of these trials has been positive on its primary endpoint, yet there is clear evidence of benefit from meta-analysis and from closer examination of the secondary endpoints or alternative analyses in most of the other trials. For marketing and drug registration reasons, there is a need to demonstrate improvement in functional outcome. Functional outcome is influenced by a number of factors that may be unrelated to the initial stroke severity or neurological improvement. The assessment of functional outcome is also open to

variability, especially where subtle distinctions need to be drawn on the basis of a short interview with the patient or carer (e.g. between Rankin scores 2 and 3).[21] The relevance of a particular cutpoint on a functional scoring system also depends on the severity of patients who are recruited. For the NINDS population, the split between Rankin 0–1 versus 2–6 proved ideal to detect the effect of treatment, whereas in ECASS II, the split between 0–2 versus 3–6 demonstrated a greater benefit.[4,14] Overall, it is unlikely that the arbitrary selection of a single endpoint such as this is either the perfect method of analysis or a major mistake. Instead, it is likely that all of these trials were relatively underpowered and that chance variation caused some to miss statistical significance on one endpoint compared with another. Both meta-analysis[22,23] and advanced statistical analysis using the bootstrap technique[24] suggest that the problem was an unfortunate choice of endpoint in the presence of an underpowered trial.

Secondary outcome measures

Despite the apparently tenuous link between functional outcome and infarct size, the alternative of using infarct size measured on CT scan as an endpoint measure seems to be disappointingly unsuccessful.[25] Perhaps because infarct size and location are inextricably linked to outcome and perhaps because measurement on CT scan is prone to error, variability in infarct size is too great to improve on clinical measures for outcome assessment. There is, however, considerable interest in using initial infarct volume or volume of 'at-risk' tissue as a covariate in such analysis, and this explains the rise in the use of diffusion-weighted MRI scanning at trial entry assessment of lesion growth as a trial endpoint.[26,27] While such measures have considerable appeal, and there has been encouragement from neuroprotection trials, there remain substantial practical difficulties in obtaining emergency MRI scans in most clinical centers, and this has severely limited the use of MRI in thrombolysis trials to date. Trials such as DIAS are, however, exploring this approach.

In addition to evaluating secondary outcome measures of effectiveness of treatment, it is also important to evaluate the *safety* of the intervention. For trials of thrombolytic and antithrombotic agents, the most important is symptomatic intracranial and extracranial hemorrhage. Trials to date suggest that treating 1000 ischemic stroke patients with thrombolysis within 6 h of onset saves 44 (95% confidence interval (CI) 15–73) overall from death or dependency despite an excess of 70 (95% CI 58–83) symptomatic intracranial hemorrhages and 44 (95% CI 34–54) fatal intracranial hemorrhages. Similarly, treating 1000 ischemic stroke patients with aspirin within 48 h of onset prevents 9 recurrent ischemic strokes yet causes 2 hemorrhagic strokes and four extracranial hemorrhages. Last, treating 1000 ischemic stroke patients with systemic anticoagulants (heparins or heparinoids) prevents 9 recurrent ischemic strokes but causes 9 hemorrhagic strokes, with no net improvement in death or dependency.

Follow-up

Prospective

All patients should be followed up prospectively at prespecified, regular intervals.

Completeness of follow-up

If patient follow-up is not complete, this can lead to attrition bias (systematic differences in withdrawals from trials) because patients who are withdrawn from or stop participating in a trial tend to differ from those who remain in the study (e.g. they may have a higher rate of complications or adverse effects from the disease or treatment, respectively). This type of bias can be minimized by performing an 'intention-to-treat' analysis, where the analysis of results at the end of the study includes every patient who was assigned to the intervention or control group, regardless of whether they received the assigned treatment or subsequently dropped out of the trial (see below).

Outcome evaluation – blinding

Avoidance of bias is essential if the results are to be reliable. It may be difficult to blind investigators (and patients and outcome evaluators) to the effects of

thrombolysis over the early hours after administration, because some oozing of blood from venepuncture sites or effects on routinely measured coagulation tests may reveal treatment allocation. To some extent, this can be controlled by ensuring that outcome is assessed by a separate investigator or even by centrally co-ordinated telephone assessment as used by MAST-I, MAST-E, and IST.[12,13] Bias can be difficult to estimate, and is not reduced by increasing the sample size. Even with the very large number of patients who participated in the IST, bias may still have affected estimates of the number of hemorrhagic transformations that occurred, since treatment allocation was open and deteriorations were more likely to be investigated by repeat CT scanning when patients were allocated to heparin and aspirin than when they were receiving neither. A design is to mandate a repeat CT scan at a fixed time after treatment: typically this would be between 24 and 72 h for a thrombolytic trial or after 7–10 days' treatment with an antiplatelet or anticoagulant drug. CT scans should be read centrally in a systematic fashion. Even here, there is the potential for bias: interpretation of a pretreatment scan can be influenced by knowledge of the second scan, and so these scans should be read in an unpaired fashion. This is particularly important when subtle early infarct signs are being sought.[11]

Sample size calculation to detect modest treatment effects reliably

Stroke is common and is responsible for an enormous burden on healthcare services in society. A small reduction in this burden would have major implications, yet most trials were designed to detect only a substantial alteration in outcome. The NINDS trial of tPA detected an absolute improvement in favorable outcome of 12%,[4] but this was under virtually ideal circumstances of early treatment with a reperfusion strategy. The likely effect size for thrombolysis will be rather smaller, but even a 5% absolute improvement is well worthwhile. Unfortunately, overoptimistic estimates of effect size have led to underpowered trials that failed to reach conventional levels of statistical significance on their primary endpoint,[11,14] and even so-called large trials such as IST-III are still targeting an effect size between 5% and 10%, where a much smaller benefit would be clinically important.

Treatments for ischemic stroke that may have such modest but important effects can be identified or excluded most reliably by means of large, blinded randomized controlled trials involving thousands of patients (not the tens or hundreds of patients in the many apparent 'negative' stroke trials). More than 58 600 patients with myocardial infarction were evaluated in clinical trials of thrombolysis before modest but important treatment effects could be reliably identified and the treatment became standard practice.[28] Similarly, more than 41 325 patients with acute ischemic stroke were randomized in clinical trials of aspirin to reliably identify a mild but worthwhile and cost-effective treatment effect (treating 1000 patients prevents 12 from death or dependency).[29] However, only 5216 patients with ischemic stroke due to several causes have been studied in clinical trials of thrombolysis.[30] While a systematic review of these trials is conclusive that thrombolysis *is* effective, it remains uncertain *in whom* it may be effective, in whom it is ineffective, and in whom it may be dangerous. Further trials are also indicated to unravel what is the optimal thrombolytic agent, dose, half-life, and route of administration, or the most effective concomitant neuroprotective, antithrombotic, and antihypertensive regime.

Meanwhile, there are now major efforts to put the raw data from trials into the public domain in a form that will allow thorough exploration of the relationship between stroke severity, outcome and effect size. Only through collaborations such as VISTA (Virtual International Stroke Trials Archive) can we learn from previous trials and optimally design our future work.

Statistical analysis

Intention-to-treat analysis

Even in a properly randomized trial, bias can be inadvertently introduced by the postrandomization exclusion of certain patients (e.g. those who are noncompliant with treatment), particularly if the outcome of those excluded from one treatment group differs from that of those excluded from another. 'On-treatment' comparisons, among only those who were compliant, are therefore potentially biased.

However, because there is always some noncompliance with allocated treatments in clinical trials, intention-to-treat analyses tend to underestimate the effects produced by full compliance with study treatments. In order to estimate the treatment effect with full compliance, it is more appropriate to avoid using potentially biased 'on-treatment' comparisons, and to apply the approximate estimate of level of compliance seen in the trial (e.g. 80%) to the estimate of the treatment effect provided by the intention-to-treat comparison (e.g. a 30% relative risk reduction (with 80% compliance). Doing this reveals a less biased estimate of therapeutic effect with full compliance (e.g. 35–40% relative risk reduction with 100% compliance).

Additional ('on treatment') analyses

An 'on-treatment' analysis may be of value in describing the frequency of specific adverse effects among only those who actually received the treatment; strictly randomized comparisons may not be needed to assess extreme relative risks.

Subgroup analyses

Because individual patients differ from each other, there is an understandable temptation to examine treatment effects in subgroups of interest, particularly if the overall trial result is negative. However, the more subgroups that are examined, the more likely it is that an effect will be identified due to chance (e.g. analyzing 20 subgroups will lead to one being statistically significant at the $p = 0.05$ level (1 out of 20) – just due to the play of chance). Post hoc subgroup analyses cannot, therefore, be regarded as anything more than hypothesis-generating. Any apparent treatment effect, such as the apparent effectiveness of danaparoid in acute ischemic stroke due to large-artery athero-thrombosis in TOAST (Trial of ORG 10172 in Acute Stroke Treatment),[10] must be studied in a further trial in which there is an a priori hypothesis that a particular subgroup of patients will benefit while other subgroups will not (e.g. the TOAST II trial). The most reliable estimate of a treatment effect, even in a subgroup, is that obtained in the whole sample of randomized patients. It can be assumed that subgroups will differ *quantitatively* in their response to treatment to some extent, but it cannot be assumed that there will be an unexpected *qualitative* difference in the direction of the treatment effect, such that treatment is harmful for one subgroup of patients but beneficial for another.

Collaboration

It is disappointing that to date so few trials have been effective: two trials with thrombolysis were positive, one with ancrod, none with heparin, and only one that used aspirin. Even that last trial (CAST: Chinese Acute Stroke Trial[31]) presented unblinded treatment results to investigators after 14 000 patients had been recruited and effectively altered the sample size in order to achieve a positive result. While this is a technique that is often criticised, greater use of Bayesian statistical methods for assessing sample sizes and adapting the sample size according to the results is a perfectly valid approach. One of the greatest difficulties is to predict in advance which endpoint should be selected for a trial, which patients should be recruited, and how large to make the trial. We have conducted many trials with antithrombotic drugs, and now have a substantial bank of data that could be used to answer these questions. Unfortunately, to a large extent, these data are held only within commercial or academic centers, without agreement to share the results. Greater collaborations are needed and are now being developed that will give opportunities for wider benefits from these data while respecting the commercial and academic rights of the original triallists. The lesson for future trials is that they should be designed on the basis of access to full information on previous analyses. As far as possible,

data should be collected in a manner that will permit pooling of data on important subgroups at the conclusion of the trial. The need for safety committees to communicate actively with each other is crucial. Had it not been for communication from MAST-E to the other streptokinase trials, it is likely that more patients would have been treated in MAST-I and the Australian Streptokinase Trial, to the detriment of a number of patients who would have died.

Summary

Numerous small lessons have been learned from the conduct of antithrombotic trials over the last decade. These and current trials were designed using the best available information and few, if any, have reached the wrong conclusion. It is much easier to criticize than to praise. Some lessons have been learned from these trials, but we must neither overemphasize the flaws in these nor underestimate the contribution that they have made to our evidence base for stroke management.

Acknowledgments

Professor Lees was an investigator in IST and TAIST and a member of the Steering Committee for MAST-E and of the SITS Thrombolysis Register, chairs the Data and Safety Monitoring Committee for the DIAS trial of desmotoplase and ECASS-III trial with alteplase, and has received fees and expenses for participation in meetings with Boehringer Ingelheim, who manufacture alteplase.

References

1. Multicentre Acute Stroke Trial – Italy (MAST-I) Group. Randomised controlled trial of streptokinase, aspirin, and combination of both in treatment of acute ischaemic stroke. Lancet 1995;346:1509–14.
2. The Multicenter Acute Stroke Trial – Europe Study Group. Thrombolytic therapy with streptokinase in acute ischemic stroke. N Eng J Med 1996;335:145–50.
3. Donnan GA, Davis SM, Chambers BR, et al. Streptokinase for acute ischemic stroke with relationship to time of administration: Australian Streptokinase (ASK) Trial Study Group. JAMA 1996;276:961–6.
4. The National Institute of Neurological Disorders and Stroke rt-PA Stroke Study Group. Tissue plasminogen activator for acute ischemic stroke. N Eng J Med 1995;333:1581–7.
5. Furlan A, Higashida R, Wechsler L, et al. Intra-arterial prourokinase for acute ischemic stroke. The PROACT II study: a randomized controlled trial.

Prolyse in Acute Cerebral Thromboembolism. JAMA 1999;282:2003–11.

6. Sherman DG, Atkinson RP, Chippendale T, et al. Intravenous ancrod for treatment of acute ischemic stroke: the STAT study: a randomized controlled trial. Stroke Treatment with Ancrod Trial. JAMA 2000; 282:2395–403.

7. Bath PMW, Lindenstrom E, Boysen G, et al. Tinzaparin in Acute Ischaemic Stroke (TAIST): a randomised aspirin-controlled trial. Lancet 2001; 358:702–10.

8. Cornu C, Boissel JP, Hommel M, et al. Protocol for the Multicenter Acute Stroke Trial – Thrombolysis Study. Clin Trials 1993;28:329–44.

9. Hommel M, Boissel JP, Cornu C, et al. Termination of trial of streptokinase in severe acute ischaemic stroke. Lancet 1995;345:57.

10. The Publications Committee for the Trial of ORG 10172 in Acute Stroke Treatment (TOAST) Investigators. Low molecular weight heparinoid, ORG 10172 (danaparoid), and outcome after acute ischemic stroke: a randomized controlled trial. The Publications Committee for the Trial of ORG 10172 in Acute Stroke Treatment (TOAST) Investigators. JAMA 1998;279:1265–72.

11. The European Cooperative Acute Stroke Study (ECASS). Intravenous thrombolysis with recombinant tissue plasminogen activator for acute hemispheric stroke. JAMA 1995;274:1017–25.

12. von Kummer R, Hacke W. Safety and efficacy of intravenous tissue plasminogen activator and heparin in acute middle cerebral artery stroke. Stroke 1992; 23:646–52.

13. International Stroke Trial Collaborative Group. The International Stroke Trial (IST): a randomised trial of aspirin, subcutaneous heparin, both, or neither among 19,435 patients with acute ischemic stroke. Lancet 1997;349:1569–81.

14. Hacke W, Kaste M, Fieschi C, et al. Randomised double-blind placebo-controlled trial of thrombolytic therapy with intravenous alteplase in acute ischemic stroke (ECASS II). Lancet 1998;652:1245–51.

15. Baron J-C. Mapping the ischemic penumbra with PET: implications for acute stroke treatment. Cerebrovasc Dis 1999;9:193–201.

16. Bozik ME, Smith JM, Douglass A, et al. POST: Double-blind, placebo controlled, safety and efficacy trials of intravenous BMS-204352 in patients with acute stroke. In: Proceedings of the 25th International Stroke Congress (AHA), New Orleans; February 10–12, 2000 (abst).

17. ISIS-3 Collaborative Group. ISIS-3: a randomised comparison of streptokinase vs tissue plasminogen activator vs anistreplase and of aspirin plus heparin vs aspirin alone among 41,299 cases of suspected acute myocardial infarction. ISIS-3 (Third International Study of Infarct Survival) Collaborative Group. Lancet 1992;339:753–70.

18. Wahlgren NG, MacMohan DG, de Keyser J, et al. Intravenous Nimodipine West European Stroke Trial (INWEST) of nimodipine in the treatment of acute ischaemic stroke. Cerebrovasc Dis 1994;4:204–10.

19. Cornu C, Boutitie F, Candelise L, et al. Streptokinase in acute ischemic stroke: an individual patient data meta-analysis: The Thrombolysis in Acute Stroke Pooling Project. Stroke 2000;31:1555–60.

20. Del Zoppo GJ, Poeck K, Pessin MS, et al. Recombinant tissue plasminogen activator in acute thrombotic and embolic stroke. Ann Neurol 1992;32:78–86.

21. Rankin J. Cerebral vascular accidents in patients over the age of 60, II: Prognosis. Scot Med J 1957;2:200–15.

22. Wardlaw JM, Sandercock PAG, Warlow CP, Lindley RI. Trials of thrombolysis in acute ischemic stroke. Does the choice of primary outcome measure really matter? Stroke 2000;31:1133–5.

23. Less KR. Thrombolysis. Br Med Bull 2000;56:389–400.

24. Stingele R, Bluhmki E, Hacke W. Bootstrap statistics of ECASS II data: Just another post hoc analysis of a negative stroke trial? Cerebrovasc Dis 2001;11:30–33.

25. Clark WM, Wissman S, Albers GW, et al. Recombinant tissue-type plasminogen activator (alteplase) for ischemic stroke 3 to 5 hours after symptom onset. The ATLANTIS Study: a randomized controlled trial. Alteplase Thrombolysis for Acute Noninterventional Therapy in Ischemic Stroke. JAMA 1999;282:2019–26.

26. Warach S. Diffusion and perfusion. MRI: Functional brain imaging. In: Eddman RR, Zlatkin MB, Hesselink JR (eds). Clinical Magnetic Resonance Imaging, 2nd edn. Philadelphia: WB Saunders, 1996:828–50.

27. Warach S, Boska M, Welch KMA. Pitfalls and potential of clinical diffusion-weighted MR imaging in acute stroke. Stroke 1997;28:481–2.

28. Collins R, Peto R, Baigent C, Steight P. Aspirin, heparin, and fibrinolytic therapy in suspected acute myocardial infarction. N Engl J Med 1997;336:847–60.

29. Sandercock P, Gubitz G, Foley P, Counsell C. Antiplatelet therapy for acute ischemic stroke. The Cochrane Database of Systematic Reviews 2003, Issue 2. Art. No.: CD000029. DOI: 10.1002/14651858;CD000029.

30. Wardlaw JM, del Zoppo G, Yamaguchi T, Berge E. Thrombolysis for acute ischemic stroke. The Cochrane Database of Systematic Reviews 2003, Issue 3. Art. No.: CD000213. DOI: 10.1002/14651858.CD000213.

31. Cast (Chinese Acute Stroke Trial) Collaborative Group. CAST: randomised placebo-controlled trial of early aspirin use in 20,000 patients with acute ischaemic stroke. Lancet 1997;349:1641–9.

8

Unfractionated heparin, low-molecular-weight-heparins, and heparinoids in acute stroke

Ángel Chamorro

Introduction

Stroke is an enormous public health problem in industrialized countries.[1] Ranking number three as a cause of mortality, it is also a major cause of morbidity and disability. Within 2 weeks of a stroke, no less than 20% and as many as 60% of stroke patients require some assistance with activities of daily living; about 20% are dead in a month, and among those alive at 6 months, about a third are more or less dependent on others for daily living.[2,3] Stroke survivors are also at high risk for a second vascular event – about 5% per annum[4] – and they are also at high risk of serious coronary events – about 3% per annum. Despite these grim figures, the treatment of acute ischemic stroke remains challenging, as no single drug has unequivocally been demonstrated to be effective, or suitable for a significant percentage of patients.

The frustrating shortage of efficacious stroke therapies is partially offset by an increasingly better understanding of the inner mechanisms that bridge brain ischemia with cell death, including the roles of excitotoxicity, inflammation, oxidative damage, and apoptosis.[5] It is also beyond doubt that to minimize the consequences of acute stroke, external interventions need to be started as diligently as possible. Nevertheless, while this advice has been strictly endorsed in most clinical trials that have evaluated the role of thrombolytic or neuroprotectant agents, it has been disregarded without exception in trials

that have assessed the value of unfractionated heparin (UFH), low-molecular-weight heparins (LMWH), or heparinoids.[6]

Rationale for the use of anticoagulants in patients with acute ischemic stroke

On theoretical grounds, anticoagulants are given to patients with acute ischemic stroke to prevent thrombus progression, facilitate collateral circulation, hinder the development of early stroke recurrence, and prevent deep venous thrombosis (DVT) and pulmonary embolism.[7] In patients with stroke complicating acute myocardial infarction, antithrombotics can also be given for the prevention of mural thrombosis, which might result in a recurrent thromboembolic event.[8] Improvement of functional outcome, and reduction of mortality, are additional endpoints included in the more recent anticoagulation trials. However, the long delay to the initiation of treatment from the onset of symptoms suggests that functional improvement was expected in most anticoagulation trials to reflect an overall reduction of thromboembolic events rather than direct neuroprotectant effects. Otherwise, it is very unlikely that therapeutic measures initiated so long after the onset of symptoms could result in a significant salvage of tissue at risk.

Table 8.1 Anticoagulant agents assessed in randomized controlled trials

Trial[a]	Agent[b]/control	Dose
FISS	Nadroparin/placebo	4100 IU anti-Xa bid
	Nadroparin/placebo	4100 IU anti-Xa/day
FISS-bis	Nadroparin/placebo	85 IU anti-Xa/kg/bid
	Nadroparin/placebo	85 IU anti-Xa/kg/day
IST	UFH/placebo/aspirin	12 550 IU bid
	UFH/placebo/aspirin	5000 IU/day
RAPID	UFH/	Bolus + 12 IU/kg/h
	aspirin	300 mg PO
TOAST	Danaparoid/placebo	0.6–0.8 IU anti-Xa
HAEST	Dalteparin/aspirin	100 IU/kg/bid
TOPAS	Certoparin	3000 IU anti-Xa/day
TOPAS	Certoparin	3000 IU anti-Xa/bid
TOPAS	Certoparin	5000 IU anti-Xa bid
TOPAS	Certoparin	8000 IU anti-Xa bid
TAIST	Tinzaparin/aspirin	175 IU anti-Xa/kg/day
TAIST	Tinzaparin/aspirin	100 IU anti-Xa/kg/day

[a]FISS, Fraxiparin in Stroke Study; IST, International Stroke Trial; RAPID, Rapid Anticoagulation Prevents Ischemic Damage; TOAST, Trial of ORG 10172 in Acute Stroke Treatment; HAEST, Heparin in Acute Embolic Stroke Trial; TOPAS, Therapy of Patients with Acute Stroke; TAIST, Tinzaparin in Acute Ischemic Stroke.
[b]UFH, unfractionated heparin.

Anticoagulation and evidence-based medicine

A systematic review of 23 427 stroke patients anticoagulated within 2 weeks from the onset of symptoms revealed that treatment was associated with about 9 fewer recurrent ischemic strokes per 1000 patients treated. However, this benefit was offset by a similar-sized 9 per 1000 increase in symptomatic intracranial hemorrhage.[9,10] Practitioners of evidence-based medicine advise strongly that anticoagulants should not be used at therapeutic doses in patients with acute ischemic stroke because they have offered no net benefits in randomized clinical trials or meta-analyses.[10] Regardless of the lack of a convincing proof of therapeutic efficacy, physicians have administered UFH to stroke patients for more than 50 years[11] and LMWH for at least two decades. Other physicians are more reluctant to put the last nail into the coffin of anticoagulants as they believe that important limitations in many anticoagulation trials mean that the hypothesis that anticoagulation in acute stroke is not beneficial has never been adequately tested.[12–14] Clinical trials of unfractionated heparin, LMWH, and heparinoids evaluated in randomized trials are listed in Table 8.1.

Unfractionated heparin (UFH)

IST (International Stroke Trial) is the largest study to date that has evaluated the role of UFH in patients with completed ischemic stroke.[15] IST found that patients allocated to UFH (12 550 IU twice daily) had significantly fewer recurrent strokes within 14 days (2.9% vs 3.8%) than patients not treated with UFH.[14] However, this benefit was offset by a similar-sized increase in hemorrhagic strokes (1.2% vs 0.4%), so the difference in death or nonfatal recurrent stroke was not significant. The study also showed that the combined incidence of intracranial hemorrhage, recurrent stroke, and pulmonary embolism was 3.4% in patients allocated to aspirin plus low-dose UFH (5000 IU twice daily), 4.4% in patients allocated to aspirin only, and 4.7% in those allocated to low-dose UFH only.

The value of adjusted high-dose intravenous UFH, which represents the most usual mode of heparin administration, has never been completely determined in a large randomized clinical trial. The RAPID (Rapid Anticoagulation Prevents Ischemic Damage) trial was the largest effort to rectify this important lack of knowledge, but the study was interrupted due to

Table 8.2   Primary and secondary endpoints of the RAPID study

| | Treatment arm[a] | | | |
	Aspirin (n =35)	UFH (n =32)	p	Odds ratio[b]
Rankin Score 0–2 at 3 months	19 (54.3)	13 (40.6)	0.26	1.74 (0.7–4.6)
NIHSS at day 7	12.3 (11.7)	12.4 (11.6)	0.97	
NIHSS <1 at day 90	9 (25.7)	8 (25.0)	0.94	1.04 (0.34–3.13)
Ischemic stroke recurrence	3 (8.6)	0 (0)	0.09	0.13 (0.01–1.39)
Hemorrhagic worsening	3 (8.6)	2 (6.3)	0.71	1.41 (0.2–9.0)
Ischemic worsening	7 (20.0)	8 (25.0)	0.62	0.75 (0.4–2.4)
DVT or pulmonary embolism	0	0		
Death, recurrence or bleeding	5 (14.3)	4 (12.5)	0.83	1.17 (0.28–4.79)

UFH, unfractionated heparin; NIHSS, National Institutes of Health Stroke Scale; DVT, deep-vein thrombosis.
[a]Mean values (SD in parentheses).
[b]95% confidence interval in parentheses.

insufficient funding when only 67 patients had been included.[16] The study compared the value of aspirin (300 mg/day) and UFH in patients with suspected nonlacunar ischemic stroke and symptoms lasting less than 12 h using a parallel-group, randomized, open, blinded endpoint assessment (PROBE) design. The primary endpoint of RAPID trial was the rate of favorable outcome, defined as a modified Rankin scale less than 2 at day 90. For sample size calculations, it was estimated that 592 patients per treatment group were required (0.05%, 80%) to detect or disprove an absolute difference of about 8% in favorable outcome. UFH was started with an intravenous bolus of 40 IU/kg followed by a weight-adjusted continuous infusion of 12 IU/kg/h aimed to achieve plasma levels of 0.3–0.5 U/ml as soon as possible. Control of UFH therapy was assessed by activated partial thromboplastin time (aPTT) ratios (patient aPTT/control aPTT). Six hours after treatment onset, or after any dose adjustment, an aPTT was obtained. Otherwise, aPTTs were ordered every 12 h. Local laboratories were requested at study onset to calibrate the aPTT ratio for their individual UFH levels. The study treatment was maintained for 6 days in stroke units of tertiary hospitals. The primary and secondary endpoints of RAPID are shown in Table 8.2. Despite the small number of patients, RAPID disclosed a trend toward a lower recurrence rate in patients allocated anticoagulation, and this was achieved without a parallel increment in bleeding complications.[16] Interestingly, ischemic worsening of at least 4 points in the National

Institutes of Health Stroke Scale (NIHSS) was associated with lower UFH levels than clinically stable strokes, and hemorrhagic worsening was associated with higher UFH levels than bland infarctions. Unfortunately, RAPID was not adequately powered to compare the outcome effects between UFH and aspirin.[16]

Nadroparin

FISS (Fraxiparin in Stroke Study) demonstrated that nadroparin was better than placebo in improving clinical outcome after ischemic stroke.[17] However, this positive finding could not be replicated in the FISS-bis trial performed in European patients. Several critics have emphasized that the beneficial effect of nadroparin was only observed 6 months after stroke onset, but not at 3 months. According to the investigators, nadroparin saved more tissue in penumbra than the placebo did, and that this effect took longer to manifest clinically.[15] In conflict with this speculation is the clinical observation that the efficacy of thrombolytics is detected a shorter time delay after treatment administration. Other possible explanations for the unconfirmed positive findings of FISS are chance (false-positive), the unexpected absence of hemorrhagic complications observed in the two nadroparin-treated groups, and the (unlikely) existence of ethnic heterogeneity in the response to nadroparin.

Danaparoid

In TOAST (Trial of ORG 10172 in Acute Stroke Treatment), a 7-day course of danaparoid (ORG 10172) or placebo was given as a bolus within 24 h of stroke.[18] At 3 months, 482 (75.2%) of 641 persons assigned to treatment with danaparoid and 467 (73.7%) of 634 patients treated with placebo had favorable outcomes (not significant); 49.5% and 47%, respectively, of patients in each group had very favorable outcomes at 3 months. Therefore, the null hypothesis of the study could not be rejected. At 7 days, 215 (33.09%) of 635 persons given danaparoid and 176 (27.8%) of 633 persons administered placebo had very favorable outcomes ($p = 0.01$). Within 10 days of treatment onset, serious intracranial bleeding occurred in 14 patients given danaparoid (15 events) and in 4 placebo-treated patients ($p = 0.05$).

Dalteparin

HAEST (Heparin in Acute Embolic Stroke Trial) was a randomized, double-blind trial on the effect of dalteparin (100 IU/kg subcutaneously twice daily) or aspirin (160 mg daily) for the treatment of 449 patients with acute ischemic stroke and atrial fibrillation.[19] The primary aim of the study was to test whether treatment with dalteparin started within 30 h of stroke onset was superior to aspirin for the prevention of recurrent stroke. The frequency of recurrent ischemic stroke during the first 2 weeks was 8.5% in dalteparin-allocated patients and 7.5% in aspirin-allocated patients (odds ratio (OR) 1.13 (95% (CI 0.57–2.24). There were no significant differences in functional outcome or death at 14 days or 3 months. There were more symptomatic cerebral hemorrhages in the dalteparin group than in the aspirin group (2.6% vs 1.7%).

Tinzaparin

The TAIST (Tinzaparin in Acute Ischemic Stroke) study expands the list of unsuccessful LMWH in ischemic stroke.[20] The proportions independent at 6 months were similar in the groups assigned tinzaparin 175 IU anti-Xa/kg daily (41.5%), tinzaparin 100 IU anti-Xa/kg daily (42.4%), or aspirin 300 mg daily (42.5%). Disability, case-fatality, and neurological deterioration rates were also similar between the treatment groups. During the in-hospital treatment period, no patients assigned high-dose tinzaparin developed a symptomatic DVT compared with none assigned aspirin. Symptomatic intracerebral hemorrhage was significantly higher in the high-dose tinzaparin group (OR vs aspirin 7.17 (95% CI 1.10–163).

Certoparin

In the TOPAS (Therapy of Patients with Acute Stroke) trial,[21] the LMWH certoparin was allocated to 404 patients in four treatment groups within 12 h of stroke onset: 3000 IU anti-Xa certoparin once daily (treatment group 1); 3000 IU anti-Xa twice daily (group 2); 5000 IU anti-Xa twice daily (group 3); and 8000 IU anti-Xa twice daily (group 4). The primary efficacy variable was the proportion of patients reaching a favorable functional outcome (Barthel Index ≥ 90) at 3 months. The proportion of patients with Barthel Index ≥ 90 did not differ between treatment arms (61.5%, 60.8%, 63.3%, and 56.3% in the four groups, respectively; intent-to-treat population). European Stroke Scale scores improved in all treatment groups within the first 14 days to a similar extent. During the follow-up of 6 months, percentages of patients with recurrent stroke/transient ischemic attack (TIA) were 11.0%, 5.9%, 9.7%, and 13.0%, respectively, in the four groups. Two parenchymal cerebral hematomas and one extracranial bleeding episode occurred in treatment group 1 versus one and none in group 2, two and nine in group 3, and four and five in group 4. During certoparin treatment, one DVT but no pulmonary embolism was observed. Based on these findings, the investigators concluded that dose increase of certoparin up to 8000 IU anti-Xa twice daily did not improve the functional outcome of patients with ischemic stroke, and that severe bleeding tended to be more frequent in the highest-dose group only.

Critique of the anticoagulation trials

IST recommended that a computed tomography (CT) scan be performed at the time of randomization to rule out a hemorrhagic infarct. However, 5600 IST patients were scanned after randomization and treatment initiation, and it is likely that approximately 500 hemorrhagic strokes were erroneously included in the trial. Another major limitation of the IST trial was the lack of monitoring of the biological effects achieved with UFH. The reason for this was that even the highest dose of UFH allocated in IST (25 000 IU) was considered safe in clinical trials conducted previously in patients with DVT. The importance of monitoring the effects of UFH was clearly emphasized in RAPID, since UFH proved at least as safe as aspirin when the effects of UFH were adequately monitored.[16]

With the exception of RAPID and TOAST, which adjusted the rate of treatment infusion to achieve the intended biological effect, the remainder of the trials evaluated the effects of different doses of LMWH or UFH without dose adjustments. This could be a major drawback, since all trials showed a direct relationship between increasing doses of active treatment and the rate of bleeding complications. There have been no randomized trials in patients with ischemic stroke nor have there been any head-to-head comparisons of LMWH versus UFH.

Whereas the severity of strokes among patients randomized to receive active treatment or placebo varied across the trials, all of the latter had a significant proportion of patients with lacunar stroke – at least a quarter of treated patients. However, it is uncertain whether antithrombotic drugs are of any use in lacunar stroke, where the ischemia is presumably not followed by arterial reperfusion.

A major limitation of most of these trials is the long delay to treatment onset: 24–48 h, a therapeutic window of opportunity well beyond the most optimistic limits for the ischemic penumbra.[22] While this treatment delay seems appropriate to reduce the possibility of pulmonary embolism or DVT, it is less likely that it provides adequate neuronal protection, as most of the events responsible for neuronal death take place in a much earlier phase. On completion of the studies, the belief arose that heparins and heparinoids have a very limited, if any, role to play in the prevention of early recurrent stroke and in the improvement of functional outcome.[10,23] However, these conclusions might be premature, especially if due attention is paid to recent data demonstrating that the inflammatory mechanisms that arise in brain ischemia could be modulated by means of rapid anticoagulation.[6,24,25]

Hemorrhagic conversion

Heparin prolongs bleeding time in humans[26] and enhances blood loss from the microvasculature in animals.[27] The interaction of heparin with platelets and endothelial cells may contribute to the risk of bleeding by a mechanism independent of its anticoagulant effect.[28] LMWH are said to cause less bleeding than UFH,[29] although LMWH and UFH were associated with similar rates of bleeding in reported clinical trials. As the result of these effects, the most feared complication of anticoagulants in patients with acute stroke is the conversion of a previously pale infarct into a symptomatic hemorrhage. Hemorrhagic worsening proved to be a crucial issue in some clinical trials, where a greater reduction of recurrent thromboembolic events was neutralized by a greater risk of hemorrhagic worsening.

A widely accepted classification of hemorrhagic conversion outlines two main types: hemorrhagic infarction (HI) and parenchymal hematoma (PH).[30] Whereas HI is generally a radiological finding without clinical repercussions,[31] PH frequently results in worsening symptoms or in death of the patient. Hemorrhagic worsening may sometimes reflect the spontaneous bleeding tendency of bland infarcts; as shown in Table 8.2, this risk can be estimated indirectly by analyzing the bleeding rate observed in placebo-treated patients assessed in recent anticoagulation trials.

The pathophysiology of hemorrhagic conversion has evolved since the seminal descriptions of Fisher et al[32] explaining this event as the result of reperfusion of the vascular bed of the infarct following relief of the occlusion, such as would occur after fragmentation and distal migration of an embolus. Currently, it is recognized that spontaneous hemorrhagic conversion can also supervene before recanalization of an occluded artery through collateral circulation.[33]

The reported incidence of hemorrhagic conversion varies depending upon the definition used for hemorrhagic conversion, the type of patient, the use of concomitant medications (frequently omitted), the timing and type of neuroimaging techniques used for diagnosis, and whether the studies were prospective or retrospective.[34,35] Although retrospective studies tend to overestimate the true incidence of bleeding, the incidence of hemorrhagic conversion in CT studies has variously been reported from a few percent to 43% of consecutive patients.[36] However, repeated neuroimaging tests are more likely in those patients with poor outcome than in those with an uneventful clinical course. In addition, the true incidence of symptomatic hemorrhagic conversion can also be obscured by the clinical situation of the patient at the time of bleeding. Thus, small parenchymal hematomas (PH type I) are more easily suspected in patients with mild ischemic symptoms or normal neurological examination before the bleeding. In contrast, large hematomas (PH type II) could pass unnoticed in patients with major stroke and severe deficits that may blur the detection of worsening symptoms. In the latter situation, complicating hematomas would only be reliably detected if neuroimaging studies were repeated during the clinical course. Unfortunately, this policy was not followed in most of the available anticoagulation trials, or in retrospective studies, in which repeated neuroimaging examinations were usually restricted to patients who developed worsening symptoms.

Several factors have been associated with a greater risk of hemorrhagic conversion, including aging,[37] cardioembolic mechanism of ischemic stroke,[30] failure of collateral flow,[38] early abnormal findings on CT scan,[39] and M1 middle cerebral artery occlusion.[34] Increased blood pressure during the acute stage of stroke has also been correlated with the incidence and severity of hemorrhagic infarction in some studies,[40] but not in others.[41] Preliminary results have emphasized the potential role of increased activation of matrix metalloproteinases (MMPs) in individuals with hemorrhagic conversion.[42]

Hemorrhagic conversion in patients treated with anticoagulants

Unquestionably, the risk of hemorrhagic conversion is increased by the use of anticoagulants in the setting of acute stroke.[43] In a meta-analysis,[10] it was estimated that the use of anticoagulants increased the risk of symptomatic hemorrhagic conversion by an odds ratio of 2.52 (95% CI 1.92–3.32). It has been suggested that bleeding is more likely to occur when a coagulation test is prolonged excessively.[44] Indeed, our group observed in patients treated with UFH that both symptomatic and asymptomatic intracerebral bleeding occurred more frequently after excessive prolongation of aPTT.[37] These findings emphasize the importance of strict biological monitoring of the effects of heparin in order to safeguard its relatively narrow therapeutic margin.

Anticoagulation of patients with large infarctions

It is controversial whether bleeding occurs more frequently in patients with severe clinical deficits or large infarctions. Thus, large-volume lesions and mass effect were found to be associated with cerebral bleeding in some studies.[45] Chamorro et al also found a greater bleeding tendency for larger infarctions.[41] However, the size of the lesion did not predict hemorrhagic worsening, since the unique factor independently associated with this complication was an excessive prolongation of aPTT.[37] Moreover, hemorrhagic transformation did not result in a significant change of previous neurological status in most patients. Pending corroboration in further studies, these findings suggest that in patients with large strokes, the crucial issue to address is not the safety of anticoagulation. Rather, the main question is whether sufficient salvageable cerebral tissue remains after the initial event to justify even a low risk of bleeding. If the answer is affirmative, the benefit/risk ratio of UFH has to be maximized through judicious administration of the agent.

Early stroke recurrence

Early stroke recurrence significantly increases the costs of stroke, prolongs hospital stay, and increases the 30-day case-fatality rate, with mortality almost three times greater after this complication. For many physicians, the individual risk that a patient has of sustaining an early recurrent stroke is a major element to ponder when evaluating the need to prescribe anticoagulant agents in the setting of acute stroke.[46] Some experts recommend a treatment delay of a few days before the initiation of anticoagulation to minimize the risk of intracerebral bleeding.[47] Accordingly, a greater risk or recurrent stroke would justify a hastier initiation of anticoagulant therapies. There are no major flaws in this theoretical rationalization if we ignore the inherent difficulties in estimating the risk of stroke recurrence in individual patients, and neglect the possibility that the main benefits of anticoagulation might be lost if treatment onset is delayed.

With few exceptions, most of the available information concerning the risks and mechanisms of stroke recurrence is based on retrospective data. While earlier studies reported a stroke recurrence rate of 10–20% in the first 10 days after the initial event,[48,49] more recent anticoagulation trials that included placebo-treated patients provide a lower figure of early stroke recurrence. The risk of early recurrence depends on the characteristics of the populations under evaluation. Lodder et al[50] estimated a risk of recurrence greater than 8% in patients with cardioembolic stroke, although Halperin and Hart[51] estimated in the same stroke subtype a 15–20% stroke recurrence rate within the first year alone. Yasaka et al[52] found the rate of recurrent embolization within the first 2 weeks after stroke to be 20.3%, and the recurrent events occurred more frequently during the first 2 days after the initial stroke. In addition, the mortality rate in patients who recurred in this study was 19.6%, compared with 8.8% in patients who did not recur. Darling et al[53] reported the rate of thromboembolism within 14 days to be 19.6% in 148 patients with valvular or nonvalvular atrial fibrillation; half of all recurrent events occurred within the first 2 weeks after the initial embolic event. van Latum et al[54] suggested that the risk of stroke recurrence depended strongly on the coexistence of variables such as history of previous embolism, enlarged cardiothoracic ratio on chest X-ray, systolic blood pressure greater than 160 mmHg, atrial fibrillation existing for more than 1 year, and evidence of an ischemic lesion on CT.

An accurate estimation of the risk of recurrence relies on many factors, of which the proper definition of stroke recurrence is not the least important. It may be relevant that the definition of recurrence requires that symptoms reappear within different vascular territories from the first event, and that it includes symptoms pertaining to the same arterial branch. The identification of a recurrent event also depends on the baseline neurological situation. Thus, it is easier to document the sudden reappearance of a new stroke in asymptomatic patients or in individuals with partially recovered deficits than to recognize this complication in patients with severe deficits, or in stuporous subjects with concomitant metabolic or infectious complications. The presence of aphasia, behavioral abnormalities, or fluctuating attentional defects may also complicate the accuracy of the clinical diagnosis of recurrence. To what extent these factors might have confounded the results of apparently well-conducted clinical trials is difficult to determine. Finally, the power to detect statistically significant differences between two drugs aimed at preventing stroke recurrence also depends on the recurrence rates identified in the groups under comparison. Therefore, only very large studies would be able to detect small differences between two therapeutic alternatives.

Factors predisposing to early stroke recurrence

It is acknowledged that early stroke recurrence could be related to a hypercoagulable state that exists for a few days following the initial ischemic brain injury.[55] In some studies,[56] but not in others,[57] a history of recent TIA was also associated with stroke recurrence. The Stroke Data Bank[53] estimated that the risk of early recurrence for cardioembolic stroke was 4.3%; however, the risk increased to 9% in patients with hypertension and hyperglycemia. Nevertheless, these risks were estimated in patients who received some form of (unreported) antithrombotic treatment, including anticoagulants. Chamorro et al[58] found no relationship between the presence of traditional risk factors and the recurrence rate. In contrast, the cumulative risk of recurrence in patients with low erythrocyte sedimentation rate (ESR) on admission was 2.9% within 2 weeks of a qualifying event, and 9.7%, in patients with higher ESR, suggesting an inflammatory component in the pathogenesis of early recurrent stroke. Nevertheless, ESR was more elevated in patients with risk factors such as diabetes or hypercholesterolemia.[54] Thus, these apparently clashing results between the presence or absence of risk factors and the rate of recurrent events could be reconciled if the concept of risk factor is switched from a dichotomous classification (yes versus no) to a mechanistic investigation of many interrelated risks.[59]

In conclusion, it is difficult at present to determine the borderline between overstimulation and understimulation of the risk of stroke recurrence in patients with acute stroke given the substantial differences in the magnitude of stroke risk in subpopulations of patients with stroke, the uncontrolled use of therapeutic measures in reported series, the variability of the definition of stroke recurrence, and the dissimilar statistical methodology used to analyze independent determinants of recurrence.[60]

Early clinical worsening

As platelets and thrombin are involved in thrombus progression, the administration of agents that block their activation is considered by many physicians an attractive therapeutic option for the prevention of early clinical worsening. By inactivating thrombin, heparin not only prevents fibrin formation but also inhibits thrombin-induced activation of platelets and of factors V and VIII. Heparin binds to platelets, and can induce or inhibit platelet aggregation in vitro.[61] Binding of heparin to von Willebrand factor (vWF) also inhibits vWF factor-dependent platelet function.[62]

Theoretically, UFH and LMWH could fail to prevent thrombus formation in clinical practice as the result of their biophysical limitations. These limitations arise because the heparin or LMWH/antithrombin III (ATIII) complex is unable to inactivate factor Xa in the prothrombinase complex, and thrombin bound to fibrin or to subendothelial surfaces.[8] Platelets limit the anticoagulant effect of heparins by protecting surface factor Xa from inhibition by heparin/ATIII,[63] and by secreting platelet factor 4 (PF4).[64] Fibrin limits the anticoagulant effect of heparin by protecting fibrin-bound thrombin from inhibition by heparin/ATIII.[65] Thrombin also binds to subendothelial matrix proteins, where it is protected from inhibition by heparin.

Atherothrombotic infarction is frequently considered to be the stroke subtype with the greatest risk of clinical worsening due to thrombus progression. However, the prediction of this risk in individual patients is difficult as clinical, neuroimaging, ultrasonographic, and biochemical predictive factors have all been invoked.[66]

Unfortunately, there have been no randomized clinical trials assessing whether an expeditious administration of anticoagulants prevents stroke progression. Duke et al[67] studied 225 stable patients for at least 48 h after clinical onset to evaluate whether UFH was more effective than placebo in the prevention of stroke progression occurring after the second day of stroke. The results of this study were disappointing because the rate of progression in anticoagulated patients was 17%, compared with 19.5% in the placebo-treated group. However, a major limitation of the study is the long delay to treatment onset. Indeed, the rates of stroke progression disclosed in current clinical trials among placebo-treated patients are very high within the first hours after stroke onset. In ECASS (European Cooperative Acute Stroke Study), 23% of patients had worsening symptoms within 8h from the onset of symptoms, and 37.5% within 30 hours. These data strongly suggest that Duke and colleagues did not select the ideal group of patients for prevention of stroke progression, as presumably the best candidates were excluded from the study. In another small nonrandomized study, Haley et al[68] failed to stop the progression of worsening symptoms in 36 consecutive patients treated with porcine heparin adjusted to mantain the aPTT at 1.5–2 times control.

Old drugs revisited: the case of UFH

Early clinical worsening could also implicate non-thrombotic mechanisms that could be influenced by the administration of anticoagulant agents. In this setting, the contribution of inflammatory processes to the progression of brain ischemia is well established.[69,70] Inhibition of inflammation could be among the beneficial effects of UFH in patients with acute ischemic stroke.[6] Additional biological effects, such as regulation of angiogenesis, lipoprotein lipase modulation, maintenance of endothelial wall competence, and inhibition of vascular smooth muscle proliferation after endothelial injury,[71–74] could have clinical implications that at present remain untested.

Increasing evidence, both experimental and clinical, indicates that UFH possesses anti-inflammatory properties.[75] Inhibition of inflammation could be among the beneficial effects of UFH in coronary heart disease.[76] In murine brain focal ischemia, higher anticoagulant doses[77] and shorter anticoagulation delays[78] were the most effective, and UFH showed better results than equivalent anticoagulant doses of LMWH.[73,74] Total leukocyte count[79] and plasma levels of proinflammatory cytokines[80] were also lower in patients anticoagulated than in those antiaggregated, and these effects were associated with greater recovery and less risk of worsening.[81] The participation of cytokines, adhesion factors, and leukocytes in cerebral ischemia occurs rapidly, since most molecules are upregulated at 1 h post ischemia and have a peak response at 6–12 h.[82] Anti-inflammatory effects include binding to Mac-1 (CD11b/CD18), inhibition of leukocyte rolling, blocking of selectins, and attenuation of inducible nitric oxide synthase (iNOS) and NO release.[83–85] Heparin also modulates the adhesion of mononuclear cells to vascular cells in vitro,[86] and in a preliminary study heparin decreased plasmatic levels of vascular cell adhesion molecule 1 (VCAM-1), which is involved in mononuclear adhesion and transmigration.[87] VCAM-1 is an adhesion factor strongly expressed by human astrocytes and endothelial cells from infarcted tissue in human cortex.[88] VCAM-1 has been shown to induce tissue factor (TF) expression, which is the initiator of the coagulation cascade in vivo.[89] UFH abrogates the endotoxin-induced increase in TF-positive monocytes in vivo and increases plasma levels of TF pathway inhibitor.[90] UFH decreases high TF plasma levels and monocyte procoagulant activity in unstable angina.[91] It has also been shown that after interacting with the cell surface, UFH protects the endothelium from damage by free radicals.[92,93] Heparin and other related polyanions, such as dermatan and heparan sulfate, are also capable of releasing diamine oxidase and superoxide dismutase (SOD) from the endothelial cell surface.[94,95] Therefore, heparin may also have antioxidant properties.

Clinical guidelines for early anticoagulation

Some clinical guidelines recommend immediate anticoagulation for patients at higher risk of stroke recurrence, whereas delaying anticoagulation for several days is preferred for patients at low risk for early recurrence.[7] Case-by-case consideration of anticoagulation is advocated by others, depending upon the underlying vascular mechanism, the size and location of the affected vessel, and the extent of the atherosclerotic process. Finally, the Cochrane Investigators disregard *any type of anticoagulant* in acute ischemic stroke.[10]

The evidence favoring or discouraging the administration of adjusted-dose UFH to patients with ischemic stroke is scanty.[30,63,96] Available data on 'immediate' anticoagulation is also inadequate, especially if it is considered that a 2-week delay outlasts the concept of treatment immediacy in ischemic stroke. Clashing with the main conclusion of the systematic review of randomized trials, a few nonrandomized studies have emphasized the relevance of dose-adjusted UFH[37] and rapid treatment.[97] In these studies, recovery was greater in patients treated within 6 h from symptom onset than in similar patients in whom treatment was started between 6 and 48 h from symptom onset. Moreover, stroke recurrence and serious bleeding were associated with inadequate or excessive anticoagulation tests, respectively.[93] While the nature of these studies makes it difficult to completely overcome the effects of confounding they represent the largest series of patients 'immediately' anticoagulated with intravenous adjusted-dose UFH. In IST, 800, 3000, and 7000 patients were randomized to treatment within 3, 6, and 12 hours, respectively, and there was no heterogeneity of effect with decreasing time to randomization. However, UFH was administered subcutaneously and at least an additional 24 h had to be added before stable anti-coagulant effects were accomplished.[8]

Stroke subtypes and anticoagulation

In ischemic stroke, current clinical practice individualizes the need for anticoagulation according to the cause of stroke and the risk of early stroke recurrence or impending clinical worsening. This attitude is firmly ingrained in the therapeutic reasoning of many practitioners – despite the failure of randomized trials, anticoagulants are still used in patients with cardioembolic stroke or clinical worsening secondary to large-vessel disease.

The clinical decision is supported, in the former case, by an expected greater risk of early stroke recurrence and, in the latter, by the assumption that coagulation results from exposure of blood to TF located in ruptured plaques, damaged subendothelium, and activated leukocytes. However, it is possible that additional factors arise in the cerebral circulation, particularly once brain ischemic damage has supervened. Thus, following the release of cytokines, TF is the primary cellular initiator of the coagulation cascade in vivo, and represents a hemostatic envelope diffusely expressed in human cortex and cerebral vessels.[98] Accordingly, when ischemic cerebral damage is produced, exposure of TF to flowing blood results in a transient prothrombotic state. Importantly, this pathogenic mechanism would follow any stroke subtype, irrespective of the cause of symptoms, given the strong and widespread expression of TF on the cerebral cortex and intracerebral vessels.

Thus – pending appropriate endorsement by an adequately powered clinical trial – there is a theoretical framework to uphold the use of anticoagulants after most ischemic strokes. Some exceptions to this theoretical recommendation would be patients with active bleeding disorders, a low platelet count, or recent thrombolysis. Ideally, anticoagulation would have to be initiated as soon as possible, before the ischemic lesion has reached the threshold of structural irreversibility. Moreover, to minimize the risk of untoward complications, a sensible administration of anticoagulants would include determination

of the therapeutic range of aPTT results,[99] close monitoring of biological effects during active treatment, and the use of drugs with high molecular weight.

Conclusions

Available evidence gathered in randomized trials of heparinoids or LMWH, and in trials in which UFH was given subcutaneously at low or medium doses to patients with ischemic stroke, is disappointing. Based on these studies, anticoagulants are not recommended in patients with acute stroke. However, these results should not be extrapolated to adjusted-dose intravenous UFH before adequate clinical testing has established its value. Recent observational studies and experimental data have provided encouraging clinical results and suggested new mechanisms by which UFH could be beneficial for patients with ischemic stroke, including blockage of inflammatory mechanisms. Obviously, firm recommendations cannot be provided until a large, well-designed clinical trial has determined the true value of anticoagulation in the setting of acute ischemic stroke. Such a clinical trial has to give appropriate credit to the importance of the therapeutic window, adjusted dose, intravenous administration, high molecular weight, and close monitoring.

Addendum

Recently, a paper has been published describing the value of intravenous heparin started within the first 3 h after onset of symptoms in patients with acute nonlacunar hemispheric cerebral infarctions.[100] The study was an outcome evaluator-blinded design trial. Patients had to display signs of a nonlacunar hemispheric infarction to be randomly allocated to receive intravenous heparin sodium or saline. Heparin was infused at a rate to maintain activated an aPTT ratio of 2.0–2.5 times control for 5 days. The primary endpoint was recovery of a modified Rankin Score of 0–2 at 90 days of stroke by telephone interview by a single physician blinded to treatment. Safety endpoints were death, symptomatic intracranial hemorrhages, and major extracranial bleeds by 90 days of stroke. A total of 418 stroke patients were included. In the heparin group, there were more self-independent patients (38.9% vs 28.6%; $p < 0.025$). In addition, in the same group, there were fewer deaths (16.8% vs 21.9%; $p < 0.189$), more symptomatic brain hemorrhages (6.2% vs 1.4%; $p < 0.008$), and more major extracerebral bleedings (2.9% vs 1.4%; $p < 0.491$). According to the authors of this paper, intravenous heparin sodium could be of help in the earliest treatment of acute nonlacunar hemispheric cerebral infarction, even taking account of an increased frequency of intracranial symptomatic brain hemorrhages. Overall, these recent findings further justify a large and appropriately designed clinical trial assessing the value of well-adjusted intravenous heparin in patients with acute stroke of very recent onset.

References

1. Taylor TN, Davis PH, Torner JC, et al. Lifetime cost of stroke in the United States. Stroke 1996;27: 1459–66.
2. Warlow CP. Epidemiology of stroke. Lancet 1998; 352(Suppl III):1–4.
3. Dobkin B. The economic impact of stroke. Neurology 1995;45(Suppl 1):S6–9.
4. European Carotid Surgery Trialists' Collaborative Group. Randomised trial of endarterectomy for recently symptomatic carotid stenosis: final results of the MRC European Carotid Surgery Trial (ECST). Lancet 1998;351:1379–87.
5. Dirnagl U, Iadecola C, Moskowitz A. Pathobiology of ischemic stroke: an integrated view. Trends Neurosci 1999;22:391–7.
6. Chamorro A. Immediate anticoagulation in acute focal brain ischemia revisited. Gathering the evidence. Stroke 2001;32:577–8.
7. Sherman DG, Dyken ML Jr, Gent M, et al. Antithrombotic therapy for cerebrovascular disorders. An update. Chest 1995;108(Suppl):444S–56S.
8. Hirsh J, Anand SS, Halperin JL, Fuster V. Mechanisms of action and pharmacology of unfractionated heparin. Arterioscler Thromb Vasc Biol 2001;21:1094–6.
9. Sandercock PAG, Van den Belt GM, Lindley IR, Slattery J. Antithrombotic therapy in acute ischemic stroke: an overview of the completed randomized trials. J Neurol Neurosurg Psychiatry 1993;56:17–25.
10. Gubitz G, Sandercock P, Counsell C. Anticoagulants for acute ischemic stroke. In: The Cochrane Library, Issue 3, 2000. Oxford: Update Software.
11. Hedenius P. The use of heparin in internal diseases. Acta Med Scand 1941;107:170–82.
12. Chamorro A. Anticoagulation and antiaggregation for acute cerebral ischemia. In: Castillo J, Dávalos A, Toni D (eds). Management of Acute Ischemic Stroke. Barcelona: Springer,1997:97–108.
13. Bousser MG. Aspirin or heparin immediately after stroke? Lancet 1997;349:1564–5.
14. Al-Sadat A, Sunbulli M, Chaturvedi S. Use of intravenous heparin by North American neurologists: Do the data matter? Stroke 2002;33:1574–7.
15. International Stroke Trial Collaborative Group. The International Stroke Trial (IST): a randomised trial of aspirin, subcutaneous heparin, both, or neither among 19 435 patients with acute ischemic stroke. Lancet 1997;349:1569–81.
16. Chamorro A , Busse O, Obach V, et al, for the RAPID Investigators. The Rapid Anticoagulation Prevents Ischemic Damage Study in Acute Stroke – final results from the Writing Committee. Cerebrovasc Dis 2005; 19:402–4.
17. Kay R, Wong KS, Yu YL, et al. Low-molecular weight heparin for the treatment of acute ischemic stroke. N Engl J Med 1995;333:1588–93.
18. The Publications Committee for the Trial of ORG 10172 in Acute Stroke Treatment (TOAST) Investigators. Low molecular weight heparinoid, ORG 10172 (danaparoid), and outcome after acute ischemic stroke. JAMA 1998;279:1265–72.
19. Berge E, Abdelnoor M, Nakstad PH, Sandset PM, on behalf of the HAEST Study Group. Low-molecular weight heparin versus aspirin in patients with acute ischemic stroke and atrial fibrillation: a double-blind randomised study. Lancet 2000;355:1205–10.
20. Bath PMW, Linderstrom E, Boysen G, et al, for the TAIST Investigators. Tinzaparin in acute ischemic stroke (TAIST): a randomised aspirin-controlled trial. Lancet 2001;358:702–10.
21. Diener HC Ringelstein EB, von Kummer R, et al. Treatment of acute ischemic stroke with the low-molecular-weight heparin certoparin: results of the TOPAS trial. Therapy of Patients With Acute Stroke (TOPAS) Investigators. Stroke 2001;32:22–9.

22. Bogousslavsky J, Brott TG, Diener HC, et al. The European Ad Hoc Consensus Group. European strategies for early intervention in stroke. A report of an Ad Hoc Consensus Group Meeting. Cerebrovasc Dis 1996;6:315–24.

23. Hankey GJ. One year after CAPRIE, IST and ESPS 2. Any changes in concepts? Cerebrovasc Dis 1998; 8(Suppl 5):1–7.

24. Chamorro A, Cervera A, Castillo J, et al. Unfractionated heparin is associated with a lower rise of serum vascular cell adhesion molecule-1 in acute ischemic stroke patients. Neurosci Lett 2002;328:229–32.

25. Cervera A, Justicia C, Reverter JC, et al. Steady plasma concentration of unfractionated heparin reduces infarct volume and prevents inflammatory damage after transient focal cerebral ischemia in the rat. J Neurosci Res 2004;15:565–72.

26. Heiden D, Mielke CH, Rodvien R. Impairment by heparin of primary hemostasis and platelet [^{14}C]5-hydroxytryptamine release. Br J Hematol 1977;36:427–36.

27. Blajchman MA, Young E, Ofosu FA. Effects of unfractionated heparin, dermatan sulfate and low molecular weight heparin on vessel wall permeability in rabbits. Ann NY Acad Sci 1989; 556:245–54.

28. Fernandez F, Nguyen P, Van Ryn J, et al. Hemorrhagic doses of heparin and other glycosaminoglycans induce a platelet defect. Thromb Res 1986;43:491–5.

29. Carter CJ, Kelton JG, Hirsh J, et al. The relationship between the hemorrhagic and antithrombotic properties of low molecular weight heparin in rabbits. Blood 1982;59:1239–45.

30. Hart RG, Easton JD. Hemorrhagic infarcts. Stroke 1986;17:586–9.

31. Horning CR, Bauer T, Simon C, et al. Hemorrhagic transformation in cardioembolic cerebral infarction. Stroke 1993;24:465–8.

32. Fisher CM, Adams RD. Observations on brain embolism with special reference to the mechanism of hemorrhagic infarction. J Neuropathol Exp Neurol 1951;10:92–4.

33. Ogata J, Yutani C, Imakita M, et al. Hemorrhagic infarct of the brain without a reopening of the occluded arteries in cardioembolic stroke. Stroke 1989;20:876–83.

34. Cerebral Embolism Task Force. Cardiogenic brain embolism. The Second Report of the Cerebral Embolism Task Force. Arch Neurol 1989;46:727–43.

35. Fiorelli M, Bastianello S, von Kummer R, et al. Hemorrhagic transformation of a cerebral infarct. Relationship with early clinical deterioration and 3-month outcome in the European Cooperative Acute Stroke Study (ECASS I). Stroke 1999;30:2280–4.

36. Lodder J. CT-detected infarction, relation with the size of the infarct, and the presence of midline shift. Acta Neurol Scand 1984;2:329–35.

37. Okada Y, Yamaguchi T, Minematsu K, et al. Hemorrhagic transformation in cerebral embolism. Stroke 1989;20:598–603.

38. Alexandrov AV, Black SE, Ehrlich LE, et al. Predictors of hemorrhagic transformation occurring spontaneously and on anticoagulants in patients with acute ischemic stroke. Stroke 1997;28:1198–202.

39. Toni D, Fiorelli M, Bastioanello S, et al. Hemorrhagic transformation of brain infarct: predictability in the first 5 hours from stroke onset and influence on clinical outcome. Neurology 1996;46:341–5.

40. Faris AA, Hardin CA, Poser CM. Pathogenesis of hemorrhagic infarction on the brain. I. Experimental investigations of role of hypertension and of collateral circulation. Arch Neurol 1963;9:468–72.

41. Chamorro A, Vila N, Saiz A, et al. Early anticoagulation after large cerebral embolic infarction: a safety study. Neurology 1995;45:861–5.

42. Montaner J, Alvarez-Sabín J, Molina CA, et al. Matrix metalloproteinase expression is related to hemorrhagic transformation after cardioembolic stroke. Stroke 2001;32:2762–7.

43. Drake ME Jr, Shin C. Conversion of ischemic to hemorrhagic infarction by anticoagulant administration. Report of two cases with evidence from serial computed tomographic brain scans. Arch Neurol 1983;40:44.

44. Levine MN, Raskob G, Landerfeld S, Kearon C. Hemorrhagic complications of anticoagulant treatment. Chest 1998;114:511–23.

45. Jorgensen L, Torvik A. Ischemic cerebrovascular diseases in an autopsy series, Part II: prevalence, location, pathogenesis, and clinical course of cerebral infarct. J Neurol Sci 1969;9:285–320.

46. Marsch EE, Adams HP Jr, Biller J, et al. Use of antithrombotic drugs in the treatment of acute ischemic stroke: a survey of neurologists in practice in the United States. Neurology 1989;39:1631–4.

47. Mohr JP, Albers GW, Amarenco P, et al. Etiology of stroke. Stroke 1997;28:1510–16.

48. Cerebral Embolism Study Group. Cardioembolic stroke, early anticoagulation, and brain hemorrhage. Arch Intern Med 1987;147:636–40.

49. Koller RL. Recurrent embolic cerebral infarction and anticoagulation. Neurology 1982;32:283–5.

50. Lodder J, Dennis MS, Van Raak L, et al. Cooperative study on the value of long-term anticoagulation in stroke patients with nonrheumatic atrial fibrillation. BMJ 1988;296:1437–8.

51. Halperin JL, Hart RG. Atrial fibrillation and stroke: new ideas, persisting dilemmas. Stroke 1988;19:937–41.

52. Yasaka M, Yamaguchi T, Oita J, et al. Clinical features of recurrent embolization in acute cardioembolic stroke. Stroke 1993;24:1681–5.

53. Darling RC, Austen WC, Linton RR. Arterial embolism. Surg Gynecol Obstet 1987;124:106–14.

54. van Latum JC, Koudstaal PJ, Venables GS, et al. The European Atrial Fibrillation Trial (EAFT) Study Group. Stroke 1995;16:801–6.

55. Ameriso SF, Wong VLY, Quismorio FP, Fisher M. Immunohematological characteristics of infection-associated cerebral infarction. Stroke 1991;22:1004–9.

56. Fon EA, Mackey A, Cote R, et al. Hemostatic markers in acute transient ischemic attacks. Stroke 1994;25:282–6.

57. Sacco RL, Foulfes MA, Mohr JP, et al. Determinants of early recurrence of cerebral infarction: the Stroke Data Bank. Stroke 1989;20:983–9.

58. Chamorro A, Vila N, Blanc R, et al. The prognostic value of the acute-phase response in stroke recurrence. Eur J Neurol 1997;4:491–7.

59. Edelman ER. On causes. Hippocrates, Aristotle, Robert Koch, and the Dread Pirate Roberts. Circulation 2001;104:2509–12.

60. Chamorro A, Vila N, Saiz A, et al. Safety of heparin in acute stroke. Neurology 1996;46:589–90.

61. Eika C. Inhibition of thrombin-induced aggregation of human platelets in heparin. Scand J Hematol 1971;8:216–22.

62. Sobel M, McNeill PM, Carlson PL, et al. Heparin inhibition of von Willebrand factor-dependent platelet function in vitro and in vivo. J Clin Invest 1991;87:1787–93.

63. Marciniak E. Factor Xa inactivation by antithrombin III: Evidence for biological stabilization of factor Xa by factor V–phospholipid complex. Br J Haematol 1973;24:391–400.

64. Lane DA, Pejler G, Flynn AM, et al. Neutralization of heparin-related saccharides by histidine-rich glycoprotein and platelet factor 4. J Biol Chem 1986;261:3980–6.

65. Weitz JI, Hudoba M, Massel D, et al. Clot-bound thrombin is protected from inhibition by heparin–antithrombin but is susceptible to inactivation by antithrombin III-independent inhibitors. J Clin Invest 1990;86:385–91.

66. Castillo J. Deteriorating stroke: diagnostic criteria, predictors, mechanisms and treatment. Cerebrovasc Dis 1999;9(Suppl 3):1–8.

67. Duke RJ, Bloch RF, Turpie AGG, et al. Intravenous heparin for the prevention of stroke progression in acute partial stable stroke: a randomised control trial. Ann Intern Med 1986;105:825–8.

68. Haley EC Jr, Kassell NF, Torner JC. Failure of heparin to prevent progression in progressing ischemic infarction. Stroke 1988;19:10–14.

69. Kochanek PM, Hallenbeck JM. Polymorphonuclear leukocytes and monocytes/macrophages in the pathogenesis of cerebral ischemic and stroke. Stroke 1992;23:1367–79.

70. Feuerstein GZ, Liu T, Barone FC. Cytokines, inflammation and brain injury: role of tumor necrosis factor α. Cerebrovasc Brain Metab Rev 1994;6:341–60.

71. Arfors KE, Key K. Sulfated polysaccharides in inflammation. J Lab Clin Med 1993;121:201–2.

72. Clowes AW, Karnowsky MJ. Suppression by heparin of smooth muscle cell proliferation in injured arteries. Nature 1977;265:625–6.

73. Diamond MS, Alon R, Parkos CA, et al. Heparin is an adhesive ligand for the leukocyte integrin Mac-1 (CD11b/CD18). J Cell Biol 1995;130:1473–82.

74. Sy MS, Schneeberger E, McCluskey R, et al. Inhibition of delayed type hypersensitivity by heparin depleted of anticoagulant activity. Cell Immunol 1983;82:23–32.

75. Tyrrell DJ, Horne AP, Holme KR, et al. Heparin in inflammation: potential therapeutic applications beyond anticoagulation. Adv Pharmacol 1999;46:151–208.

76. Ott I, Neumann FJ, Gawaz M, et al. Increased neutrophil–platelet adhesion in patients with unstable angina. Circulation 1996;94:1239–46.

77. Yanaka K, Spellman SR, McCarthy JB, et al. Reduction of brain injury using heparin to inhibit leukocyte accumulation in a rat model of transient focal cerebral ischemia. I. Protective mechanism. J Neurosurg 1996;85:1102–7.

78. Yanaka K, Spellman R, McCarthy JB, et al. Reduction of brain injury using heparin to inhibit leukocyte accumulation in a rat model of transient focal cerebral ischemia. II. Dose–response effect and the therapeutic window. J Neurosurg 1996;85:1108–12.

79. Chamorro A, Obach V, Vila N, et al. A comparison of the acute-phase response in patients with ischemic stroke treated with high-dose heparin or aspirin. J Neurol Sci 2000;178:18–22.

80. Vila N, Castillo J, Dávalos A, Chamorro A. Proinflammatory cytokines and early stroke progression. Stroke 2000;31:2325–9.

81. Chamorro A, Cervera A, Castillo J, et al. Unfractionated heparin is associated with a lower rise of serum vascular cell adhesion molecule-1 in acute ischemic stroke patients. Neurosci Lett 2002;16(328):229–32.

82. Feuerstein GZ, Wang X, Yue TL, Barone FC. Inflammatory cytokines and stroke: emerging new strategies

for stroke therapeutics. In: Moskwitz MA, Caplan LR (eds). Cerebrovascular Disease: Nineteenth Princeton Stroke Conference. Newton, MA: Butterworth–Heinemann, 1995:75–91.

83. Kitamura N, Yamaguchi M, Shimabukuro K, et al. Heparin-like glycosaminoglycans inhibit leukocyte adhesion to endotoxin activated human vascular endothelial cells under nonstatic conditions. Eur Surg Res 1996;28:428–35.

84. Nelson RM, Cecconi O, Roberts WG, et al. Heparin oligosaccharides bind L- and P-selectin and inhibit acute inflammation. Blood 1993;11:3253–8.

85. Bazzoni G, Nuñez AB, Mascellani G, et al. Effect of heparin, dermatan sulfate, and related oligo-derivatives on human polymorphonuclear leukocyte functions. J Lab Clin Med 1992;121:268–75.

86. Smailbegovic A, Lever R, Page CP. The effects of heparin on the adhesion of human peripheral blood mononuclear cells to human stimulated umbilical vein endothelial cells. Br J Pharmacol 2001;134: 827–36.

87. Osborn L, Hession C, Tizard R, et al. Direct expression cloning of vascular cell adhesion molecule 1 (VCAM 1), a cytokine-induced endothelial protein that binds to lymphocytes. Cell 1989;1203–11.

88. Blann A, Kumar P, Krupinski J, et al. Soluble intercellular adhesion molecule-1, E-selectin, vascular cell adhesion molecule-1 and von Willebrand factor in stroke. Blood Coagul Fibrinolysis 1999;10:277–84.

89. McGilvray ID, Lu Z, Bitar R, et al. VLA-4 integrin crosslinking on human monocytic THP-1 cells induces tissue factor expression by a mechanism involving mitogen-activated protein kinase. J Biol Chem 1997; 272:10287–94.

90. Pernerstorfer T, Hansen JB, Knechtelsdorfer M, et al. Heparin blunts endotoxin-induced coagulation activation. Circulation 1999;100:2485–90.

91. Gori AM, Pepe G, Attanasio M, et al. Tissue factor reduction and tissue factor pathway inhibitor release after heparin administration. Thromb Haemost 1999;81:589–93

92. Hiebert LM, Liu J. Heparin protects cultured endothelial cells from damage by toxic oxygen metabolites. Atherosclerosis 1990;83:47–51.

93. Hiebert LM, Liu J. The protective action of polyelectrolytes on endothelium. Semin Thromb Hemost 1991;17(Suppl 1):42–6.

94. Robinson-White A, Baylin SB, Olivecrona T, Beaven MA. Binding of diamine oxidase activity to rat and guinea pig microvascular endothelial cells: comparison with lipoprotein lipase binding. J Clin Invest 1985;76:93–100.

95. Karlsson K, Marklund SL. Heparin-induced release of extracellular superoxide dismutase to human blood plasma. Biochem J 1987;242:55–9.

96. Dobkin BH. Heparin for lacunar stroke in progression. Stroke 1983;14:421–3.

97. Chamorro A, Vila N, Ascaso C, Blanc R. Heparin in acute stroke with atrial fibrillation. Clinical relevance of very early treatment. Arch Neurol 1999;56: 1098–102.

98. Drake TA, Morrissey JH, Edgington TS. Selective cellular expression of tissue factor in human tissues. Implications for disorders of hemostasis and thrombosis. Am J Pathol 1989;134:1087–97.

99. Brill-Edwards P, Ginsberg JS, Johnston M, Hirsh J. Establishing a therapeutic range for heparin therapy. Ann Intern Med 1993;119:104–9.

100. Camerlingo M, Salvi P, Belloni G, et al. Intravenous heparin started within the first 3 hours after onset of symptoms as a treatment for acute nonlacunar hemispheric cerebral infarctions. Stroke 2005;36:2415–20.

9
Aspirin in acute stroke

Eivind Berge and Peter Sandercock

Introduction

It is estimated that there will be 8.5 million patients with acute ischemic stroke in Europe and the USA over this decade,[1–3] and of these, about one half will die within 6 months of stroke onset.[4] Of those who survive, about one-third will depend on other people for help with their activities of daily living.[5] Ischemic stroke is therefore a most significant health burden, for patients, their carers, and society.

Treatments with modest or even small relative effects can produce important health benefits to the population, provided they can be given to a large number of patients. If some widely practicable therapies could be shown to prevent death or dependence for 'just' 10 or 20 of every 1000 patients, it would, for every million stroke patients so treated, ensure that an extra 10 000 were alive and independent. If such benefits exist, they must not, therefore, be overlooked. Aspirin is one such candidate. It is inexpensive, easy to administer, and widely used in cardiovascular disease.

Rationale for aspirin in acute ischemic stroke

Aspirin prevents platelet aggregation, and reduces the release of thromboxane and other thrombogenic eicosanoids in the circulation.[6–9] Taken for a few years after a myocardial infarction (MI), ischemic stroke, or transient ischemic attack (TIA), aspirin typically prevents about 40 serious vascular events (MI, stroke, and vascular death) per 1000 patients treated.[10] In patients with ischemic stroke or TIA, long-term antiplatelet therapy prevents 36 serious vascular events for every 1000 patients treated for 3 years.[10] In the venous circulation, among patients at high risk of venous thromboembolism (chiefly as a result of general or orthopedic surgery), antiplatelet drugs also reduce deep venous thrombosis (DVT) by 39% and pulmonary embolism (PE) by 64%.[11]

Aspirin is also effective in the treatment of acute myocardial infarction (AMI), preventing about 40 serious vascular events per 1000 patients treated for just 1 month.[10] In acute stroke, there is substantial platelet activation,[12,13] and aspirin therapy might therefore also be beneficial for this disease. The rationale for the use of aspirin in acute ischemic stroke is to suppress or halt the ongoing thrombotic process, which may reduce the volume of infarcted cerebral tissue and reduce the risk of neurological deficits, disability, and death. Aspirin can also be given to prevent stroke recurrence (secondary prophylaxis), and to prevent or treat other thromboembolic complications (e.g. DVT or PE) in patients who have had a stroke (tertiary prophylaxis).

Until few years ago, there was no reliable evidence of the effects of aspirin therapy for acute ischemic stroke, and clinical practice in the use of aspirin still varies considerably around the world. In the UK, a 1995 survey showed that 50% of physicians who routinely treated patients with acute stroke started antiplatelet therapy within 48 h of the onset of stroke, if they thought that it was likely to have been a cerebral infarct.[14] An updated review in 1998 found that this number had increased to 77%.[15] In the USA, physicians often use anticoagulant therapy with heparin, and aspirin is not frequently used for the treatment of acute ischemic stroke.[16]

Intracranial hemorrhage

One of the risks of aspirin therapy in the acute phase of stroke is that it might exacerbate any tendency to hemorrhagic transformation of the infarct, which might offset any benefits. It is therefore unwise to extrapolate directly from the results of the secondary prevention trials. Aspirin is associated with an excess of intracerebral hemorrhage in animal models,[13] and antiplatelet drugs are consistently associated with a small but definite excess of intracranial and extra-cranial hemorrhages.[10]

The clinical impact of hemorrhagic transformation is difficult to assess in an individual patient. Minor degrees of transformation can occur without any clinical deterioration, whereas the development of a large parenchymatous hematoma may be fatal. In a review of the trials of thrombolytic therapy within 6 h of onset, 1.0% of the patients allocated control had a fatal intracranial hemorrhage.[17]

However, even if a specific category of patients were at especially high risk of symptomatic hemorrhagic transformation, this does not necessarily mean that the net result will be adverse for this group of patients. By analogy with carotid endarterectomy for carotid stenosis, some patients may be at high risk of stroke with surgery, but even higher risk without it, so that the balance of adverse and beneficial effects may be favorable.

As well as increasing the risk of hemorrhagic transformation, aspirin could both increase the risk of symptomatic intracranial hemorrhage arising de novo (as intracerebral, subarachnoid, or subdural bleeding) and the risk of bleeding at other, extra-cranial sites. The key question is, therefore, whether or not the benefits of treatment outweigh the adverse outcomes. Randomized-controlled trials provide the best means to assess this balance.

Evidence from randomized-controlled trials and systematic reviews

Data available

The first randomized trial of antiplatelet drugs in the *prevention* of stroke was reported in 1969.[18] A systematic review in 1988 of all of the trials proved that antiplatelet drugs, given long term, reduce the risk of stroke, MI, and vascular death in high-risk individuals.[19] The benefit of aspirin as treatment for AMI was established in the same year.[20] The lack of data about the effects of antiplatelet drugs as a treatment for the acute phase of stroke led to two large-scale randomized controlled trials of aspirin – IST (International Stroke Trial) and CAST (Chinese Acute Stroke Trial) – which together randomized over 40 000 patients.[5,21] In IST, patients were allocated, in an open factorial design, to treatment policies of aspirin 300 mg daily, heparin, the combination, or to 'avoid both aspirin and heparin' for 14 days. In CAST, patients were allocated, in a double-blinded design, to 1 month of 160 mg daily aspirin or matching placebo.

Two systematic reviews of these data are available. The Cochrane review includes all of the completed randomized trials of any antiplatelet drug in acute stroke, and examines their effects on a variety of clinical outcomes.[22] The second review is a meta-analysis of individual patient data from CAST and IST to examine the effects of aspirin in particular categories of patient during the scheduled treatment period.[23] Both reviews report the frequency of events during the scheduled treatment period (2–4 weeks), and the Cochrane review also reports events and outcomes at the end of scheduled follow-up (at 6 months in IST and 1 month in CAST).[22]

Since over 99% of the randomized evidence relates to aspirin, we shall refer to aspirin, rather than 'antiplatelet drugs', for the rest of this section.

Recurrent ischemic stroke during the treatment period

Aspirin significantly reduced the odds of recurrent ischemic stroke during the treatment period by 30% (95% confidence interval (CI) 20–40%) – from 2.3% in controls to 1.6% in treated patients – i.e. avoiding 7 events per 1000 patients treated[23] (Figure 9.1).

Symptomatic intracranial hemorrhage during the treatment period

There was a small excess of symptomatic intracranial hemorrhage with aspirin (including symptomatic transformation of an infarct). It occurred in 0.8% of

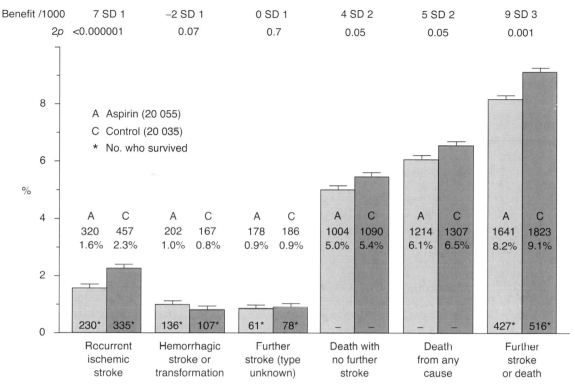

Benefit /1000	7 SD 1	−2 SD 1	0 SD 1	4 SD 2	5 SD 2	9 SD 3
2p	<0.000001	0.07	0.7	0.05	0.05	0.001

A Aspirin (20 055)
C Control (20 035)
* No. who survived

	Recurrent ischemic stroke		Hemorrhagic stroke or transformation		Further stroke (type unknown)		Death with no further stroke		Death from any cause		Further stroke or death	
	A	C	A	C	A	C	A	C	A	C	A	C
	320	457	202	167	178	186	1004	1090	1214	1307	1641	1823
	1.6%	2.3%	1.0%	0.8%	0.9%	0.9%	5.0%	5.4%	6.1%	6.5%	8.2%	9.1%
	230*	335*	136*	107*	61*	78*	–	–	–	–	427*	516*

Figure 9.1
Absolute effects in CAST and IST. Numbers and percentages of patients with various outcomes during the scheduled treatment period. The percentages are plotted as bars (with the SD of each bar plotted at the top). The difference between aspirin and control is given as the benefit per 1000, along with its SC and statistical significance (2p). Reproduced with permission from reference 23.

controls versus 1.0% of treated patients, a nonsignificant 21% relative increase in odds (95% CI 1% reduction to 49% increase); this is an excess of about 2 per 1000 patients treated[23] (Figure 9.1).

Death during the treatment period

Aspirin significantly reduced the relative odds of death (without further stroke) during the treatment period by 8% (95% CI 1–16%) – from 5.4% in controls to 5.0% in treated patients – i.e. avoiding 4 deaths for every 1000 patients treated[23] (Figure 9.1).

Further stroke or death during the treatment period

This outcome event summarizes the overall balance of benefits and adverse events within the treatment

period: recurrent ischemic stroke, recurrent stroke of unknown type, symptomatic intracranial hemorrhage, symptomatic hemorrhagic transformation of the infarct, and death from any cause. We refer to this composite outcome event as 'further stroke or death'. Aspirin significantly reduced the relative odds of further stroke or death by 11% (95% CI 5–15%) – from 9.1% to 8.2%; for every 1000 patients treated, 9 avoid further stroke or death during the treatment period[23] (Figure 9.1).

Death by the end of the scheduled follow-up

The benefit seen during the treatment period was still evident, so the difference in deaths from all causes, at the end of follow-up at least 1 month later, was about 8 deaths for every 1000 patients treated.[22]

Functional outcome at 1 month or later (death, dependency, or full recovery)

Aspirin significantly reduced the odds of being dead or dependent at final follow-up by 6% (95% CI 2–8%) – from 47.1% in controls to 45.8% in treated patients – i.e. an additional 13 patients were alive and independent for every 1000 patients treated. Aspirin also significantly increased the odds of making a complete recovery by 6% (95% CI 1–11%), an extra 10 patients making a complete recovery for every 1000 patients treated.[22]

Deep venous thrombosis and pulmonary embolism

Two trials including 136 patients reported data on DVT. Only 35 patients developed 'symptomatic or asymptomatic DVT' during the treatment period: 29% of those allocated to control and 24% of those allocated to treatment. There was a nonsignificant 22% relative reduction in the odds of DVT (95% CI 64% reduction to 67% increase), but it is potentially important. If confirmed, it would imply that for 1000 patients treated, about 50 would avoid DVT.[22]

However, data on 40 000 patients were available for the effects of aspirin on PE. Aspirin significantly reduced the relative odds of PE by 29% (95% CI 4–47%) – from 0.5% in controls to 0.3% in treated patients – i.e. for every 1000 patients treated, two avoided PE. Underascertainment of events in both groups may mean that the *absolute* benefit has been underestimated (the *proportional* reduction is not likely to be biased by underascertainment); if the true rate of PE were 3% in the controls, and the same proportional reduction were applied, then for every 1000 patients given aspirin, 12 might avoid PE (estimate of control PE risk from Davenport et al[24]). These benefits are consistent with those seen in the systematic review of aspirin in prevention of PE in surgical patients and in the PEP (Pulmonary Embolism Prevention) trial.[11,25]

These data therefore strengthen the rationale for the routine use of aspirin in the acute phase of a stroke and for continuing it long term; aspirin is likely to be adequate thromboprophylaxis for patients at low and moderate risk of DVT and PE. For patients at high risk of DVT, perhaps because of a history of a previous episode of venous thromboembolism or the presence of thrombophilia, the question is 'what to add to aspirin?' Graded compression stockings are one option and low-dose subcutaneous heparin another; both are supported by reasonable evidence (chiefly from trials in higher-risk patients, but not from trials in stroke patients). The SIGN (Scottish Intercollegiate Guidelines Network) guideline on prevention of DVT has been updated, and is a useful reference work[26] (www.show.scot.nhs.uk/sign/home.htm).

Subgroup analyses

The individual patient data meta-analysis, based on over 40 000 patients with acute ischemic stroke, did not identify any group in which the benefits – or the adverse outcomes – were significantly greater than or less than the averages reported above.[23] For the one-third reduction in recurrent ischemic stroke, the overall treatment effect ($2p < 0.0000001$) was large enough for the subgroup analyses to be informative. The recurrence rate among control patients was similar in all 28 subgroups, so the absolute reduction of 7 per 1000 did not differ substantially with respect to age, sex, conscious level, atrial fibrillation, computed tomography (CT) findings, blood pressure, stroke subtype, or concomitant heparin use. There was no good evidence that the 11% reduction in relative odds of death without further stroke was reversed in any subgroup, or that in any subgroup the increase in hemorrhagic stroke was much larger than the average of about 2 per 1000, and there was no heterogeneity between the reductions in further stroke or death during the scheduled treatment period (Figure 9.2).

Aspirin in patients without CT or magnetic resonance imaging (MRI) or in patients with hemorrhagic stroke

Among the 9000 patients randomized without a prior CT scan in IST and CAST, aspirin appeared to be of net benefit, with no unusual excess of hemorrhagic stroke, and among the 800 who had inadvertently been randomized after a hemorrhagic stroke, there was no evidence of net hazard (further stroke or death: 67 allocated control vs 63 allocated aspirin).[23]

These data are reassuring in that they establish that the patients inadvertently entered in the trials with a hemorrhagic stroke were not, on average, harmed as a result. However, they do not establish the safety of continued aspirin treatment in patients with primary intracerebral hemorrhage, nor do they establish the safety of giving aspirin in patients who are not CT-scanned at all. There is little point CT scanning after a week or so, since, at that stage, CT is decreasingly able to differentiate infarction from haemorrhage.

Guidelines for clinical practice

Which patients should be treated with aspirin?

Early aspirin is of benefit for a wide range of patients, so all patients with suspected acute ischemic stroke should receive it unless there is a clear contraindication. Implementing a hospital policy or guideline of 'immediate aspirin for all patients with acute ischemic stroke' requires considerable effort – it is of course part of a well-organized stroke service. Several different strategies may be required to maintain a high level of compliance with the policy.[27–29] Such a policy will also reduce the risk of venous thromboembolism.

These benefits are consistent with those seen when antiplatelet therapy is used in long-term secondary prevention after a stroke. Antiplatelet therapy given for 3 years avoids about 40 serious vascular events (stroke, MI, and vascular death) for every thousand patients treated.[10] More specifically, long-term antiplatelet use results in a significant reduction in the absolute risk of recurrent stroke (20 prevented per 1000), while the risk of intracranial hemorrhage with long-term antiplatelet use remains low, with an excess of 2 hemorrhages for every 1000 patients treated over an average of 2 years.[10]

Patients with atrial fibrillation

IST and CAST included 4500 patients who had atrial fibrillation at the time of randomization. In these patients, the risk of recurrent stroke in hospital was 2.9% in the controls and 2.0% in patients allocated aspirin. The one-third reduction in the relative odds of recurrent ischemic stroke with aspirin was no different to that seen in patients without atrial fibrillation.[23] HAEST (Heparin in Acute Embolic Stroke Trial) was a small trial comparing a low-molecular-weight heparin (LMWH) with aspirin in 449 patients with acute ischemic stroke and atrial fibrillation, and did not show evidence of an advantage to LMWH over aspirin.[30] All such patients should therefore be started on aspirin in the acute phase, and continued on oral anticoagulant therapy when the risk of hemorrhagic transformation of the infarct is decreased (after a week or so).[31]

Patients already on antiplatelet drugs

The priority is to perform a brain CT or MRI scan to determine whether the stroke is hemorrhagic or ischemic; if it is hemorrhagic, then antiplatelet drugs should be stopped. In IST, 4000 patients were already on aspirin or other antiplatelet drugs at randomization. The question of what to do for long-term secondary prevention in patients who have a stroke while already on antiplatelet drugs is discussed elsewhere in this book.

Patients already receiving anticoagulants

Recurrent ischemic stroke in patients receiving oral anticoagulants may be due to an inadequate dose, but infective endocarditis must first be ruled out. If it has been ruled out, then more careful supervision to maintain the International Normalized Ratio (INR) above 2.0 (or whatever target range has been chosen for that specific patient) should minimize the risk of further ischemic strokes.[31] However, recurrent ischemic stroke despite an adequate INR may necessitate the addition of low-dose aspirin, although this is likely to increase the risk of intracranial hemorrhage.[32,33]

Who should not be given aspirin?

It should go without saying that a patient with proven primary intracerebral hemorrhage should not have

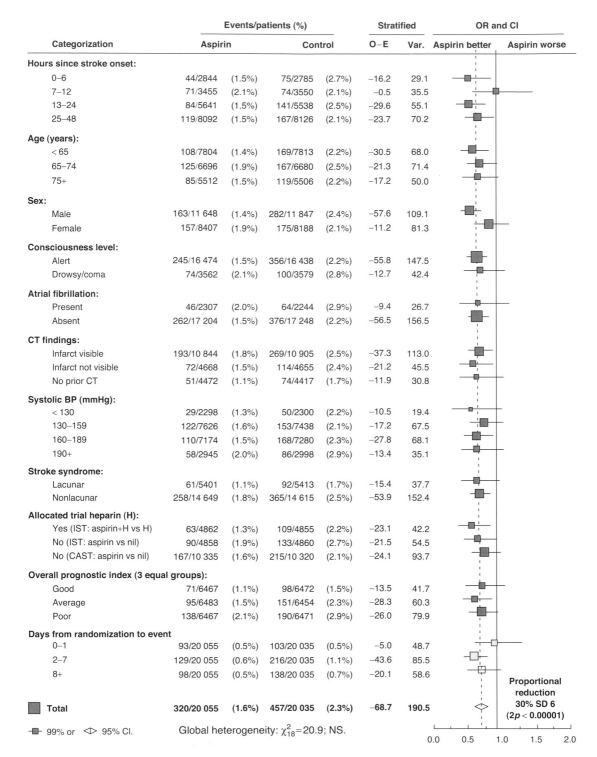

| | Events/patients (%) | | | | Stratified | | OR and CI | |
Categorization	Aspirin		Control		O−E	Var.	Aspirin better	Aspirin worse
Hours since stroke onset:								
0–6	44/2844	(1.5%)	75/2785	(2.7%)	−16.2	29.1		
7–12	71/3455	(2.1%)	74/3550	(2.1%)	−0.5	35.5		
13–24	84/5641	(1.5%)	141/5538	(2.5%)	−29.6	55.1		
25–48	119/8092	(1.5%)	167/8126	(2.1%)	−23.7	70.2		
Age (years):								
< 65	108/7804	(1.4%)	169/7813	(2.2%)	−30.5	68.0		
65–74	125/6696	(1.9%)	167/6680	(2.5%)	−21.3	71.4		
75+	85/5512	(1.5%)	119/5506	(2.2%)	−17.2	50.0		
Sex:								
Male	163/11 648	(1.4%)	282/11 847	(2.4%)	−57.6	109.1		
Female	157/8407	(1.9%)	175/8188	(2.1%)	−11.2	81.3		
Consciousness level:								
Alert	245/16 474	(1.5%)	356/16 438	(2.2%)	−55.8	147.5		
Drowsy/coma	74/3562	(2.1%)	100/3579	(2.8%)	−12.7	42.4		
Atrial fibrillation:								
Present	46/2307	(2.0%)	64/2244	(2.9%)	−9.4	26.7		
Absent	262/17 204	(1.5%)	376/17 248	(2.2%)	−56.5	156.5		
CT findings:								
Infarct visible	193/10 844	(1.8%)	269/10 905	(2.5%)	−37.3	113.0		
Infarct not visible	72/4668	(1.5%)	114/4655	(2.4%)	−21.2	45.5		
No prior CT	51/4472	(1.1%)	74/4417	(1.7%)	−11.9	30.8		
Systolic BP (mmHg):								
< 130	29/2298	(1.3%)	50/2300	(2.2%)	−10.5	19.4		
130–159	122/7626	(1.6%)	153/7438	(2.1%)	−17.2	67.5		
160–189	110/7174	(1.5%)	168/7280	(2.3%)	−27.8	68.1		
190+	58/2945	(2.0%)	86/2998	(2.9%)	−13.4	35.1		
Stroke syndrome:								
Lacunar	61/5401	(1.1%)	92/5413	(1.7%)	−15.4	37.7		
Nonlacunar	258/14 649	(1.8%)	365/14 615	(2.5%)	−53.9	152.4		
Allocated trial heparin (H):								
Yes (IST: aspirin+H vs H)	63/4862	(1.3%)	109/4855	(2.2%)	−23.1	42.2		
No (IST: aspirin vs nil)	90/4858	(1.9%)	133/4860	(2.7%)	−21.5	54.5		
No (CAST: aspirin vs nil)	167/10 335	(1.6%)	215/10 320	(2.1%)	−24.1	93.7		
Overall prognostic index (3 equal groups):								
Good	71/6467	(1.1%)	98/6472	(1.5%)	−13.5	41.7		
Average	95/6483	(1.5%)	151/6454	(2.3%)	−28.3	60.3		
Poor	138/6467	(2.1%)	190/6471	(2.9%)	−26.0	79.9		
Days from randomization to event								
0–1	93/20 055	(0.5%)	103/20 035	(0.5%)	−5.0	48.7		
2–7	129/20 055	(0.6%)	216/20 035	(1.1%)	−43.6	85.5		
8+	98/20 055	(0.5%)	138/20 035	(0.7%)	−20.1	58.6		
Total	320/20 055	(1.6%)	457/20 035	(2.3%)	−68.7	190.5		

■ 99% or ◇ 95% CI.

Global heterogeneity: $\chi^2_{18} = 20.9$; NS.

Proportional reduction 30% SD 6 ($2p < 0.00001$)

0.0   0.5   1.0   1.5   2.0

Figure 9.2
Proportional effects of early aspirin on recurrent ischemic stroke. Fatal and nonfatal events are included. For each particular subgroup, the observed − expected (O − E) number of events among aspirin-allocated

antiplatelet drugs as a treatment for their stroke. However, patients with intracerebral hemorrhage who have a very clear and pressing indication to continue aspirin (e.g. unstable angina) and are thought – for whatever reason – to have a low risk of further intracerebral bleeding can continue aspirin. The pathophysiology of aneurysmal subarachnoid hemorrhage is rather different, and here there have been a few small inconclusive trials in which the primary aim was to prevent ischemic deficits after a ruptured aneurysm had been clipped.[10]

Patients with a history of definite aspirin sensitivity (e.g. wheeze or skin rash on exposure to aspirin) should not be given aspirin.

When should aspirin treatment be started?

There was no clear evidence of a 'time window' for the benefit of aspirin; the relative benefits among those randomized late (24–48 h after stroke onset) were as great as those randomized early (within the first 0–6 h).[23] IST and CAST tested a policy of 'start aspirin immediately'. Aspirin should therefore be started as soon as a CT or MRI scan has been performed and has excluded intracranial hemorrhage as the cause of the stroke. If the doctor who admits the patient to hospital writes the prescription for aspirin immediately, the patient is more likely to receive long-term aspirin. If writing the aspirin prescription is left for later, it can be forgotten.

If CT scanning is not immediately available and the clinician feels, on clinical grounds, that the patient is unlikely to have a hemorrhagic stroke (i.e. there was no 'apoplectic onset', with early headache or vomiting, the patient is fully conscious, etc.), then aspirin can be started while the CT or MRI scan is being organized. This policy does not appear to reduce the benefits from aspirin.[23]

The risk of intracranial hemorrhage with thrombolysis may be increased if this is given together with aspirin.[17,34] In the highly selected few patients to be treated with thrombolysis, it is probably best to delay starting aspirin. Starting aspirin the next day, probably around 24h after thrombolytic treatment, is unlikely to reduce the benefit of early aspirin.[23]

Which agent, dose, and route of administration?

Based on the available randomized evidence, the appropriate dose of aspirin for use in acute ischemic stroke is between 160 and 300 mg daily. The former is the lowest dose that has been shown to be effective in AMI.[10,35] Lower doses of aspirin are effective for long-term secondary stroke prevention, but have not been evaluated in acute stroke. There is some (but not abundant) evidence that at least 120 mg of aspirin is needed to acetylate all circulating platelets within a short period of time.[36,37] There is also some experimental evidence that a dose of 160–300 mg of aspirin daily is required in the acute phase of an ischemic cerebral or cardiac event in order to achieve rapid inhibition of thromboxane biosynthesis.[7,12,35] For patients who cannot swallow safely, aspirin can be given rectally by suppository, by nasogastric tube, or by intravenous injection (as 100 mg of the lysine salt, infused over 10 min).

Adverse effects

Major extracranial hemorrhage (defined as bleeding serious enough to cause death or require transfusion) is the most frequent serious adverse event. In the trials, the relative increase in odds with aspirin

Figure 9.2 (continued)
patients, its variance (Var.), the odds ratio (OR) (dark square, with area proportional to the total number of patients with an event), and its 99% confidence interval (CI) are given. The diamond indicates the overall result and its 95% CI. Summation of the 10 separate χ^2 heterogeneity test statistics (one for each baseline characteristic, but not for 'days') yields the global test for heterogeneity between the 28 subgroups: $\chi^2_{18} = 20.9$, NS. Results for those with missing information on particular characteristics are not listed separately (except for CT finding), but numerators and denominators for them can be obtained through subtraction of the subgroup results from the total. Reproduced with permission from reference 23.

was large (68%; 95% CI 34–109%), but the absolute excess was small: four additional major extracranial hemorrhages for every 1000 patients treated.[22] The excess was greater among patients allocated heparin (0.9% heparin alone vs 1.8% allocated aspirin plus heparin, an excess of 9 per 1000 treated) than among other patients (0.5% among those allocated to avoid aspirin and 0.7% among those allocated aspirin, an excess of 2 per 1000).[23] The risk of adverse events with aspirin can therefore be kept to a minimum by avoiding anticoagulants.

Suggestions for future research

Other antiplatelet agents

The overall treatment effect of aspirin in acute ischemic stroke is not large, and better acute therapies are therefore necessary. There are no reliable data as yet on whether any other antiplatelet regimen looks more promising than aspirin in the treatment of acute ischemic stroke. The data from the Cochrane review showed no significant differences between aspirin alone, ticlopidine alone, or the combination of aspirin and dipyridamole,[22] but the data from the non-aspirin regimens were extremely limited, and such indirect comparisons are unreliable.[10]

Combination of aspirin and other antiplatelet agents

There are many different pathways involved in the aggregation of platelets, and a combination of two effective antiplatelet agents working through different mechanisms might be more effective than a single agent. However, particularly large trials will be needed to test whether the addition to aspirin of ticlopidine, dipyridamole, or clopidogrel can produce significantly greater clinical benefit than aspirin alone.[38]

Combination of aspirin and low-dose heparin

As part of a systematic review of anticoagulants versus antiplatelet agents for acute ischemic stroke, we sought to assess whether the addition of anticoagulants to antiplatelet agents offers any net advantage over antiplatelet agents alone.[39] The data from this review suggested that the combination of low-dose unfractionated heparin (UFH) and aspirin might be associated with net benefits over aspirin alone, and this might be worth testing in further large-scale randomized-controlled trials.

Summary

Aspirin 160–300 mg daily, started within 48 h of onset of presumed ischemic stroke, reduces the risk of early recurrent ischemic stroke without a major risk of early hemorrhagic complications, and improves long-term outcome. Patients with acute stroke in whom intracranial hemorrhage has been excluded or is thought to be unlikely should therefore receive aspirin as soon as is practicable, provided no definite contraindications exist. In those who cannot tolerate aspirin, an alternative antiplatelet agent should be considered, although the evidence for other agents is inadequate at present. Aspirin is effective in the long-term prevention of recurrent ischemic stroke and other major vascular events, and should therefore be continued after hospital discharge.

References

1. Bamford J, Sandercock P, Dennis M, et al. A prospective study of acute cerebrovascular disease in the community: the Oxfordshire Community Stroke Project – 1981–86. 2. Incidence, case fatality rates and overall outcome at one year of cerebral infarction, primary intracerebral and subarachnoid haemorrhage. J Neurol Neurosurg Psychiatry 1990;53:16–22.

2. Broderick JP, Phillips SJ, Whisnant JP, et al. Incidence rates of stroke in the eighties: the end of the decline in stroke? Stroke 1989;20:577–82.

3. Homer D, Whisnant JP, Schoenberg BS. Trends in the incidence rates of stroke in Rochester, Minnesota, since 1935. Ann Neurol 1987;22:245–51.

4. Sandercock P, Celani MG, Ricci S. The likely public health impact of simple treatments for acute ischaemic stroke. Cerebrovasc Dis 1992;2(Suppl):234.

5. International Stroke Trial Collaborative Group. The International Stroke Trial (IST): a randomised trial of aspirin, subcutaneous heparin, both, or neither among 19 435 patients with acute ischaemic stroke. Lancet 1997;349:1569–81.

6. Antiplatelet Trialists' Collaboration. Collaborative overview of randomised trials of antiplatelet therapy – II: Maintenance of vascular graft or arterial patency by antiplatelet therapy. BMJ 1994;308:159–68.

7. van Kooten F, Ciabattoni G, Patrono C, et al. Platelet activation and lipid peroxidation in patients with acute ischemic stroke. Stroke 1997;28:1557–63.

8. Riepe MW, Kasischke K, Rapuach A. Acetylsalicylic acid increases tolerance against hypoxic and chemical hypoxia. Stroke 1997;28:2006–11.

9. Bednar MM, Gross CE. Antiplatelet therapy in acute cerebral ischemia. Stroke 1999;30:887–93.

10. Antiplatelet Trialists' Collaboration. Collaborative overview of randomised trials of antiplatelet therapy – I: Prevention of death, myocardial infarction, and stroke by prolonged antiplatelet therapy in various categories of patients. BMJ 1994;308:81–106.

11. Antiplatelet Trialists' Collaboration. Collaborative overview of randomised trials of antiplatelet therapy – III: Reduction in venous thrombosis and pulmonary embolism by antiplatelet prophylaxis among surgical and medical patients. BMJ 1994;308:235–46.

12. van Kooten F, Ciabattoni G, Patrono C, et al. Evidence for episodic platelet activation in acute ischaemic stroke. Stroke 1994;25:278–81.

13. Koudstaal P, Ciabattoni G, van Gijn J. Increased thromboxane biosynthesis in patients with acute cerebral ischaemia. Stroke 1993;24:219–23.

14. Lindley RI, Amayo EO, Marshall J, et al. Acute stroke treatment in UK hospitals: the Stroke Association survey of consultant opinion. J R Coll Physicians Lond 1995;29:479–84.

15. Ebrahim S, Redfern J. Stroke Care – A Matter of Chance. A National Survey of Stroke Services. London: The Stroke Association, 1999.

16. Marsh EE III, Adams HP Jr, Biller J, et al. Use of antithrombotic drugs in the treatment of acute ischemic stroke: a survey of neurologists in practice in the United States. Neurology 1989;39:1631–4.

17. Wardlaw JM, del Zoppo G, Yamaguchi T, Berge E. Thrombolysis for acute ischaemic stroke. The Cochrane Database of Systematic Reviews 2003, Issue 3. Art. No.: CD000213. DOI: 10.1002/14651858. CD000213.

18. Acheson J, Danta G, Hutchinson EC. Controlled trial of dipyridamole in cerebral vascular disease. BMJ 1969;i:614–15.

19. Antiplatelet Trialists' Collaboration. Secondary prevention of vascular disease by prolonged antiplatelet treatment. BMJ 1988;296:320–31.

20. ISIS-2 (Second International Study of Infarct Survival) Collaborative Group. Randomised trial of intravenous streptokinase, oral aspirin, both, or neither among 17,187 cases of suspected acute myocardial infarction: ISIS-2. Lancet 1988;ii:349–60.

21. CAST (Chinese Acute Stroke Trial) Collaborative Group. CAST: randomised placebo-controlled trial of early aspirin use in 20,000 patients with acute ischaemic stroke. Lancet 1997;349:1641–9.

22. Sandercock P, Gubitz G, Foley P, Counsell C. Antiplatelet therapy for acute iscaemic stroke. The Cochrane Database of Systematic Reviews 2003, Issue 2. Art. No.: CD000029. DOI: 10.1002/14651858. CD000029.

23. Chen ZM, Sandercock P, Pan HC, et al. Indications for early aspirin use in acute ischemic stroke: a combined analysis of 40 000 randomized patients from the Chinese acute stroke trial and the international stroke trial. On behalf of the CAST and IST collaborative groups. Stroke 2000;31:1240–9.

24. Davenport R, Dennis M, Wellwood I, Warlow C. Complications after acute stroke. Stroke 1996;27:415–20.

25. Prevention of pulmonary embolism and deep vein thrombosis with low dose aspirin: Pulmonary Embolism Prevention (PEP) trial. Lancet 2000;355:1295–302.

26. Scottish Intercollegiate Guidelines Network. Prevention of Venous Thromboembolism. A National Clinical Guideline. Edinburgh: Scottish Intercollegiate Guidelines Network, Royal College of Physicians, 2000.

27. Bero LA, Grilli R, Grimshaw JM. Closing the gap between research and practice: an overview of systematic reviews of interventions to promote the implementation of research findings. BMJ 1998;317: 465–8.

28. Scottish Intercollegiate Guidlines Network. Antithrombotic Therapy. A National Clinical Guideline. Edinburgh: Scottish Intercollegiate Guidelines Network, Royal College of Physicians, 1999.

29. Woolf SH, Grol R, Hutchinson A, et al. Clinical guidelines: potential benefits, limitations and harms of clinical guidelines. BMJ 1999;318:530.

30. Berge E, Abdelnoor M, Nakstad PH, Sandset PM. Low molecular-weight heparin versus aspirin in patients with acute ischaemic stroke and atrial fibrillation: a double-blind randomised study. Lancet 2000; 355:1205–10.

31. EAFT (European Atrial Fibrillation Trial) Study Group. Secondary prevention in non-rheumatic atrial fibrillation after transient ischaemic attack or minor stroke. Lancet 1993;342:1255–62.

32. Turpie AGG, Gent M, Laupacis A, et al. A comparison of aspirin with placebo in patients treated with warfarin after heart-valve replacement. N Engl J Med 1993;329:524–9.

33. Hart RG, Benavente O, Pearce LA. Increased risk of intracranial hemorrhage when aspirin is combined with warfarin: a meta-analysis and hypothesis. Cerebrovasc Dis 1999;9:215–17.

34. Multicentre Acute Stroke Trial – Italy (MAST-I) Group. Randomised controlled trial of streptokinase, aspirin, and combination of both in treatment of acute ischaemic stroke. Lancet 1995;346:1509–14.

35. Patrono C, Coller B, Dalen JE, et al. Platelet-active drugs: the relationships among dose, effectiveness, and side effects. Chest 1998;114(Suppl 5):470S–88S.

36. Patrono C. Aspirin as an antiplatelet drug. N Engl J Med 1994;330:1287–94.

37. van Gijn J. Aspirin: dose and indications in modern stroke prevention. Neurol Clin 1992;10:193–209.

38. Born GVR, Collins R. Aspirin versus clopidogrel: the wrong question? Lancet 1997;349:806.

39. Berge E, Sandercock P. Anticoagulants versus antiplatelet agents for acute ischaemic stroke. The Cochrane Database of Systematic Reviews 2002, Issue 4. Art. No.: CD003242. DOI: 10.1002/14651858. CD003242.

10

Platelet glycoprotein IIb/IIIa antagonists

Jacques R Leclerc and Julien Bogousslavsky

Introduction

Giulio Bizzozero (1816–1901) was first to recognize platelets as independent cellular elements of blood.[1] He pointed out their likely role in hemostasis, thrombosis in particular. The clinical observation of a normal clotting time in the face of severe thrombocytopenia remained an enigma for several decades, elucidated only upon discovery of the enzymatic cascade of coagulation in the late 1950s. Interest in platelets rekindled in the 1960s, as the field of hemostasis moved towards interactions between platelets and blood coagulation. Evidence of platelet activation in atherothrombosis was documented in the early 1970s.[2] Trials of secondary prevention with antiplatelet agents provided the first line of evidence on the role of platelets in arterial thromboembolism.[3]

An important milestone occurred in 1974, when Nurden and Caen identified the molecular defect of Glanzmann's thrombasthenia, namely deficiency of the glycoprotein (GP)IIb/IIIa membrane receptor.[4,5] Glanzmann's thrombasthenia is a rare congenital disorder characterized by a lifelong mild bleeding disorder, reduced platelet aggregation, and normal platelet adhesion. Subsequent work involving purification, cloning and expression of GPIIb/IIIa advanced the field of platelet signaling, and led to the development of pharmacological antagonists.

The role of antiplatelet therapy in the acute phase of arterial thromboembolism is a more recent concept, perhaps first underscored by the landmark International Study of Infarct Survival (ISIS-2),[6] which compared in a 2 × 2 factorial design systemic streptokinase, aspirin (160 mg daily), both agents, or neither of them. The study showed that aspirin started within 24 h of onset of acute myocardial infarction (AMI) had the same treatment benefit as systemic streptokinase for improving 1-month mortality (i.e. about 2.5% absolute improvement for each agent; 5% combined).

In spite of the overwhelming impact of antiplatelet therapy in coronary artery disease, it received much less attention among the neurologists until publication of IST (International Stroke Trial)[7] and CAST (Chinese Acute Stroke Trial).[8] These two trials, with nearly 20 000 patients, showed a small benefit of aspirin when started within 48 h of stroke onset, for reducing early stroke recurrence and improving functional dependency (i.e. 1% absolute improvement at 6 months). Given the low cost and wide availability of aspirin worldwide and the rising stroke incidence, particularly among developing nations, the small therapeutic effect observed in IST and CAST remain clinically meaningful.

Multifaceted role of platelets

Platelets are the smallest corpuscular elements of blood (0.5 μm × 3 μm), and are formed by the fragmentation of megakaryocytes in the bone marrow.[9] Platelets are anuclear, and hence are unable to divide and have limited capacity for de novo protein synthesis. They provide the primary line of defense against hemorrhage along the estimated 65 000 square miles of vascular surface area in the human body.

Under normal physiological conditions, platelets circulate in the bloodstream without interacting with the vessel wall or with each other.[10,11,12] The reasons for this lack of platelet reactivity involve several factors, among which are the net electrical charge of blood components, the biophysical properties of flowing blood, and secretion of nitric oxide (NO) by the endothelium.[10,13] After activation, platelets provide a catalytic surface for coagulation factor activation, leading to thrombin generation and fibrin formation.

Platelet responses cannot differentiate between traumatic injury and pathological process.[14,15] Hence, a process conditioned to guard against hemorrhage throughout evolution may trigger occlusive thrombi at sites of atherosclerotic lesions with the same diligence and efficiency to halt hemorrhage. In brief, platelet thrombus formation involves dynamic interactions among the various components of hemostatic response, including the endothelium, leukocytes, fibrinolysis, inhibitors of blood coagulation, adhesion molecules, and inflammatory cytokines.[16–18]

The traditional mechanism of platelet function in hemostasis involves a multistep process that includes: (1) activation upon contact with constituents of the extracellular matrix (ECM) or with adhesion receptors on activated endothelial cells; (2) shape change from a tiny disc to a sphere with extending filopodia; (3) adhesion and spreading, leading to a monolayer deposit at the site of injury; (4) platelet–platelet aggregation, leading to a growing thrombus through successive layers of an interwoven lattice.

Beyond hemostasis and thrombosis, platelets participate in other biological mechanisms, including phagocytosis, inflammation, immune reactions, and interactions with tumor cells.[18–20] Many of the proteins contained in α-granules are inflammatory mediators, such as P-selectin, thrombospondin-1, platelet factor 4 (PF4), CD40 ligand (CD40L/CD154), NO, and the T-cell cytokine RANTES ('regulated upon activation normally T-cell expressed and secreted').

CD40 ligand is present in atheroma specimens and may contribute to macrophage tissue factor (TF) expression in atherosclerotic lesions.[21–23] (CD40L/CD154) is a transmembrane protein structurally related to tumor necrosis factor α (TNF α), originally identified on stimulated CD4$^+$ T cells, and later on stimulated mast cells, basophils, and

vascular smooth muscle cells. Its receptor, CD40, is constitutively expressed on B cells, monocytes, macrophages, endothelial cells, and dendritic cells. CD40 ligand is contained in platelets and expressed within seconds after platelet activation, and it can induce an inflammatory reaction in endothelial cells.[24]

TF factor expression on macrophages may be the predominant thrombogenic factor in the lipid-rich core of atherosclerotic plaques.[25] TF is a 47 kDa membrane-bound glycoprotein and is an important activator of blood coagulation via the factor VII/VIIa pathway. TF–factor VIIa complexes, in turn, activate circulating factors X and IX by limited proteolysis, culminating in thrombin generation and deposition of insoluble fibrin.

Integrins

Integrins are heterodimeric, asymmetric, transmembrane receptors that belong to the family of adhesion molecules.[26–31] The primary function of integrins is to regulate the dynamic interactions between the ECM and cell signaling. Integrins are ubiquitous to a large variety of cells, blood cells in particular. They are highly expressed on hematopoietic precursors, and endothelial cells, taking part in hematopoiesis, hemostasis, inflammation, and cell trafficking. The term 'integrin' was coined because of their role as membrane proteins coupling ECM interactions to cell signaling pathways.

Structure

Integrin structure consists in the non-covalent assembly of a single alpha (α) - (128-80 kDa) and beta (β) - (90-110 kDa) subunit. Each subunit consists of: 1) a long N-terminal extracellular domain with a globular head; 2) single transmembrane domain, and; 3) signaling region, consisting in a short carboxy-terminal cytoplasmic linked to cytoskeleton (Figure 10.1). The ligand-binding sites seem to occupy epitopes within in the globular head of the extracellular domain, in each of the α- and β-subunit. Normal ligand binding requires both subunits and the presence

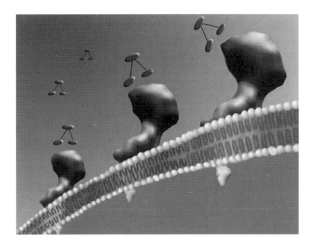

Figure 10.1
GPIIb/IIIa integrins embedded in the platelet membrane.

of divalent cations. The cation-binding sites are located in the β-subunit.

The cytoplasmic tail of each subunit interacts with a number of cytoskeletal proteins and signaling molecules. Integrins have no intrinsic enzymatic activity carry and function their signaling via downstream molecules (e.g. pp125 focal adhesion kinase (FAK), GTPases Rho or Rac, cytoskeletal components including talin, paxilin, and p130^{CAS}).

Classification

At least 24 paired integrin receptors, eight β-subunits (β$_1$–β$_8$), and 18 α-subunits have been cloned or identified in mammals. The α-subunit constitutes the backbone of the structure, while the β-subunit conveys the binding specificity for each integrin (Table 10.1). There are five known platelet integrins: three in the α$_1$ class and two in the β$_3$ class. In general, α$_1$-integrins mediate cell–matrix interactions, whereas β$_3$ integrins are primarily involved in cell–cell interactions.

Function

Cells modulate their adhesive properties via selective expression of integrins. Further versatility is conditioned by the dynamic interactions between integrins and their respective ligands.[32] Integrins are able to bind multiple ligands and are conformationally labile. Conformational change appears to be one of the key mechanisms utilized by integrins to modulate affinity for their counterligands. In contrast to most membrane receptors, integrins have a relatively low affinity for their ligands and therefore require a minimum cell-surface concentration for ligand binding to occur. Hence, cells attach to the ECM via multiple weak adhesions to several ligands. Cells migrate through their environment through repeated cycles of focal attachment and detachment,

Table 10.1   Platelet adhesion receptors

Family Integrins		Function	Ligands
β$_1$	α$_2$	Adhesion	Collagen
	α$_5$	Adhesion	Fibronectin
	α$_6$	Adhesion	Laminin
β$_3$	α$_{IIb}$	Aggregation, adhesion	Fibrinogen, vitronectin, fibronectin, thrombospondin, vWF
	α$_v$	Aggregation	Vitronectin
Non-integrins			
GPIb/V/IX		vWF	vWF
GPIV		Collagen	Collagen
GPVI		Collagen	Collagen
P-selectin		Adhesion	PSGL-1 on neutrophils and monocytes

PSGL-1, P-selectin glycoprotein ligand 1; vWF, von Willebrand factor.

modulated by affinity changes of integrins for their counter-ligands. Integrins are known to signal in both directions across cell membranes (i.e. inside–out and outside–in signaling).

Platelet GPIIb/IIIa ($\alpha_{IIb} \beta_3$)

Function

GPIIb/IIIa, termed $\alpha_{IIb} \beta_3$ in the integrin nomenclature, was among the first integrins to be expressed in complete recombinant form.[28] Benchmark research on $\alpha_{IIb} \beta_3$ has been instrumental in mapping the ligand-binding sites of integrins in general. $\alpha_{IIb} \beta_3$ is the most abundant platelet integrin, with approximately 80 000 copies expressed on the surface of a resting platelet.[33–36] Additional $\alpha_{IIb} \beta_3$ molecules reside within α-granules, and can translocate to the surface upon platelet activation.

The primary role of $\alpha_{IIb} \beta_3$ is to sustain platelet aggregation, the final step in the formation of platelet thrombus. A number of stimuli contribute to platelet activation, including rolling under high-shear flow conditions over perturbed endothelium, interactions between von Willebrand factor (vWF), platelet adhesion receptors (e.g. GPIb/IX/V, GPVI, $\alpha_{IIb} \beta_3$) over denuded endothelium, and exposure to thrombin and other clotting factors in the presence of atherothrombosis.[15] On resting platelets, $\alpha_{IIb} \beta_3$ has very low affinity for fibrinogen and other soluble ligands, but can bind to immobilized fibrinogen. The affinity of $\alpha_{IIb} \beta_3$ for fibrinogen and other soluble ligands increases severalfold upon platelet activation.[32]

Activated $\alpha_{IIb} \beta_3$ binds to other RGD (Arg–Gly–Asp)-containing adhesive proteins, including vWF, thrombospondin, fibronectin and vitronectin.[33] While vWF and fibrinogen are important for mediating initial platelet adhesion and aggregation, thrombospondin and fibronectin are involved in further strengthening these interactions. Vitronectin appears to regulate thrombus growth by attracting and binding onto plasminogen activator inhibitor 1 (PAI-1) locally. Recent additions to the list of $\alpha_{IIb} \beta_3$ ligands include cyr61, Fisp12, L1-Ig6, and prothrombin.[28] Prothrombin binding to $\alpha_{IIb} \beta_3$ appears to be involved in the generation of platelet procoagulant activity.[28]

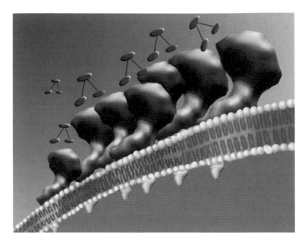

Figure 2
Avidity modulation with clustering of GPIIb/IIIa integrins during platelet activation.

The exact mechanisms of the platelet activation-dependent increases in the affinity and avidity of $\alpha_{IIb} \beta_3$ for its counter ligands are not known, but are thought to involve inside–out and outside–in signaling.[32]

Inside–out signaling

Inside–out signaling refers to the path of excitatory or inhibitory platelet agonists for initiating intracellular signals that modulate the affinity and avidity of $\alpha_{IIb} \beta_3$. The exact molecular mechanisms underlying modulation of $\alpha_{IIb} \beta_3$ activity are not entirely known. The cytoplasmic domains of both subunits are likely involved, since both mutations and deletions in these domains yield $\alpha_{IIb} \beta_3$ receptors that either cannot be activated or remain permanently activated.

Affinity modulation is the process that exposes the ligand-binding sites. It presumably occurs via an interaction between microskeletal proteins (e.g. spectrin) and the integrin, which triggers a conformational change of the receptor and exposes its ligand-binding sites.[34,37]

Avidity modulation presumably arises from the clustering of integrin heterodimers within the plane of the membrane (Figure 10.2). The available data suggest that avidity modulation occurs via the release of a subpopulation of $\alpha_{IIb} \beta_3$ from cytoskeletal constraints that maintain the receptor as an unclustered heterodimer in resting platelets. Affinity modulation appears to be the main factor responsible for the initial, reversible phase of ligand binding to $\alpha_{IIb}\beta_3$, whereas receptor clustering appears to mediate the later, irreversible phase of fibrinogen binding, and initiation of outside–in signaling.

Outside–in signaling

Outside–in signaling refers to platelet stimulation through $\alpha_{IIb}\beta_3$-mediated reverse signaling. A working model for outside–in signaling indicates that adhesive protein binding onto $\alpha_{IIb}\beta_3$, together with clustering, induce a change in the cytoplasmic domain structure that triggers signaling reactions within the platelet. Tyrosine phosphorylation of cytoplasmic domains of $\alpha_{IIb}\beta_3$ is thought to be a key mechanism for outside–in signaling.[31] Outside–in signaling induces a number of important vessel-wall events, including platelet protein phosphorylation, increased cytoplasmic Ca^{2+}, calpain activation, release of α-granule proteins and dense body constituents, release of membrane microparticles, cytoskeletal protein polymerization causing platelet contraction and clot retraction, and translation of Bcl 3. Clot retraction is a well-described phenomenon that involves outside–in signals through interactions among fibrin, $\alpha_{IIb}\beta_3$, cytoskeleton and contractile proteins.[38,39]

GPIIb/IIIa antagonists

Parenteral agents

Abciximab (ReoPro), eptifibatide (Integrelin) and tirofiban (Aggrastat) are the three parenteral agents currently available for the prevention of ischemic complications after percutaneous coronary interventions (PCI) and in the management of acute coronary syndromes (Table 10.2).[40]

Abciximab is the Fab fragment of a chimeric human/mouse monoclonal antibody directed against the human GPIIb/IIIa receptor. Eptifibatide is a cyclic heptapeptide based on the KGD (Lys–Gly–Asp) sequence of the snake venom barbourin, a natural disintegrin.[33,34] Cyclic RGD peptides have been engineered to be more resistant to enzymatic breakdown than synthetic linear peptides, by replacing Arg with amidino or benzamidino groups. Tirofiban is a tyrosine derivative nonpeptide mimetic of the RGD cell recognition sequence. All three agents are administered by intravenous bolus followed by a continuous intravenous infusion.

There are important differences in the mechanism of action and pharmacology of these agents that, theoretically, may pertain to therapeutic effect in ischemic brain syndromes. Eptifibatide and tirofiban are highly selective for inhibiting ligand binding onto activated GPIIb/IIIa receptors. In contrast, abciximab is not specific for $\alpha_{IIb}\beta_3$ and shares binding affinity for the vascular integrin $\alpha_v\beta_3$ and the leukocyte integrin $\alpha_M\beta_2$.[41–44] The clinical significance of cross-reactivity of abciximab with these other integrins, however, is not entirely clear.

$\alpha_{IIb}\beta_3$ is the major integrin expressed on activated endothelial cells and mediates platelet–endothelium adhesion.[45] Data also suggest that $\alpha_{IIb}\beta_3$ is also involved in other processes, including angiogenesis, apoptosis of proliferating vascular cells, smooth muscle cell migration, neointimal hyperplasia, and restenosis after angioplasty.[48] The leukocyte integrin Mac-1 (CD11b/CD18) is involved in monocyte– and neutrophil–platelet interactions, and could potentially play a role in the inflammatory response associated with reperfusion injury.[41]

Abciximab exerts high binding affinity for $\alpha_{IIb}\beta_3$. After a bolus dose 0.25 mg/kg, approximately two-thirds of the agent binds to platelets, resulting in a greater than 80% blockade of receptors and a greater than 80% blockade of ADP-induced platelet aggregation (5–20 μM).[45,46] Abciximab has a higher binding affinity for $\alpha_{IIb}\beta_3$ than does soluble fibrinogen, and hence can displace the latter from the receptor. This property underlies the phenomenon of 'dethrombosis' observed in vitro and during coronary angioplasty. Abciximab dissociates slowly from $\alpha_{IIb}\beta_3$ with an 'off-rate' of approximately 10–30 min, and the level of free plasma abciximab drops rapidly thereafter. Some abciximab is internalized within α-granules after administration. Flow cytometry mixing studies show that abciximab redistributes among platelets over a time course of minutes to hours. This phenomenon underlies the use of platelet concentrates for antidote,

Table 10.2 Parenteral GPIIb/IIIa antagonists

Feature	Abciximab	Eptifibatide	Tirofiban
Structure	Fab fragment of a chimeric human/mouse monoclonal antibody	Synthetic peptide	Small molecule
MW (Da)	47 615	832	495
Mechanism of action	Irreversible antagonist of fibrinogen binding to GPIIb/IIIa by steric hindrance and/or conformational effects	Reversible antagonist of fibrinogen binding to GP IIb/IIIa	Reversible antagonist of fibrinogen binding to GPIIb/IIIa
$\alpha_{2b}\beta_3$-binding epitope	??	KGD recognition sequence	RGD recognition sequence
Cross-reactivity with other integrins	$\alpha_v\beta_3$ $\alpha_M\beta_2$	No	No
Mode of administration	IV bolus followed by continuous infusion	IV bolus followed by continuous infusion	IV bolus followed by continuous infusion
Pharmacokinetics	Plasma $T_{1/2}\approx 10$–30 min	Plasma $T_{1/2}\approx 2.5$ h	Plasma $T_{1/2}\approx 2$ h
Platelet off-rate	Slow (≈ 90 min)	Rapid	Rapid
PD	>80% occupancy >90% inhibition of platelet aggregation Platelet aggregation return to $\approx 50\%$ baseline < 48 h of stopping infusion	135 µg/kg bolus +0.5 µg/kg/min: • 40–50% inhibition of platelet aggregation at steady state • <30% inhibition of platelet aggregation 4 h after infusion discontinuation 180 µg/kg bolus +12.0 µg/kg/min: • >90% inhibition of platelet aggregation at steady state • <50% inhibition of platelet aggregation 4 h after infusion discontinuation	>90% inhibition of platelet aggregation by end of 30 min infusion Platelet aggregation returns to near baseline <4–8 h
Elimination route	Senescent platelets	$\approx 50\%$ renal	Mostly renal
FDA-approved indications	• PCI • Refractory UA[a]	• PCI • ACS[b]	• ACS[b]
FDA-approved dosing regimens	PCI: 0.25 mg/kg bolus + 0.125 mg/kg/min (max. 10 µg/min) × 12 h Refractory UA: 0.25 mg/kg bolus + 10 µg/min × 18–24 h before PCI and continued 1 h thereafter	PCI: 180 µg/kg double-bolus (10 min apart) +2.0 µg/kg/min × 18–24 h ACS: 180 µg/kg bolus + 2.0 µg/kg/min up to 72 h	0.4 µg/kg/min × 30 min + 0.1 µg/kg/min × 48–108 h, 12–24 h post PCI

MW: molecular weight. PD: pharmacodynamics; PK: pharmacokinetic; PCI = percutaneous coronary intervention; ACS = acute coronary syndrome (i.e., UA or non-Q wave myocardial infarction); UA = unstable angina.
[a]PCI planned within 24 hours.
[b]Medical treatment of ACS, PCI.

as the redistribution of abciximab among the entire platelet pool yields a lower number of blocked receptors per platelet. Sufficient platelets should be given to reduce receptor occupancy to below 50%. Heterozygotes for Glanzmann's thrombasthenia who have 50–60% of functional copies of the receptor do not have excess bleeding. Abciximab is probably not eliminated in significant amounts in the urine, but rather via antibody degradation of senescent platelets. The infusion regimen of 0.125 µg/kg/h maintains greater than 80% receptor blockade in the majority of patients over the 12 h infusion course. Following cessation of infusion, the bleeding time returns to normal within 2 h and hemostasis is returned to normal over the following 48 h. The sustained and constant level of platelet inhibition and a gradual tapering of the antiplatelet effect after the end of infusion, theoretically, may be beneficial in ischemic brain syndromes in term of prolonged effect within the ischemic lesion.

In contrast, eptifibatide and tirofiban have a lower binding affinity than abciximab for $\alpha_{IIb}\beta_3$ and dissociate more rapidly from the receptor. Hence, these agents depend on higher plasma levels to sustain a target receptor blockade level above 80%. Renal clearance is thought to be the main route of elimination of both of these agents. The pharmacodynamic half-life of eptifibatide and tirofiban is approximately 2–2.5 h. Thus, platelet transfusion may not completely reverse the pharmacodynamic effect of these agents, since newly transfused platelets will be rapidly inhibited. Instead, reversal of the effect relies mainly on discontinuing the infusion.

Oral agents

Although the development of oral GPIIb/IIIa antagonists has been discontinued and they do not directly pertain to ischemic stroke, data accrued during their evaluation phase provide useful insight into the physiology of $\alpha_{IIb}\beta_3$ and integrins in general.[48–50] The underlying premise for the development of these agents was to provide extended secondary prevention following initial systemic treatment, somewhat analogous to warfarin sodium treatment after systemic heparin for venous thromboembolism.

In contrast with the success of parenteral agents, however, oral GPIIb/IIIa antagonists have encountered major setbacks. Dosing regimens were designed to achieve high-grade inhibition of platelet aggregation with twice-daily or thrice-daily dosing regimens. In comparison, aspirin inhibits ADP-induced platelet aggregation (20 µM) by approximately 10%, and the thienopyridine antagonists such as ticlopidine and clopidogrel produce inhibition by up to 30%. Unfortunately, all trials of oral GPIIb/IIIa antagonists were halted in view of failed efficacy or due to serious adverse events, increased mortality amongst others. Based on the experience with systemic agents, the principle of more intense receptor blockade for chronic use appears logical. However, the global overview of clinical trials brought forward new hypotheses pertaining to platelet physiology. Possible explanations for the failure of oral agents include receptor activation from outside–in signaling and the rapid off-rate of some agents from the receptor.[50] Conversely, dual blockade of the arachidonic acid pathway with aspirin and of the ADP P2Y1 purine receptor with clopidogrel has yielded noticeable results in the secondary prevention of acute coronary syndromes.[51]

Acute GPIIb/IIIa blockade in ischemic stroke

Rationale

The rationale for the use of a GPIIb/IIIa antagonist in this setting can be summarized as follows. First, the proof of concept of more intense platelet blockade than is achievable with aspirin has been demonstrated with parenteral GPIIb/IIIa antagonists in the setting of PCI and with the combination of aspirin and thienopyridine ADP receptor antagonists in the prevention of coronary stent thrombosis and ischemic complications post acute coronary syndrome.[51–66] Studies in experimental stroke models have documented reductions in platelet accumulation, fibrin accretion, and infarct volume with GPIIb/IIIa blockade. Second, the apparent relationship between efficacy and time from stroke onset in the pooled analysis of IST, CAST,[8] and MAST-I (Multicenter Acute Stroke Trial – Italy)[67] suggests that earlier blockade of platelet function may improve overall efficacy results. Third, there are a few additional mechanisms that are unique to abciximab or have been better substantiated with this agent. These additional effects include 'dethrombosis' and cross-reactivity with the $\alpha_v \beta_3$ and $\alpha_M \beta_2$ integrins.

Reversal of ADP-induced platelet aggregation by abciximab has been documented in vitro, and 'dethrombosis' has been observed in studies of PCI for the treatment of ST–T segment elevation myocardial infarction. In the ADMIRAL trial (a randomized comparison of Abciximab Before Direct Angioplasty and Stenting in Myocardial Infarction Regarding Acute and Long-Term Follow-Up), 17% of patients in the abciximab treatment group had restored complete coronary flow before PCI, compared with 5% of placebo patients.[68] Dethrombosis may be due to the competitive displacement of fibrinogen by abciximab, which has much greater affinity for $\alpha_{IIb} \beta_3$ (than fibrinogen).

There may also be an enhancement of endogenous fibrinolysis by reducing the release of platelet activation inhibition 1 (PAI-1) from platelet α-granules. Abciximab cross-reactivities with $\alpha_v \beta_3$ and $\alpha_M \beta_2$ integrins may reduce endothelial reactivity and leukocyte-platelet interactions, respectively.

From the *microvascular* standpoint, GP IIb/IIIa antagonists may prevent further platelet aggregation, fibrin formation and lesion growth in the ischemic penumbra.[69] Cross-reactivity with $\alpha v\beta 3$ may reduce endothelial reactivity and with $\alpha M\beta 2$ may reduce leukocyte-platelet interactions.

Studies in experimental models have documented reductions in platelet accumulation, fibrin accretion and infarct volume with GP IIb/IIIa blockade, hence providing a supporting rationale. GP IIb/IIIa antagonists may improve stroke outcome via an effect both on the macro- and micro-circulation.[70–74]

Clinical results

There are two published studies on the use of abciximab in the treatment of acute ischemic stroke.[75,76] Preliminary safety data were obtained in a randomized, dose-escalation study involving 74 patients treated within 24 h of stroke onset. None of the patients sustained symptomatic parenchymal hemorrhage and there were trends of improved functional

recovery at 3 months in favor of abciximab.[75] Notwithstanding the limited sample size of the study, these data open the prospect for future studies evaluating the administration of abciximab beyond 6 h of stroke onset.

A follow-up randomized, double-blinded trial of 400 patients treated within 6 h of onset was undertaken to obtain additional efficacy and safety data.[76]

Studies of eptifibatide in ischemic brain syndromes are also underway.[77,78]

Summary

Platelets are crucial cellular elements of blood and are involved in several processes, including primary hemostasis, inflammation, atherosclerosis and pathophysiology of atherothrombosis. Careful observations of patients with congenital bleeding disorders over the years, along with translation of clinical trials results and advances in vascular biology, have brought platelet research to a new era. Contemporary platelet research focuses, among other things, on the elucidation of signaling mechanisms in response to a variety of stimuli, including exposure to ECM constituents, soluble agonists, and growth factors. The evidence linking platelets to atherothrombosis is overwhelming, as evidenced by the results of clinical trials of antiplatelet agents in a variety of disease states. The effect of aspirin in the treatment of acute coronary syndromes and ischemic stroke is intriguing, particularly since it has yielded improved outcomes despite the start of therapy several hours after symptom onset. Parenteral platelet GPIIb/IIIa antagonists are currently under investigation in the treatment of ischemic stroke, and the initial results have been encouraging.

Disclosure

Dr Leclerc is a full-time employee and shareholder, Eli Lilly and Co., codeveloper and distributor of abciximab (ReoPro).

References

1. Bizzozero J. Über einen Formbestandteil des Blutes und die Rolle bei der Thrombose und der Blutgerinnung. Virchows Arch Pathol Anat 1882;90:261.

2. Mustard JF, Rowsell HC, Murphy EA. Reversible platelet aggregation and myocardial ischemia. Circulation 1964; 30(Suppl III):III-23.

3. Antiplatelet Trialists' Collaboration. Collaborative overview of randomised trials of antiplatelet therapy – I: Prevention of death, myocardial infarction, and stroke by prolonged antiplatelet therapy in various categories of patients. BMJ 1994;308:81–106.

4. Nurden AT, Caen JP. Specific roles for platelet surface glycoproteins in platelet function. Nature 1975;255: 720–2.

5. Caen J, Levy-Toledano S. Interaction between platelets and von Willebrand factor provides a new scheme for primary hemostasis. Nature 1972;244:159–60.

6. ISIS-2 (Second International Study of Infarct Survival) Collaborative Group. Randomized trial of intravenous streptokinase, oral aspirin, both or neither among 17 187 cases of suspected acute myocardial infarction: ISIS-2. Lancet 1988;ii:349–60.

7. Sandercock P, for the International Stroke Trial Collaborative Group. The International Stroke Trial (IST): a randomized trial of aspirin, subcutaneous heparin, both, or neither among 19 435 patients with acute ischemic stroke. Lancet 1997;349:1569–81.

8. Chinese Acute Stroke Trial (CAST). Randomized placebo-controlled trial of early aspirin use in 20 000 patients with acute ischaemic stroke. Lancet 1997,349. 1641–9.

9. Bithell TC. The physiology of primary hemostasis. In: Lee GR, Bithell TC, Foerster J, et al (eds). Wintrobe's Clinical Hematology, 9th edn. Philadelphia: Lea & Febinger, 1993.

10. Andrews RK, Lopez JA, Berndt MC. Molecular mechanisms of platelet adhesion and activation. Int J Biochem Cell Biol 1997;29:91–105.

11. Ware JA, Heistad DD. Platelet–endothelium interactions. N Engl J Med 1993;328:628–635.

12. Vane JR, Anggard EE, Botting RM. Regulatory functions of the vascular endothelium. N Engl J Med 1990; 323:27–36.

13. Moncada S, Palmer RMJ, Higgs EA. Nitric oxide: physiology, pathophysiology, and pharmacology. Pharmacol Rev 1991;43:109–42.

14. Goto S, Ikeda Y, Salvidar E, Ruggeri ZM. Distinct mechanisms of platelet aggregation as a consequence of different shearing flow conditions. J Clint Invest 1998;101:479–86.

15. Kulkarni S, Dopheide SM, Yap CL, et al. A revised model of platelet aggregation. J Clin Invest 2000; 105:783–91.

16. Folts JD, Gallagher K, Rowe GG. Blood flow reductions in stenosed canine coronary arteries. Circulation 1982;65:248–55.

17. Webb DJ. Endothelin receptors cloned, endothelin converting enzyme characterized and pathophysiological roles for endothelin proposed. Trends Pharmacol Sci 1991;12:43–6.

18. Reed GL, Fitzgerald ML, Polgar J. Molecular mechanisms of platelet exocytosis: insights into the 'secret' life of thrombocytes. Blood 2000;96:3322–8.

19. Marcus AJ. Review: Stratton Lecture 1989: Thrombosis and inflammation as multicellular processes: pathophysiological significance of Tran cellular metabolism. Blood 1990;76:1903–7.

20. Libby P. Molecular bases of the acute coronary syndromes. Circulation 1995;91:2844–50.

21. Schonbeck U, Libby P. CD40 and plaque instability. Circ Res 2001;89:1092–103.

22. Lederman S, Yellin MJ, Krichevsky A, et al. Identification of a novel surface protein on activated CD4⁺ T cells that induces contact-dependent B cell differentiation (help). J Exp Med 1992;175:1091–101.

23. Mach F, Schonbeck U, Sukhova GK, et al. Functional CD40 ligand is expressed on human vascular endothelial cells, smooth muscle cells, and macrophages: implications for CD40–CD40 ligand signaling in atherosclerosis. Proc Natl Acad Sci USA 1997;94:1931–6.

24. Houston DS, Shepard JT, Vanhoutte PM. Aggregating human platelets cause direct contraction and endothelium-dependent relaxation of isolated canine coronary arteries: role of serotonin, thromboxane A_2, and adenine nucleotides. J Clin Invest 1986;78: 539–44.

25. Slupsky JR, Kalbas M, Willuweit A, et al. Activated platelets induce tissue factor expression on human umbilical vein endothelial cells by ligation of CD40. Thromb Haemost 1998;80:1008–14.

26. Hynes JO. Integrins: versatility, modulation, and signaling in cell adhesion. Cell 1992;69:11–25.

27. Green LJ, Mould AP, Humphries MJ. The integrin β subunit. Int J Biochem Cell Biol 1998;30:179–84.

28. Plow EF, Cierniewski CS, Haas TA, Byzova TV. $\alpha_{IIb}–\beta_{IIIa}$ and its antagonism at the new millennium. Thromb Hemostat 2001;86:34–40.

29. Nurden AT, Caen JP. Specific roles for platelet surface glycoproteins in platelet function. Nature 1975;255: 720–2.

30. Caen J, Levy-Toledano S. Interaction between platelets and von Willebrand factor provides a new scheme for primary hemostasis. Nature 1972;244:159–60.

31. Phillips DR, Nannizzi-Alaimo N, Srinivasa Prasad KS. B3 tyrosine phosphorylation in α_{IIb}-β_{III} signaling (platelet membrane GPIIb–IIIa) outside-in integrin signaling. Thromb Haemostat 2001;86:246–58.

32. Shattill SJ, Kashiwagi H, Pampori N. Integrin signaling: the platelet paradigm. Blood 1998;8:2645–57.

33. Lefkovits J, Plow EF, Topol EJ. Platelet glycoprotein IIb/IIIa receptors in cardiovascular medicine. N Engl J Med 1995;332:1553–9.

34. Topol EJ, Byzova TV, Plow EF. Platelet GP IIb–IIIa blockers. Lancet 1999;353:227–31.

35. Madan M, Berkowitz SD, Tcheng JE. Glycoprotein IIb/IIIa integrin blockade. Circulation 1998;98: 2629–35.

36. Roe MT, Sapp SK, Lincoff MA. Glycoprotein IIb/IIIa inhibitors in acute coronary syndromes. Cleveland Clin J Med 2000;67:131–40.

37. Brass LF, Hoxie JA, Manning DR. Signaling through G protein and G-protein-coupled receptors during platelet activation. Thromb Haemost 1993;70:217–23.

38. Ichinose A. Physiopathology and regulation of factor XIII. Thromb Haemost 2001;86:57–65.

39. Cox AD, Devine DV. Factor XIIIa binding to activated platelets is mediated through activation of glycoprotein IIb–IIIa. Blood 1994;83:1006–16.

40. de Queiroz JO, Araújo F, Horta Veloso HH, et al. Efficacy and safety of abciximab on acute myocardial infarction treated with precutaneous coronary interventions: a meta-analysis of randomized, controlled trials. Am Heart J 2004;148:937–43.

41. Altieri D, Edgington TS. A monoclonal antibody reacting with distinct adhesion molecules defines a transition in the functional state of the receptor CD11b/CD18 (Mac-1). J Immunol 1998;141:2656–60.

42. Piccardoni P, Rita Sideri R, Manarini S, et al. Platelet/polymorphonuclear leukocyte adhesion: a new role for SRC kinases. Blood 200;98:108–16.

43. Tam SH, Sassoli PM, Jordan RE, Nakada MT. Abciximab (ReoPro, Chimeric 7E3 Fab) demonstrates equivalent affinity and functional blockade of glycoprotein IIb/IIIa and $\alpha_v\beta_3$ integrins. Circulation 1998;141:1085–91.

44. Gawaz M, Neumann FJ, Dickfeld T, et al. Vitronectin receptor ($\alpha_v\beta_3$) mediates platelet adhesion to the luminal aspect of endothelial cells. Implications for reperfusion in acute myocardial infarction. Circulation 1997;96:1809–18.

45. Coller BS. Blockade of platelet GPIIb–IIIa receptors as an antithrombotic strategy. Circulation 1995;92: 2373–80.

46. Mascelli MA, Lance ET, Damajaru L, et al. Pharmacodynamic profile of short-term abciximab treatment demonstrates prolonged platelet inhibition with gradual recovery from GPIIb/IIIa receptor blockade. Circulation 1998;97:1680–8.

47. Coller BS. Monitoring platelet GPIIb–IIIa antagonist therapy. Circulation 1998; 97:5–9.

48. The SYMPHONY Investigators. Comparison of sibrafiban with aspirin for prevention of cardiovascular events after acute coronary syndromes: a randomised trial. Lancet 2000;355:337–45.

49. O'Neill WW, Serruys P, Knudtson M, et al. Design and objectives of the evaluation of oral xemilofiban in controlling thrombotic events (EXCITE) study. J Intervent Cardiol 1999;12:109–15.

50. Cannon CP, McCabe CH, Borzak S, et al. Randomized trial of an oral platelet glycoprotein IIb/IIIa antagonist, sibrafiban, in patients after an acute coronary syndrome. Results of the TIMI 12 trial. Circulation 1998;97:340–9.

51. The Clopidogrel in Unstable Angina to Prevent Recurrent Events Trial Investigators. Effects of clopidogrel in addition to aspirin in patients with acute coronary syndromes without ST-segment elevation. N Engl J Med 2001;345:494–502.

52. Lefkovits J, Plow EF, Topol EJ. Platelet glycoprotein IIb/IIIa receptors in cardiovascular medicine. N Engl J Med 1995;332:1553–9.

53. The EPIC Investigators. Use of a monoclonal antibody directed against the platelet glycoprotein IIb/IIIa receptor in high-risk coronary angioplasty. N Engl J Med 1994;330:956–61.

54. The EPISTENT Investigators. Randomized placebo-controlled and balloon angioplasty-controlled trial to assess safety of coronary stenting with use of platelet glycoprotein-IIb/IIIa blockade. Lancet 1998;352: 87–92.

55. Brown DL, Fann CSJ, Chee JC. Meta-analysis of effectiveness and safety of abciximab versus eptifibatide or tirofiban in percutaneous coronary intervention. Am J Cardiol 2001;87:537–41.

56. Karvouni E, Katritsis DG, Ioannidis JP. Intravenous glycoprotein IIb/IIIa receptor antagonists reduce mortality after percutaneous coronary interventions. J Am Coll Cardiol 2003; 41:26–32.

57. de Queiroz Fernandes Araujo JOQ, Veloso HH, Braga De Paiva JM, et al. Efficacy and safety of abciximab on acute myocardial infarction treated with percutaneous coronary interventions: a meta-analysis of randomized, controlled trials. Am Heart J 2004;148:937–43.

58. Karvouni E, Demosthenes GK, Ioannidis JPA. Intravenous glycoprotein IIb/IIIa receptor antagonists reduce mortality after percutaneous coronary interventions. J Am Coll Cardiol 2003;41:26–32.

59. Al Suwaidi J, Holmes DR, Salam AM, et al. Impact of coronary artery stents on mortality and nonfatal myocardial infarction: meta-analysis of randomized trials comparing a strategy of routine stenting with that of balloon angioplasty. Am Heart J 2004;147–8.

60. Montalescot G, Borentain M, Payot L, et al. Early vs. late administration of glycoprotein IIb/IIIa inhibitors in primary percutaneous coronary intervention of acute ST-segment elevation myocardial infarction. A meta-analysis. JAMA 2004;292:362–6.

61. Antman EM, Giugliano RP, Gibson CM, et al. Abciximab facilitates the rate and extent of thrombolysis: results of the Thrombolysis in Myocardial Infarction (TIMI) 14 trial. The TIMI 14 Investigators. Circulation 1999;99:2720–32.

62. Herrmann HC, Moliterno DJ, Ohman EM, et al. Facilitation of early percutaneous coronary intervention after reteplase with or without abciximab in acute myocardial infarction: results from the SPEED (GUSTO-4 pilot) trial. J Am Coll Cardiol 2000;36: 1489–96.

63. Kleiman NS, Ohman EM, Califf RM, et al. Profound inhibition of platelet aggregation with monoclonal antibody 7E3 Fab after thrombolytic therapy: results of the Thrombolysis and Angioplasty in Myocardial Infarction (TAMI) 8 pilot study. J Am Coll Cardiol 1993;22:381–9.

64. Ohman EM, Kleiman NS, Gacioh G, et al. Combined accelerated tissue-plasminogen activator and platelet glycoprotein IIb/IIIa integrin receptor blockade with integrilin in acute myocardial infarction: results of a randomized, placebo-controlled, dose-ranging trial. IMPACT-AMI Investigators. Circulation 1997; 95:846–85.

65. Topol EJ, Investigators TG. Reperfusion therapy for acute myocardial infarction with fibrinolytic therapy or combination reduced fibrinolytic therapy and platelet glycoprotein IIb/IIIa inhibition: the GUSTO V randomized trial. Lancet 2001;357: 1905–14.

66. Krucoff MW, Green CL, Langer A, et al. The Abciximab ST-Recovery on AMI (ASTRONAMI) GUSTO-V substudy: enhanced early speed, stability, quality of reperfusion with anti-platelet augmented thrombolytic therapy for ST-elevation AMI. J Am Coll Cardiol 2002:39(5 Suppl 2):306.

67. Multicenter Acute Stroke Trial – Italy (MAST-I) Group. Randomised controlled trial of streptokinase, aspirin, and combination of both in treatment of acute ischaemic stroke. Lancet 1995;346:1509–1514.

68. Montalescot G, Barragan P, Wittenberg O, et al. ADMIRAL investigators. Platelet glycoprotein IIb/IIIa inhibition with coronary stenting for acute myocardial infarction. New Engl J Med 2001;344:1895–903.

69. Choudri TF, Hoh BL, Zerwes HG, et al. Reduced microvascular thrombosis and improved outcome in acute murine stroke by inhibiting GP IIb –IIIa receptor-mediated platelet aggregation. J Clin Invest 1998;102: 1301–1310.

70. Seitz R, Hamzavi M, Junghans U, et al, Thrombolysis with recombinant tissue plasminogen activator and tirofiban in stroke. Preliminary observations. Stroke 2003;34:1932–5.

71. The Abciximab in Ischemic Stroke Investigators. Abciximab in acute ischemic stroke. A randomized, double-blind, placebo-controlled, dose-escalation study. Stroke 2000;31:601–9.

72. Abciximab Emergent Stroke Treatment Trial (AbESTT) Investigators. Patients with acute ischemic stroke. Results of a randomized phase 2 trial. Stroke 2005;36:880–90.

73. Kopp CW, Steiner S, Nasel C, Seidinger D. Abciximab reduces monocyte tissue factor in carotid angioplasty and stenting. Stroke 2003;34:2560–7.

74. Lapchak PA, Araujo DM, Song D, et al. The non-peptide glycoprotein IIb/IIIa platelet receptor antagonist SM-20302 reduces tissue plasminogen activator induced intracerebral hemorrhage after thromboembolic stroke. Stroke 2002;33:147–52.

75. The Abcixmab in Ischemic Stroke investigators. Abcixmab in acute ischemic stroke. A randomized, double-blind, placebo-controlled, dose-escalation study. Stroke 2000;31:601–609.

76. Abcixmab Emergent Stroke Treatment Trial (AbESTT) Investigators. Patients with acute ischemic stroke. Results of a randomized phase 2 trial. Stroke 2005;36:880–890.

77. Pancioli AM, Brott TG. Therapeutic potential of platelet glycoprotein IIb/IIIa receptor antagonists in acute ischaemic stroke: Scientific rationale and available evidence. Adis 2004;18(14):981–988.

78. McDonald CT, O'Donnell J, Bemporad J, et al. The clinical utility of intravenous Integrilin combined with intraarterial tissue plasminogen activator in acute ischemic stroke: the MGH experience [abstract]. Stroke 2002;96:359A.

11

New antithrombotics and their potential use

Patrik Michel

Thrombosis and antithrombotics in acute stroke: current knowledge

Arterial thrombi consist of platelet aggregates held together by small amounts of fibrin, so medications that act on platelet activation and aggregation, on fibrin formation resulting from activation of the coagulation pathway, or on fibrin degradation and fibrinolysis should be effective in the treatment and prevention of early recurrences in acute ischemic stroke.

The first two mechanisms are inhibited by antithrombotic medications (antiplatelet agents and anticoagulants); in acute stroke, they may be effective by stabilizing the clot or by preventing progression of clot formation, reocclusion after recanalization, and early recurrence. A drug acting on one of these subsystems may also potentiate the effect of medications or physiological substances (such as intrinsic tissue-type plasminogen activator (tPA)) acting on one of the other subsystems.

In ischemic stroke, the mechanism of thrombus formation and the risk of early recurrence are heterogeneous. This, and the tendency of antithrombotic medications to facilitate hemorrhagic transformation, have rendered their success less spectacular than in acute coronary syndromes or venous thromboembolic disease. For the same reasons, an antithrombotic treatment that is effective in another vascular disease may not be effective in acute stroke.

Chronic prevention trials have shown that some combination antiplatelet treatments may work, but not others,[1,2] and that the effectiveness of anticoagulation for secondary prevention depends largely on the stroke mechanism.[3–5] Interestingly, drugs that are effective in the acute stage of a disease might be harmful in the chronic stage, and vice versa, as shown for glycoprotein (GP)IIb/IIIa antagonists[6,7] (Table 11.1).

Table 11.1   Lessons learned from antithrombotic trials in acute stroke and acute coronary syndromes

- The effectiveness of an antithrombotic treatment in acute stroke cannot be inferred from its effect in vitro or in other acute vascular diseases
- Because of their heterogeneity, higher intracranial hemorrhage rate, and shorter time window for effective treatment, stroke patients may benefit less from antithrombotics than patients with other vascular diseases
- A drug or combination that is effective in the acute stage of stroke might be harmful in the chronic stage, and vice versa
- Trials of antithrombotic agents may be more likely to show a benefit if they are targeted at specific stroke mechanisms
- For maximal benefit from antithrombotics, the patients most likely to suffer clot progression, reocclusion, or early recurrence should be selected
- For maximal safety with antithrombotics, patients at low risk of hemorrhagic transformation should be selected
- Drugs preventing hemorrhagic transformation may increase the benefits from antithrombotics

Table 11.2 New antiplatelet drugs in clinical development (stage II and/or III) with potential for use in cerebrovascular diseases (CVD). Approval status is indicated for Europe and/or North America

Main target	Drug	Route	Highest status reached	Highest status for CVD	Currently approved indications	Being evaluated for use in:
COX	Triflusal	PO	Approved	Approved	Cardiovascular and stroke prevention, DVT prevention (certain European countries)	Secondary cardiovascular and stroke prevention: equally effective as aspirin, fewer hemorrhages. Atrial fibrillation: effective in combination with low-dose oral anticoagulation
COX and NO receptor	NCX-4016	PO	II	—	—	PAD
Phospho-diesterase	Cilostazol	PO	Approved	III	PAD (USA, UK)	Secondary stroke prevention: more effective then placebo Progression of symptomatic intracranial stenosis: more effective than aspirin Secondary stroke prevention in comparison with aspirin: ongoing phase III trial
ADP P2Y12 receptor	AZD-6140 Prasugrel (CS-747)	PO PO	II III	— —	— —	ACS PCI in ACS: ongoing phase III trial
TxA$_2$ receptor	S-18886	PO	II	—	—	Secondary prevention of cardiovascular diseases
TxA$_2$ synthase and receptor	Picotamide	PO	II	—	—	Vascular mortality in diabetics with PAD: more effective than aspirin

GPIIb/IIIa inhibitors are discussed in Chapter 10. Other new antiplatelets in preclinical development include cangrelor (AR-C69931MX), MRS-2179, GPG-290, ifetroban (BMS-180291), solutroban (BM13,177), GR32191, ecraprost, liprostin, pamicogrel, gantofiban, Z-335, KDI-792, YM-337, TA-993, SL-65.0472, BGC-728, and the GPIb (vWF receptor) antagonist 6B4.

COX, cyclo-oxygenase; NO, nitric oxide; ADP, adenosine diphosphate; TxA$_2$, thromboxane A$_2$; DVT, deep venous thrombosis; PAD, peripheral artery disease; ACS, acute coronary syndrome; PCI, percutaneous coronary intervention.

So far, the only antithrombotic for acute stroke for which the benefit has been shown to be higher than the added risk of bleeding is aspirin in doses of 160–300 mg daily.[8,9] Currently available anticoagulants, such as heparins, low-molecular-weight heparins (LMWH), and heparinoids, have no net effect, mainly because the small benefits are offset by an increased bleeding rate;[10] however, given in small doses, they seem to be effective in the prevention of venous thromboembolism after an acute stroke.[11] In large-volume strokes, this increased risk of bleeding in the form of hemorrhagic transformation of the ischemic stroke ('hemorrhagic infarct') occurs in the first days or weeks – unfortunately precisely when ischemic recurrences tend to occur.[12–14] One way to deal with this conundrum might be the development of more specific antithrombotic agents with a higher efficacy-to-safety index. Examples are direct thrombin inhibitors, factor Xa inhibitors, and P2Y(12) ADP receptor blockers (Tables 11.2 and 11.3). Another way to increase the effectiveness of antithrombotics would be prevention of hemorrhagic transformation by protecting the blood–brain barrier, for example with matrix metalloproteinase (MMP) inhibitors.[15,16]

Although combination therapy with an antiplatelet agent, anticoagulants, and fibrinolytics theoretically makes sense in certain stroke types or with certain (invasive) interventions, this has to be carefully tested in clinical trials. Past trials have shown high bleeding rates with various combinations of these drugs.[8,17–19]

Other ongoing antithrombotic trials are mentioned below. The potential use of new heparin-like substances is discussed in Chapters 2 and 8, that of fibrinolytics in Chapter 3, and that of GPIIb/IIIa inhibitors in Chapter 10.

The effectiveness for acute ischemic stroke of many antithrombotics already on the market is unknown, as no randomized phase II or III trials have been completed. Examples are the platelet-antiaggregating agents clopidogrel and dipyridamole and the anticoagulants ximelagatran, argatroban, lepirudin, and bivalirudin (Tables 11.2 and 11.3). Of the antiplatelet agents, clopidogrel is now being tested as an add-on to aspirin for acute secondary prevention after transient ischemic attacks (TIA) (FASTER, the Fast Assessment of Stroke and Transient ischemic attack (TIA) to prevent Early Recurrence trial, and ATARI, Antithrombotic Therapy in Acute Recovered cerebral Ischaemia, trials).[20,21]

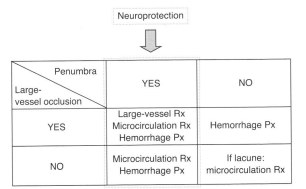

Figure 11.1
Acute ischemic stroke treatment strategies based on noninvasive assessment of penumbra and vessels. Independently of imaging results, all patients should be treated with general measures (control of oxygen, temperature, blood pressure, glucose, etc.). Rx, treatment; Px, prevention.

With increasing expertise, more efficient emergency room management, and increased availability of stroke experts, more complex treatments may be realistically applied in the future. Over the next decade, improved acute vascular and neuroimaging will allow treatment to become more pathophysiology-based and individualized (Figure 11.1).

Given these specific characterisitics of acute stroke patients, randomized controlled trials of already existing and new antithrombotics, of new treatment strategies, and of combination therapies are urgently needed and potentially rewarding.

New antithrombotic agents

Three main strategies aiming at restoring and maintaining blood flow in the macro- and microcirculation will be further developed in the future: (1) noninvasive recanalization; (2) invasive recanalization; and (3) acute clot and plaque stabilization leading to prevention of progression, reocclusion, and early stroke recurrence. Established and new antithrombotics may be used to achieve these goals. Continuous monitoring by vascular and neuroimaging (such as transcranial ultrasound) may allow the adjustment of treatment during the acute phase.

Ideally, the identification of new targets for acute therapy should lead to the development of agents that

Table 11.3 New anticoagulant drugs in clinical development (stage II and/or III) with potential for use in cerebrovascular diseases (CVD). Approval status is indicated for Europe and North America

Main target	Drug	Route	Highest status reached	Highest status for CVD	Currently approved indications	Being evaluated for use in:
TF/factor VIIa complex	Recombinant nematode anticoagulant peptide (rNAPc2)	SC	II	—	—	DVT prevention. PCI in ACS
	Active site-blocked factor VIIa (VIIai)	SC	II	—	—	Elective PCI: intervention: no better than heparin. Not further developed.
	Recombinant tissue factor pathway inhibitor (rTFPI)	IV	III	—	—	Sepsis: one negative trial Pneumonia
Factor Va/VIIIa complex (through protein C)	Recombinant human activated protein C	IV	Approved	—	Sepsis	Sepsis in children
	Protein C concentrates	IV	II	—	—	Meningococcal sepsis
	Recombinant soluble thrombomodulin (ART-123)	SC	II	—	—	DVT prevention
Factor Xa: indirect inhibitors	Fondaparinux	SC	Approved	—	DVT prevention	DVT treatment ACS
	Idraparinux	SC	III	III	—	DVT treatment Atrial fibrillation: ongoing phase III trial (AMADEUS)
Factor Xa: direct inhibitors	DX-9065a	IV	II	—	—	Stable coronary artery disease
	DPC-906	PO	II	—	—	PCIDVT prevention
	Razaxaban	PO	II	—	—	DVT prevention
Factor IIa: direct thrombin inhibitors	Ximelagatran	PO	Approved then withdrawn	III	—	Was found to be effective in atrial fibrillation and DVT prophylaxis, but withdrawn from market because of increased risk of liver toxicity

Table 11.3 (Continued)

Main target	Drug	Route	Highest status reached	Highest status for CVD	Currently approved indications	Being evaluated for use in:
	Melagatran	SC	Approved	—	DVT prevention (certain European countries only)	—
	Argatroban	IV	Approved	II	Heparin-induced thrombocytopenia HITTS PCI (USA, Japan, Switzerland only)	Acute stroke: phase II study with trend to more bleeding, no difference in outcome compared with placebo (ARGIS-I). Pilot study in combination with IV thrombolysis: ongoing (TARTS) Unstable angina and coronary angioplasty
	Dabigatran	PO	II	—	—	DVT prevention
	Lepirudin (recombinant hirudin)	IV	Approved	—	Heparin-induced thrombocytopenia	ACS DVT prevention and treatment
	Bivalirudin	IV	Approved	II	PCI	ACS

Heparinoids, low-molecular-weight heparins, and dermatan sulfate are discussed in Chapters 2 and 4. Fibrinolysis is discussed in Chapter 3.

Other thrombin inhibitors in early clinical development include BAY 59-7939 FXV-673, H-MR-2905, RPR-130737 YM-60828, JTV-803, GW-473178, BIBR-1048, BIBR-953ZW, BIBR-1048MS, SanOrg-12378, DPC-423, and LY-51,7717.

Other thrombin inhibitors in early development include desirudine, DuP 714, S-18326, and 3DP-4815.

Other antithrombotics in early development are SB249417 (anti-factor IX monoclonal antibody) and SB424323 (indirect thrombin inhibitor).

TF, tissue factor; DVT, deep venous thrombosis; PCI, percutaneous coronary intervention; ACS, acute coronary syndrome; HITTS, heparin-induced thrombocytopenia–thrombosis syndrome;

Table 11.4 Desirable features of new antithrombotics for use in acute stroke[a]

- Improve short- and long-term outcome
- High efficacy-to-safety index
- Rapid onset of action
- Administration by parenteral and oral routes, in a once- or twice-daily dosing schedule
- Availability of a safe antidote
- No need for laboratory monitoring
- Minimal interaction with other drugs

[a]Adapted from Hirsh et al.[26]

are more effective and/or safer than aspirin or heparin (Table 11.4). New antithrombotic agents may be more effective by having a better antithrombotic action or causing less hemorrhage through a more specific mechanism of action, or may provide more effective combination therapy. Thus, clinical outcome in acute coronary syndromes has been improved by replacing heparin with LMWH[22] or by adding clopidogrel to aspirin.[23] Similar strategies have not yet worked in acute stroke.[24,25] Such discrepancies between different arterial diseases and between the theoretical and clinical benefit emphasize the need for randomized phase III trials for each antithrombotic agent in specific stroke pathophysiologies.

In terms of antiplatelet agents, clopidogrel has not yet been tested in the acute phase of ischemic stroke; the same is true for triflusal, an antiaggregant chemically related to aspirin and with a similar efficacy in long-term stroke prevention.[27,28] Cilostazol,[29] a phosphodiesterase inhibitor, is currently undergoing phase III trials for secondary stroke prevention. This drug and other new antiaggregants listed in Table 11.2 have not yet been tested in the acute phase of stroke.

Regarding new agents acting on the coagulation pathway, the furthest developed are the direct thrombin (factor II) inhibitors (DTIs). Thrombin, the enzyme that converts fibrinogen to fibrin, can be inhibited indirectly or directly. Indirect thrombin inhibitors act by catalyzing the activation of antithrombin III (ATIII) and/or heparin cofactor II. In contrast, DTIs bind directly to thrombin and block its interaction with substrates, thus preventing fibrin formation, thrombin-mediated activation of factors V, VIII, XI, and XIII, and thrombin-induced platelet aggregation.[30] There are no antidotes for DTIs. In contrast to heparin, DTIs produce a more predictable anticoagulant response and usually require no

monitoring. Three parenteral DTIs (lepirudin, argatroban, and bivalirudin) and one oral DTI (ximelagatran) have been licensed for specific indications (Table 11.3). The only DTI so far tested for acute stroke in a phase II study is argatroban.[31] Used within 12 h after stroke onset, it proved to be safe but not clinically effective in this small group of patients. Another safety study (TARTS Tpa Argatroban Stroke Study) involving argatroban used together with recombinant tPA (rtPA) within 3 h of stroke onset is almost completed.[20] The oral DTI ximelagatran that was shown to be non-inferior to warfarin for stroke prevention in patients with atrial fibrillation.[32] It has not been approved in the United States and Europe for this indication because of concerns of liver toxicity, however, and has been withdrawn from the European market where it was previously approved for DVT prevention after orthopedic surgery. Bivalirudin is now recognized as an alternative to GPIIb/IIIa antagonists in patients undergoing percutaneous coronary intervention (PCI), and seems to reduce bleeding risk.[22,33]

New factor Xa inhibitors include agents that block factor Xa indirectly or directly. Synthetic pentasaccharides (fondaparinux and idraparinux) inhibit factor Xa indirectly by activating ATIII. Idraparinux is being tested in a large phase III trial (AMADEUS, Atrial Fibrillation Trial of Monitored, Adjusted Dose Vitamin K Antagonist, Comparing Efficacy and safety with Unadjusted SanOrg 34006/idraparinux) for stroke prevention in atrial fibrillation;[34] it is injected subcutaneously once a week and does not require monitoring. Of the direct factor Xa inhibitors, parenteral active (DX-9065a) and orally active (DPC-906 and razaxaban) agents are currently undergoing phase II clinical trials. As with the DTIs, there are no antidotes. None of the factor Xa inhibitors is undergoing clinical trials for acute stroke. The same is true for most of the other new agents acting on the coagulation pathway listed in Table 11.3.

Potential use of current and new antithrombotics in acute stroke

Patient selection based on stroke pathophysiology may be as important as selection of the right type of new antithrombotic agent. New antithrombotics or new uses of existing antithrombotics probably have

Table 11.5 Potential uses of established and new antithrombotics. Any of these treatments may be combined with neuroprotection and/or treatments preventing hemorrhagic transformation

- Non-invasive recanalization:
  - Adjunct to fibrinolysis and defibrinogenation (with rtPA, desmoteplase, ancrod, etc.)
  - Adjunct to ultrasound-enhanced clot lysis

- Invasive recanalization:
  - Adjunct to mechanical recanalization (with clot retrievers, intravascular ultrasound, acute thrombendarterectomy, etc.)
  - Adjunct to intravascular fibrinolysis and defibrinogenation (with urokinase, rtPA, etc.)
  - Maintenance of patency after recanalization (with balloon angioplasty, stenting, intraarterial fibrinolysis, etc.)

- Acute clot and plaque stabilization, thereby preventing progression, reocclusion, and early recurrence:
  - Antiplatelet agents: alone or in combination with the above
  - Anticoagulants: alone or in combination with the above

the highest chance of being effective in acute stroke if used for patients with:

- a high risk of early recurrence, such as acutely symptomatic carotid stenosis
- a low risk of hemorrhagic transformation, such as TIA patients
- a high risk of progression, such as lacunar motor hemiparesis
- a high risk of reocclusion, such as after large vessel recanalization or intravascular procedures (balloon angioplasty and stenting)
- a short stroke-to-treatment time

An example of such a pathophysiology-based treatment approach is symptomatic carotid artery stenosis, in which the number of emboli reaching the brain can be significantly reduced by the use of two antiplatelet agents, rather than one.[35] Similarly, current trials randomizing patients to carotid stenting in the subacute phase of an ischemic event use double platelet anti-aggregants for a limited period (ICSS, International Carotid Stenting Study; SPACE, Stent-Protected Percutaneous Angioplasty of the Carotid vs Endarterectomy; EVA-3S, Endarterectomy Versus Angioplasty in Patients with Severe Symptomatic Carotid Stenosis; and CREST, Carotid Revascularisation Endarterectomy vs Stenting Trial). Unselected TIA patients have a lower risk for hemorrhagic transformation than patients with strokes, and are therefore appropriate candidates for testing acute double antiaggregants (FASTER[20] and ATARI[21]) or even triple antiaggregants (phase II trial; Professor P Bath, Nottingham, personal communication). Again, even though these approaches may be effective in

vitro,[36] this may not be the case in vivo.[37] The use of GPIIb/IIIa receptor antagonists in combination with fibrinolysis is also being studied (ROSIE, Reopro-reteplase Reperfusion of Stroke Safety Study; and CLEAR, The Combined Approach to Lysis Utilizing Eptifibatide and rt-PA in Acute Ischemic Stroke).[20]

In addition to the above-mentioned combinations of new antithrombotics, they may be used during or after invasive recanalization or ultrasound-enhanced clot lysis, together with neuroprotection or with agents preventing hemorrhagic transformation (Table 11.5).

Finally, the availability of new antithrombotics with diverse mechanisms of action may allow selection of a treatment strategy based on an individual's drug-response profile with the help of genomics and proteomics.[38]

Conclusions

New antithrombotic drugs have the potential to improve short- and long-term outcome in acute ischemic stroke. Higher antithrombotic specificity and the selection of patients with a high risk of early recurrence will increase their efficacy. Their safety may be increased by dose adjustment, avoiding the treatment of large-volume strokes, and the development of drugs acting on the blood–brain barrier to prevent hemorrhagic transformation. Antithrombotics may also be particularly useful in combinations or during a short high-risk period and after acute recanalization procedures.

References

1. Diener HC, Cunha L, Forbes C, et al. European Stroke Prevention Study. 2. Dipyridamole and acetylsalicylic acid in the secondary prevention of stroke. J Neurol Sci 1996;143:1–13.
2. Diener HC, Bogousslavsky J, Brass LM, et al. Aspirin and clopidogrel compared with clopidogrel alone after recent ischaemic stroke or transient ischaemic attack in high-risk patients (MATCH): randomised, double-blind, placebo-controlled trial. Lancet 2004;364:331–7.
3. Saxena R, Koudstaal PJ. Anticoagulants versus antiplatelet therapy for preventing stroke in patients with nonrheumatic atrial fibrillation and a history of stroke or transient ischemic attack. Stroke 2005;36: 914–15.
4. Mohr JP, Thompson JL, Lazar RM, et al. A comparison of warfarin and aspirin for the prevention of recurrent ischemic stroke (WARSS). N Engl J Med 2001;345:1444–51.
5. Chimowitz MI, Lynn MJ, Howlett-Smith H, et al. Comparison of warfarin and aspirin for symptomatic intracranial arterial stenosis. N Engl J Med 2005;352: 1305–16.
6. Chew DP, Bhatt DL, Sapp S, Topol EJ. Increased mortality with oral platelet glycoprotein IIb/IIIa antagonists: a meta-analysis of phase III multicenter randomized trials. Circulation 2001;103:201–6.
7. Topol EJ, Easton D, Harrington RA, et al. Randomized, double-blind, placebo-controlled, international trial of the oral IIb/IIIa antagonist lotrafiban in coronary and cerebrovascular disease (BRAVO). Circulation 2003;108:399–406.
8. IST Collaborative Group. The International Stroke Trial (IST): a randomised trial of aspirin, subcutaneous heparin, both, or neither among 19 435 patients with acute ischaemic stroke. Lancet 1997;349:1569–81.
9. CAST Collaborative Group. The Chinese Acute Stroke Trial (CAST): randomised placebo-controlled trial of early aspirin use in 20 000 patients with acute ischaemic stroke. Lancet 1997;349:1641–9.
10. Berge E, Sandercock P. Anticoagulants versus antiplatelet agents for acute ischaemic stroke. Cochrane Database Syst Rev 2002;(4):CD003242.
11. Sandercock P, Counsell C, Stobbs SL. Low-molecular-weight heparins or heparinoids versus standard unfractionated heparin for acute ischaemic stroke. Cochrane Database Syst Rev 2005;(2):CD000119.
12. Lovett JK, Dennis MS, Sandercock PA, et al. Very early risk of stroke after a first transient ischaemic attack. Stroke 2003;34:e138–40.
13. Rothwell PM, Eliasziw M, Gutnikov SA, et al. Endarterectomy for symptomatic carotid stenosis in relation to clinical subgroups and timing of surgery. Lancet 2004;363:915–24.
14. Toni D, Fiorelli M, Bastianello S, et al. Hemorrhagic transformation of brain infarct: predictability in the first 5 hours from stroke onset and influence on clinical outcome. Neurology 1996;46:341–5.
15. Montaner J, Molina CA, Monasterio J, et al. Matrix metalloproteinase-9 pretreatment level predicts intracranial hemorrhagic complications after thrombolysis in human stroke. Circulation 2003;107: 598–603.
16. Lapchak PA, Chapman DF, Zivin JA, Hsu CY. Metalloproteinase inhibition reduces thrombolytic (tissue plasminogen activator)-induced hemorrhage after thromboembolic stroke. Editorial Comment. Stroke 2000;31:3034–40.
17. Multicentre Acute Stroke Trial – Italy (MAST-I) Group. Randomised controlled trial of streptokinase, aspirin, and combination of both in treatment of acute ischaemic stroke. Lancet 1995;346:1509–14.
18. Donnan GA, Hommel M, Davis SM, McNeil JJ. Streptokinase in acute ischaemic stroke. Steering Committees of the ASK and MAST-E trials. Australian Streptokinase Trial. Lancet 1995;346:56.
19. MAST-E Study Group. Thrombolytic therapy with streptokinase in acute ischemic stroke (MAST-E). N Engl J Med 1996;335:145–50.
20. www.stroketrials.org.
21. Hankey GJ. Ongoing and planned trials of antiplatelet therapy in the acute and long-term management of patients with ischaemic brain syndromes: setting a new standard of care. Cerebrovasc Dis 2004;17(Suppl 3): 11–6.
22. Kelly RV, Steinhubl S. Changing roles of anticoagulant and antiplatelet treatment during percutaneous coronary intervention. Heart 2005;91(Suppl 3):iii16–19.
23. Sabatine MS, Cannon CP, Gibson CM, et al. Addition of clopidogrel to aspirin and fibrinolytic therapy for myocardial infarction with ST-segment elevation. N Engl J Med 2005;352:1179–89.
24. Sherman DG. Antithrombotic and hypofibrinogenetic therapy in acute ischemic stroke: What is the next step? Cerebrovasc Dis 2004;17(Suppl 1):138–43.
25. Sandercock P, Counsell C, Stobbs SL. Low-molecular-weight heparins or heparinoids versus standard unfractionated heparin for acute ischaemic stroke. Cochrane Database Syst Rev 2005;(2):CD000119.

26. Hirsh J, O' Donnell M, Weitz JI. New anticoagulants. Blood 2005;105:453–63.

27. Matias-Guiu J, Ferro JM, Alvarez-Sabin J, et al. Comparison of triflusal and aspirin for prevention of vascular events in patients after cerebral infarction: the TACIP study: a randomized, double-blind, multicenter trial. Stroke 2003;34:840–8.

28. Culebras A, Rotta-Escalante R, Vila J, et al. Triflusal vs aspirin for prevention of cerebral infarction: a randomized stroke study. Neurology 2004;62: 1073–80.

29. Kwon SU, Cho YJ, Koo JS, et al. Cilostazol prevents the progression of the symptomatic intracranial arterial stenosis: the multicenter double-blind placebo-controlled trial of cilostazol in symptomatic intracranial arterial stenosis. Stroke 2005;36:782–6.

30. Weitz JI, Hirsh J, Samama MM. New anticoagulant drugs: the Seventh ACCP Conference on Antithrombotic and Thrombolytic Therapy. Chest 2004;126 (3 Suppl):265S–86S.

31. LaMonte MP, Nash ML, Wang DZ, et al. Argatroban anticoagulation in patients with acute ischemic stroke (ARGIS-1): a randomized, placebo-controlled safety study. Stroke 2004;35:1677–82.

32. Hankey GJ, Klijn CJM, Eikelboom JW. Ximelagatran or warfarin for stroke prevention in patients with atrial fibrillation? Stroke 2004;35:389–91.

33. Lincoff AM, Bittl JA, Harrington RA, et al. Bivalirudin and provisional glycoprotein IIb/IIIa blockade compared with heparin and planned glycoprotein IIb/IIIa blockade during percutaneous coronary intervention: REPLACE-2 randomized trial. JAMA 2003;289:853–63.

34. www.clinicaltrials.gov.

35. Markus HS, Ringelstein EB. The effect of dual antiplatelet therapy compared with aspirin on asymptomatic embolisation in carotid stenosis: the CARESS trial. Cerebrovasc Dis 2004;17(Suppl 5):39.

36. Zhao L, Bath PM, Fox S, et al. The effects of GPIIb–IIIa antagonists and a combination of three other antiplatelet agents on platelet–leukocyte interactions. Curr Med Res Opin 2003;19:178–86.

37. Zhao L, Fletcher S, Weaver C, et al. Effects of aspirin, clopidogrel and dipyridamole administered singly and in combination on platelet and leucocyte function in normal volunteers and patients with prior ischaemic stroke. Thromb Haemost 2005;93:527–34.

38. Meschia JF. Clinically translated ischemic stroke genomics. Stroke 2004;35(11 Suppl 1):2735–9.

12

Fibrin-degrading drugs in acute stroke

László Csiba, György Németh, and Michael Hennerici

Introduction

Fibrinogen-depleting agents reduce fibrinogen in blood plasma, reduce blood viscosity, and hence increase blood flow. This may help remove a blood clot blocking an artery and re-establish blood flow to the affected area of the brain after an ischemic stroke. The risk of hemorrhage may be less than with thrombolytic agents.

Ancrod, a glycosylated 234-amino-acid thrombin-like enzyme (serine proteinase) obtained from the venom of the Malayan pit viper is highly specific to fibrinogen, producing anticoagulation by defibrinogenation. Other extracts from pit viper venom (e.g. batroxobin) have also been shown to cleave circulating fibrinogen rather than fibrin. These agents may be beneficial in patients with acute ischemic stroke, and indeed they are used to treat such patients in some countries.[1] Ancrod cleaves fibrinogen by splitting off A-fibrinopeptides (A, AY, and AP), but not B-fibrinopeptide. The resulting fibrin polymers are imperfectly formed and much smaller ($1–2\,\mu m$ long) than the fibrin polymers produced by the action of thrombin. These ancrod-induced micropolymers are friable, unstable, and urea-soluble, and have significantly degraded α-chains. They do not crosslink to form solid thrombi.

The extravascular diffusion volume of ancrod is approximately twice the volume of the intravascular space. Ancrod appears to be catabolized in the intravascular compartment; the resulting degradation products are excreted in the urine. Data suggest that phagocytosis followed by hydrolysis may take place in the reticuloendothelial system. Only a small percentage of the administered ancrod dose is excreted unchanged in the urine. After infusions of 0.5 IU/kg ancrod over 3 h, concentrations decrease with an estimated half-life of 20 h. Once the state of hypofibrinogenemia has been achieved with the induction dose, it can be maintained by giving intravenous injections at 12 h intervals or continuous intravenous infusions.

Ancrod does not directly degrade preformed, fully crosslinked fibrin polymers. Consequently, unlike fibrinolytic agents, it can be used after surgery. However, ancrod contributes to a reduction in the level of plasminogen activator inhibitor 1 (PAI-1) and a stimulation of the release of tissue-type plasminogen activator (tPA) from the endothelium. The profibrinolytic effect of these two actions appears to be limited to local microthrombus degradation. However, the extent and clinical significance of these effects remain to be established. Unlike thrombin, ancrod does not directly activate factor XIII, nor does it affect platelets or cause the release of ADP, ATP, potassium, or serotonin from platelets.

In patients receiving ancrod, blood viscosity is progressively reduced by 30–40% of pretreatment levels. The diminished viscosity is directly attributable to the lowered fibrinogen levels and leads to an important improvement in blood flow and microcirculation. Erythrocyte flexibility is not affected by normal doses of ancrod. The rheological changes are readily sustained, and viscosity approaches pretreatment values very slowly (in about 10 days) after stopping ancrod.

General toxicology studies in a variety of laboratory animals have not displayed any evidence of target organ

Table 12.1   The most important clinical trials of ancrod in ischemic stroke

| Authors | No. of patients treated | Route duration | Bleeding | | Deaths |
			Major	Minor	
Hossmann et al[2] (single-blinded)	15 ancrod and dextran + mannitol	SC 14 days IV 10 days	0	0	2 (within 2 weeks)
	15 Placeabo and dextran + mannitol	SC, 14 days, IV, 10 days	0	0	5 (within 2 weeks)
Olinger et al[6]; Pollack et al[7] (double-blinded)	10 ancrod 10 placebo	IV, 7 days IV, 7 days	0 0	0 0	0 0
Ancrod Study investigators; (double-blinded)	64 ancrod 68 placebo	IV, NR IV, NR	0 2	23 events 11 events	8[a] (12%) 14[a] (21%)
STAT(Stroke Treatment with Ancrod Trial)[9,10] (double-blinded)	248 ancrod[b] 252 placebo[b]	IV, 72 h followed by intermittent infusions at 96 h (±6 h) and 120 h (±6 h) after start of therapy	27[c] (10.9%) 13[c] (5.2%)	186[c] (75%) 157[c] (62.3%)	63[d] (25.4%) 58[d] (23.0%)
ESTAT (European Stroke Treatment with Ancrod Trial)[11]	604 ancrod 618 placebo	72 h continuous + 48 h intermittent fibrinogen-adjusted ancrod IV	Symptomatic or asymptomatic bleeding: 12.7% ancrod 3.7% placebo ($p < 0.01$)		251 ancrod (1 year) 231 placebo (1 year)

NR, not reported.
[a]1-year mortality.
[b]1 patient in the ancrod group had a seizure; 1 patient in the placebo group had a new stroke at 3 months.
[c]Study drug + 28-day period.
[d]Mortality at 3 months.

or systemic toxicity of ancrod. Being a protein, ancrod induces immunological reactions resulting in the formation of neutralizing antibodies that lead to the development of resistance to ancrod. No mutagenic potential has been verified.

The principal side-effect of ancrod is bleeding. Ancrod may cause hematuria, and in rare cases melena, epistaxis, and hematemesis. Bleeding at puncture and instrumentation sites may occur. Fibrinogen values below 20 mg/dl have been reported to be associated with increased bleeding.

Other, less frequent, side-effects include headache and skin rash or urticaria. Fever, chills, and arthritis have rarely been reported. Hepatic, renal, and pancreatic function are not altered by ancrod.

In this chapter, we wish to summarize the most important clinical observations about the effectiveness and safety of ancrod in acute ischemic stroke trials, with special emphasis on the following questions:

- Does ancrod reduce the long-term risk of death and disability, without an increased risk of early death?
- Does the risk of hemorrhage outweigh the benefits?

Clinical data in ischemic stroke

Experimental and clinical studies have demonstrated that changes in blood viscosity affect cerebral blood flow.[2] Since fibrinogen is a major contributor to blood viscosity,[3] its reduction is associated with a decrease in apparent blood viscosity and enhancement of local blood flow.[4,5]

Ancrod plus dextran plus mannitol therapy[2]

A randomized, single-blinded study was undertaken to investigate the effectiveness of ancrod in acute cerebrovascular ischemic stroke. Thirty patients were treated within 48 h of stroke onset. The patients group received 1 IU/kg ancrod daily until plasma fibrinogen was between 100 and 130 mg/dl; thereafter a maintenance dose of ancrod was administered to keep fibrinogen within the target range for 14 days. The control group (15 subjects) received daily infusions of low-molecular-weight dextran and mannitol over the first 10 days, while the treatment group (15 subjects) received the above in combination with subcutaneous ancrod.

The combined therapy with ancrod added to low-molecular-weight dextran and mannitol produced a significant reduction in viscosity and plasminogen, but had no effect on coagulation and platelet function tests.

The placebo group improved by a mean of 1.1 AU (arbitrary unit of neurological score) and the ancrod group by 2.4 AU, and a reduction in mortality (5 of 15 in the control group vs 2 of 15 in the ancrod group) could also be observed, but the differences were not significant. While no overall difference was noted between the groups, survival at 14 days in patients with severe neurological deficits was higher in the ancrod group (4 of 6) than in the control group (2 of 6).

The results demonstrate that combined therapy reduces blood viscosity. The positive effects of ancrod were possibly related to its anticoagulant and fibrinolytic activity, since clinical improvement preceded the observed reduction in viscosity. A more rapid improvement of neurological deficits and a decrease in mortality were observed in the ancrod group.

Fibrin-degrading therapy initiated within 48 h after stroke onset[6,7]

Twenty acute ischemic stroke patients were randomized and treated either with placebo or 0.5 IU/kg ancrod on the first day of ischemic stroke. For the next 6 days, ancrod or placebo was given intravenously once or twice, titrated to maintain the plasma fibrinogen level at approximately 1.0 g/l. The mean fibrinogen level was 116 mg/dl at 6 h, 52 mg/dl at 24 h, and 67–110 mg/dl on days 2–8.

There was no evidence of bleeding, abnormal laboratory results, or rethrombosis during ancrod administration. A modified stroke scale showed a nonsignificant 30% difference in average neurological outcome at 3 months, with the ancrod group showing better outcomes than the controls. In moderate and severe stroke, subgroup improvement in the ancrod-treated group was three times better than that in the placebo group.

Fibrin-degrading therapy initiated within 6 h after stroke onset[8]

A multicenter, double-blinded randomized trial was performed to determine whether ancrod conferred improved neurological outcome that exceeded any adverse consequences of the therapy. One hundred and thirty-two ischemic stroke patients were treated with intravenous ancrod or placebo within 6 h of the onset of an acute ischemic event. Patients with mild strokes (Scandinavian Stroke Scale (SSS) ≥40) or with hemorrhagic stroke on computed tomography (CT) scan were excluded, but patients with CT signs of evolving brain infarction were not. The initial infusion of ancrod was 0.5 IU/kg over 6 h, followed by daily, 30 min infusions to maintain fibrinogen at 70–100 mg/dl. The primary endpoint was an improvement in neurological deficits assessed by the SSS Score, excluding gait at 3 months. Neurological outcome, disability, and brain infarct volume were measured.

Although the baseline-corrected 3-month SSS Score was higher in ancrod-treated than in placebo-treated patients, *this difference was not significant*. The median 3-month Barthel Index was better in ancrod than in placebo patients. Ancrod patients attaining 6 h fibrinogen levels at or below the median value of 130 mg/dl had a median Barthel Index at 3 months of 95 (a perfect score in this study), compared with a median of 75 for ancrod patients with fibrinogen levels above the median.

The 1-year mortality appeared to be somewhat lower in the ancrod group (8 of 64) than in the placebo group (14 of 68). The infarct volume on CT was significantly less in the ancrod group (13.3 cm³) compared with the placebo one (30.6 cm³). Clinically important bleeding complications were not increased

Table 12.2 Clinical scales and infarct volumes in the ancrod and placebo groups in STAT

	Ancrod	Placebo	P
Scandinavian Stroke Scale Score	36.7	33.6	0.159
Barthel Index	79.5	66.5	0.057
Infarct Volume (cm³)	31.9	42.0	0.135

in the ancrod-treated group. There was no statistically significant differences in neurological stroke scale scores between the two groups. In the ancrod-treated patients with plasma fibrinogen levels below the median of 130 mg/dl, the difference favoring ancrod for SSS Score, mortality, and Barthel Index just missed significance.

Fibrin-degrading therapy initiated within 3 h after stroke onset[9,10]

STAT (Stroke Treatment with Ancrod Trial) was a multicenter, parallel-group, sequential, double-blinded, randomized, placebo-controlled study of safety and efficacy of intravenous ancrod given within 3 h after the onset of acute, ischemic stroke. Five hundred patients were enrolled in the study. Ischemic stroke patients had a neurological deficit lasting longer than 30 min and occurring within 3 h prior to drug administration.

The study involved a 5-day treatment period followed by a 3-month follow-up. The target fibrinogen range was 40–69 mg/dl.

Defibrinogenation was induced with one of three initial infusion rates based on the pretreatment fibrinogen level: 0.083 IU/kg/h, 0.125 IU/kg/h, and 0.167 IU/kg/h. The infusion was continued for 72 h, followed by intermittent infusions administered at 96 (±6) and 120 (±6) h after the start of blinded therapy. The dosing regimen permitted frequent regulation of infusion rates on the basis of fibrinogen levels in order to achieve controlled defibrinogenation to levels of 40–69 mg/dl.

The primary efficacy variable was defined as survival for 90 days with a Barthel Index (BI) of 95–100, or at least as high as the prestroke BI. Secondary efficacy variables were the Barthel Index (at 3 months), Scandinavian Stroke Scale (SSS) Score (at 3 days and

3 months), and CT infarct volume (at 7–10 days). (Table 12.2). Safety variables were mortality, adverse events, laboratory evaluations, vital signs, electocardiogram (ECG), neurological examination, and CT/magnetic resonance imaging (MRI) findings. The mean age of patients was 72.8 years; 63.8% had a moderate to severe stroke as indicated by a SSS Score of 0–29.

Ancrod was shown to be effective in improving functional outcome, defined as Barthel Index ≥95 in patients with acute ischemic stroke. Based on the prespecified primary efficacy endpoint, ancrod was superior to placebo ($p = 0.041$).

Ancrod-treated patients had a greater improvement in neurological function than placebo-treated patients at 3 months. A higher proportion of ancrod patients achieved treatment success than placebo patients in all patient subsets characterized by age category, pretreatment SSS category, sex, early infarct signs on pretreatment CT scan, and time to treatment. There was a strong association between treatment success and fibrinogen levels 130 mg/dl or less at 6 h ($p = 0.079$) or less than 70 mg/dl at 9 h (target fibrinogen; $p = 0.073$), independent of the effects of age and pretreatment stroke severity.

In general, the incidence of serious adverse events for the two treatment groups was similar (31.9% ancrod vs 29.0% placebo) (Table 12.3). Bleeding adverse events occurred more often in ancrod patients, with women appearing to have more bleeding adverse events than men.

In summary, the use of ancrod appeared to be associated with an increased risk of bleeding, including intracranial hemorrhage, especially if fibrinogen levels were reduced to below 40 mg/dl. This bleeding risk, however, was not associated with an increase in mortality.

ESTAT (European Stroke Treatment with Ancrod Trial)[11]

This study was a multicenter, prospective, randomized, double-blinded, placebo-controlled, parallel-group comparison to determine the therapeutic efficacy and safety of intravenous ancrod in patients with acute ischemic (nonhemorrhagic) cerebral infarction, with the drug being given within 6 h after the onset of acute ischemic stroke. It was planned to

Table 12.3   Intracranial hemorrhage and mortality in the ancrod and placebo groups in STAT

	Ancrod	Placebo
Intracranial hemorrhage	59	32
Discontinuation of study drug	30	22
7-day mortality rate	8.9%	9.5%
30-day mortality rate	19.0%	19.8%
1-year mortality rate	32.7%	32.5%
Symptomatic intracranial hemorrhage	13	5

randomize 1680 eligible patients with a treatment ratio of 1:1 (ancrod : placebo). The study course comprised four different periods:

- a 72 h in-house period with continuous infusions
- a 48 h in-house period with intermittent infusions
- a 24 h in-house post-treatment observation period
- a 1-year outpatient follow-up period, including a 3-month follow-up visit

A CT scan was performed, and all patients underwent a complete neurological examination and standardized SSS assessment.

- The initial infusion schedule was based on baseline plasma fibrinogen level and body weight. Plasma fibrinogen levels were measured after 3 h and 6 h, and infusion schedules were adjusted to the measured fibrinogen levels. The goal was to lower plasma fibrinogen levels successively to the range 40–70 mg/dl.
- Within the first 6 h, ancrod infusion was started; plasma fibrinogen measurements, neurological examination, and standardized SSS assessment were performed during the visits at 24, 48 and 72 h. In total, continuous infusion lasted for 72 h.
- Following the 72 h continuous infusion, the schemes were adjusted according to the measured fibrinogen levels, and blood pressure/vital sign measurements, physical/neurological examination, and standardized SSS assessment were performed.
- During the visit at day 7, an additional CT scan was performed; activities of daily living, Rapid

Disability Rating Scale, and handicap were assessed; and blood for baseline laboratory tests was drawn.
- The 1-year outpatient follow-up period included a 3-month follow-up visit and a 1-year final visit.

Primary efficacy variable

This was:
- day-90 Barthel Index ≥ 95; or, if not,
- day-90 Barthel Index ≥ prestroke value

Secondary efficacy variables

These were:
- 3-month SSS (excluding gait)
- 3 month death rates
- success in the Rankin Scale at 3 months – specifically success defined as achievement of a score of 1

Results

A total of 1222 patients were enrolled in this study: 604 were randomized to ancrod and 618 to placebo. All 1222 randomized patients took at least one dose of study medication and were included in the full analysis set. The treatment groups were similar regarding pretreatment systolic and diastolic blood pressures and heart rate. With regard to the baseline assessments of the efficacy parameters Barthel Index, SSS, etc., both treatment groups were comparable, without showing a statistically significant difference in any of the parameters. There was no statistically significant difference between the treatment groups concerning previous and concomitant medication.

Treatment success, defined as survival and a Barthel Index of 95 or more, or return to at least the prestroke level, did not differ between treatment with ancrod and placebo ($p = 0.7710$). Success rates were similar (ancrod 43.6% vs placebo 44.4%), and, therefore, an active treatment effect was not detected.

When analyzing functional success in different selected subgroups (baseline fibrinogen class, prestroke performance class, and time to treatment), statistically significant superiority of a treatment with ancrod was not obtained in any of these groups.

Secondary and other efficacy parameters

Analysis of the secondary efficacy parameter Rankin Scale did not show statistically significant superiority of ancrod versus placebo. This was the case for both the overall evaluation and the analysis of any of the predefined subgroups.

The SSS Scores were comparable between the treatment groups at baseline. After 3 months' treatment, higher scores were observed in both groups, but the improvements in the placebo group exceeded those of the active treatment (Table 12.4).

Barthel Index total score

The statistical analysis of the Barthel Index total score at day 7, 7 months, or 1 year did not reveal statistically significant differences between the treatment groups (Table 12.5).

Mortality (3 months and 1 year)

Analysis of mortality showed that at 1 year, the difference between the treatment groups was not statistically significant, but mortality was higher in the ancrod group when compared with placebo (Table 12.6).

Efficacy conclusions

In ESTAT, no superiority of ancrod versus placebo in improving functional outcome in patients with acute ischemic stroke was detectable. Treatment success (survival and a Barthel Index ≥ 95 or return to at least the prestroke level at 3 months) did not differ between treatment with ancrod and placebo ($p = 0.7710$), either in the overall evaluation or in selected subgroups.

The findings regarding the secondary parameters of efficacy did not differ from the analysis of the primary parameter. With respect to Rankin Scale, SSS, Barthel Index total score, and Rapid Disability Rating Scale, no statistically significant differences in the sense of a superiority of the active treatment were found.

Safety conclusions

The frequency of serious adverse events was similar in both groups, while bleeding events were higher in

Table 12.4   Scandinavian Stroke Scale (SSS) Scores in ESTAT

SSS Score	Ancrod	Placebo
Baseline	26.6 ± 9.5	27.0 ± 9.1
Day 7	30.1 ± 14.4	31.1 ± 13.7
3 months	30.3 ± 17.7	32.4 ± 16.1
1 year	29.1 ± 19.3	30.7 ± 18.4

Table 12.5   Barthel Index changes in ESTAT

Barthel Index	Ancrod	Placebo
Baseline (prestroke)	98.3 ± 8.3	98.5 ± 7.4
Day 7	45.6 ± 39.3	48.9 ± 39.3
3 months	60.2 ± 42.7	63.2 ± 41.2
1 year	59.9 ± 45.0	62.0 ± 43.7

Table 12.6   One-year mortality in ESTAT

	Ancrod	Placebo	Total
Dead	151	131	282
Lost to follow-up	19	17	36
Alive	434	470	904
			($p = 0.2462$)[a]

[a]p-value of χ^2 test: ancrod vs placebo.

the ancrod group when compared with placebo. This was also the case for symptomatic and asymptomatic intracranial hemorrhage, where statistically significant higher frequencies were documented for ancrod (Table 12.7).

The whole-study mortality rate in the ancrod group exceeded the placebo mortality rate. No treatment-specific differences were found with respect to the hematological parameters analyzed or for ECG parameters.

Comments

The objective of ESTAT was to determine the therapeutic efficacy and safety of intravenously administered ancrod (given within 6 h after the onset of acute ischemic stroke) in patients with acute ischemic (non-hemorrhagic) cerebral infarction.

Table 12.7 Symptomatic or asymptomatic intracranial hemorrhage (ICH) in ESTAT

	Ancrod	Placebo	Total
No. of patients	604	618	1222
Patients with symptomatic or asymptomatic ICH	12.7%	3.7%	($p<0.01$)

Similar dosing schedules in 500 patients had been investigated in a previous clinical study without revealing safety concerns. In this study, which was performed partly in parallel, the efficacy of ancrod in improving functional outcome in patients with acute ischemic stroke was shown and was superior to placebo with statistical significance. Ancrod-treated patients had a significantly higher model-adjusted treatment success rate (Barthel index) at 3 months than placebo.

The design of ESTAT was similar to the design of the previous study, but the positive results obtained there could not be repeated.

The improvement in functional outcome in patients with acute ischemic stroke treated with ancrod was not superior to that in those treated with placebo. The results with regard to survival, a Barthel Index of 95 or more (or a return to at least the pre-stroke level at 3 months), Rankin Scale, SSS, Barthel Index total score, and Rapid Disability Rating Scale were in no case in favor of ancrod.

The overall evaluation was negative for ancrod concerning the main parameter of efficacy. In addition, none of the secondary parameters was in favor of ancrod. Furthermore, it was not possible to find positive effects of ancrod versus placebo in any of the subgroups analyzed. These negative results, which were also associated with higher mortality rates and higher frequencies of bleeding events and symptomatic and asymptomatic intracranial hemorrhage, made it necessary to stop the study following the results of an interim analysis.

Recent observations

Recent efforts have attempted to identify new thrombolytics that might improve the benefit/risk ratio in treating stroke.[12] Second-generation derivatives of alteplase have attempted to counteract the side effects of the drug by increasing fibrin specificity (tenecteplase, TNK-tPA) or half-life (lanoteplase, SUN-9216).[13] New recombinant DNA methodology has led to the revival of plasmin or a truncated form of plasmin (microplasmin), a direct-acting thrombolytic with non-thrombolytic related neuroprotective activities.[13] Other promising approaches for the treatment of stroke include the development of novel plasminogen activators, such as recombinant *Desmodus rotundus* salivary plasminogen activator (rDSPA) α_1 (desmotoplase) and a mutant fibrin-activated human plasminogen (BB10153).[14]

Tenecteplase is a genetically engineered mutant tPA that has a longer half-life, is more fibrin-specific, and is more resistant to PAI-1 than recombinant tPA (rtPA). A pilot dose-escalation safety study of tenecteplase in patients with acute ischemic stroke demonstrated its safety and tolerability at several doses.[15] No symptomatic intracranial hemorrhages were observed among any of the 75 patients treated with 0.1 mg/kg, 0.2 mg/kg, or 0.4 mg/kg tenecteplase, a fourfold range of doses begun with a dose calculated to be bioequivalent to the approved dose of rtPA for stroke. The modified Rankin Scores at 3 months were similar to those of controls treated with rtPA and not significantly different between treatment groups. Tenecteplase doses of 0.1–0.4 mg/kg are safe in ischemic stroke.

Because of its high fibrin specificity, nonactivation by β-amyloid, and long terminal half-life, desmoteplase is an attractive thrombolytic agent.[14] Another possible advantage is the absence of neurotoxicity compared with rtPA.

The DIAS (Desmoteplase In Acute Ischemic Stroke) study suggested that intravenous thrombolysis with desmoteplase 3–9 h after stroke onset is safe in patients selected according to perfusion/diffusion mismatch on MRI and that dose-dependent reperfusion on MRI is correlated with clinical outcome.[16] The symptomatic intracranial hemorrhage rate with desmoteplase was low, using doses up to 125 mg/kg.

General conclusions

The principal hypothesis that defibrinogenation leads to improved clinical outcome has not been fully tested in present study designs. The studies did not assess recanalization. The studies reviewed here only partly and inconclusively suggest potential benefits.[17] No direct comparison with thrombolytic drugs has been performed – this is obviously an important area for further evaluation.

The North American database suggests efficacy and safety with ancrod to 3.5 h after stroke onset. The European database requires further exploration; overdosing probably explains the disappointing results.

Recently, the nihilistic attitude toward treatment of acute ischemic stroke has been decreasing, and much of this progress is directly attributable to innovative, high-quality clinical trials. However, the important studies provide equally compelling lessons and much needed cautions regarding extending thrombolytic therapy for stroke to routine clinical practice. Patients will derive optimal benefit from hyperacute treatment of stroke only with careful patient selection, individualized therapy according to the causative lesion, strict adherence to treatment guidelines, and evidence-based therapeutic decision making and drug administration by physicians with experience using these new agents and interventions.

References

1. Chen ZM, Sandercock P, Xie JX, et al. Hospital management of acute ischemic stroke in China. J Stroke Cerebrovasc Dis 1997;6: 361–7.
2. Hossmann V, Heiss WD, Bewermeyer H, Wiedemann G. Controlled trial of ancrod in ischemic stroke. Arch Neurol 1983;40:803–8.
3. Dormandy JA, Reid HL. Controlled defibrination in the treatment of peripheral vascular disease. Angiology 1978;29:80–8.
4. Schmid-Schonbein H, Wells RE Jr. Rheological properties of human erythrocytes and their influence upon the 'anomalous' viscosity of blood. Ergeb Physiol 1971; 63:146–219.
5. Ehrly AM. Improvement of the flow properties of blood: a new therapeutical approach in occlusive arterial disease. Angiology 1976;27:188–96.
6. Olinger CP, Brott TG, Barsan WG, et al. Use of ancrod in acute or progressing ischemic cerebral infarction. Ann Emerg Med 1988;17:1208–9.
7. Pollak VE, Glas-Greenwalt P, Olinger CP, et al. Ancrod causes rapid thrombolysis in patients with acute stroke. Am J Med Sci 1990;299:319–25.
8. Ancrod for the treatment of acute ischemic brain infarction. The Ancrod Study Investigators. Stroke 1994; 25:1755–9.
9. Sherman DG, for the STAT Writers Group. Defibrinogenation with Viprinex™ (ancrod) for the treatment of acute ischemic stroke. Presented at 24th International Joint Conference of Stroke and Cerebral Circulation, Nashville, TN, February 4, 1999. Stroke 1999;30:234.
10. Sherman DG, Atkinson RP, Chippendale T, et al. Intravenous ancrod for treatment of acute ischemic stroke: the STAT study: a randomized controlled trial. Stroke Treatment with Ancrod Trial. JAMA 2000;283: 2395–403.
11. Orgogozo JM, Verstraete M, Kay R, et al. Outcomes of ancrod in acute ischemic stroke. Independent Data and Safety Monitoring Board for ESTAT. Steering Committee for ESTAT. European Stroke Treatment with Ancrod Trial. JAMA 2000;284:1926–7.
12. Lapchak PA. Development of thrombolytic therapy for stroke: a perspective. Expert Opin Invest Drugs 2002;11:1623–32.
13. Sheehan JJ, Tsirka SE. Fibrin-modifying serine proteases, thrombin, tPA, and plasmin in ischemic stroke: a review. Glia 2005;50:340–50.
14. Grandjean C, McMullen PC, Newschwander G. Vampire bats yield potent clot buster for ischemic stroke. J Cardiovasc Nurs 2004;19:417–20.
15. Haley EC Jr, Lyden PD, Johnston KC, Hemmen TM (TNK in Stroke Investigators). A pilot dose-escalation safety study of tenecteplase in acute ischemic stroke. Stroke 2005;36:607–12.
16. Hacke W, Albers G, Al-Rawi Y, et al. The Desmoteplase in Acute Ischemic Stroke Trial (DIAS): a phase II MRI-based 9-hour window acute stroke thrombolysis trial with intravenous desmoteplase. DIAS Study Group. Stroke 2005;36:66–73.
17. Sherman DG. Antithrombotic and hypofibrinogenetic therapy in acute ischemic stroke: what is the next step? Cerebrovasc Dis 2004, 17 Suppl 1:138–43.

13

Thrombolytic therapy for acute stroke: the studies

Peter D Schellinger, Jochen B Fiebach, and Peter A Ringleb

Introduction

The characterization of potentially reversible versus irreversible loss of function is based on the concept of the ischemic penumbra.[1] Until recently, only positron emission tomography (PET) and single photon emission computed tomography (SPECT) imaging could approximately define ischemia and penumbra thresholds. This is, however, not feasible for emergency services for broad populations, where imaging in an acute setting is confined to computed tomography (CT) and also increasingly magnetic resonance imaging (MRI). Only the advent of new imaging techniques such as novel MRI sequences and continuing improvement of imaging hardware allows improvement in diagnostic yield. An adequate therapy demands an adequate diagnostic workup first. For readers interested in a more detailed coverage of this topic, including the basics of the novel imaging techniques presented in this overview, two textbooks are now available, both published in 2003.[2,3]

Thrombolytic therapy for ischemic stroke: the data

The underlying rationale for the introduction and application of thrombolytic agents is the lysis of a thrombus and subsequent re-establishment of cerebral blood flow by cerebrovascular recanalization.[4,5] The local delivery of thrombolytic agents, at or within the thrombus (intra-arterial thrombolysis), has the advantage of providing a higher concentration of the particular thrombolytic agent where it is needed while minimizing the concentration systemically. Hence, local intra-arterial thrombolysis has the potential for greater efficacy with higher arterial recanalization rates and greater safety with lower risk of hemorrhage. The technique involves performing a cerebral arteriogram, localizing the occluding clot, navigating a microcatheter to the site of the clot, and administering the lytic agent at or inside the clot with or without mechanical destruction of the thrombus.

Randomized trials of intravenous thrombolysis

The first anecdotal report of thrombolytic therapy for ischemic stroke dates back to the early 1960s.[6] Three trials in the early 1980s investigated the effect of low-dose intravenous urokinase for the therapy of acute ischemic stroke.[7–9] These trials differ from others for several reasons, such as a late timepoint of inclusion (up to 5 or 14 days after stroke onset, respectively), the exclusion of presumed cardioembolic stroke, application of low doses of urokinase given daily for a period of several days, and the lack of assessment of clinical outcome except death and intracranial hemorrhage (ICH). In the early 1990s, three small trials of intravenous thrombolysis with recombinant tissue-type plasminogen activator (rtPA) were carried out, two of them in Japan.[10–12] Although not large enough to prove efficacy, they clearly showed the feasibility of early thrombolytic therapy and also suggested a reasonable degree of safety and a potential benefit. All of these trials were blinded or double-blinded, randomized, and placebo-controlled.

One pilot study and three large trials investigated the efficacy of streptokinase for acute ischemic stroke.[13–16] In summary, all of the trials using streptokinase for acute ischemic stroke were stopped prematurely due to a high rate of early death, mostly due to ICH, and because of a lack of benefit at outcome in a meta-analysis as well.[17] In the streptokinase trials together, there were 92 (95% confidence interval (CI) 65–120) additional fatal ICH per 1000 treated patients (odds ratio (OR) 6.03, 95% CI 3.47–10.47).[18] The higher bleeding rate may be due to pharmacological properties of streptokinase other than, for instance, those of rtPA, additional anticoagulation (in MAST-E: Multicenter Acute Stroke Trial – Europe), a rather small fraction of patients treated within 3 h, and a rather high dose of 1.5 MU, which is identical to the dose used in myocardial infarction (MI), whereas the rtPA studies (see below) chose approximately two-thirds the dose used in MI. Other side-effects of streptokinase are a decrease in systolic blood pressure of more than 20 mmHg in 33% (only 6% in the placebo group), as well as anaphylaxis in 2.2% of the patients. Therefore, intravenous administration of streptokinase, outside the setting of a clinical investigation, is dangerous and not indicated for the management of patients with ischemic stroke.

In 1995, the results of ECASS I (European Cooperative Acute Stroke Study) and the NINDS (National Institute of Neurological Disorders and Stroke) trial of intravenous rtPA for acute ischemic stroke were published,[19,20] and were followed by ECASS II in 1998[21] and the ATLANTIS (Alteplase Thrombolysis for Acute Noninterventional Therapy in Ischemic Stroke) study in 1999.[22] These four trials randomized a total of 2657 patients to treatment with placebo (1316 patients) or intravenous rtPA (1341 patients) within 0–3 h (NINDS), 3–5 h (ATLANTIS), or 0–6 h (ECASS I and II) after symptom onset. All four studies required a baseline CT scan to exclude ICH, and, except for the NINDS study, all others also established CT exclusion criteria such as major early signs of infarction. All trials used the 0.9 mg/kg bodyweight dose up to a maximum of 90 mg rtPA,

except ECASS I, in which 1.1 mg/kg up to a maximum dose of 100 mg was given. Ten percent of the total dose was given as a bolus; the rest was infused over 1 h in all four trials.

The NINDS trial randomized 624 patients (312 each placebo and intravenous rtPA) within a time window of 3 h after stroke symptom onset.[19] Half of the patients were treated within 0–90 min and the other half within 91–180 min. A good outcome was defined as a National Institutes of Health Stroke Scale (NIHSS) Score ≤ 1, Glasgow Outcome Score (GOS) = 1, Barthel Index (BI) ≥ 95, and modified Rankin Score (mRS) ≤ 1. The median baseline NIHSS Score was 14 (rtPA group) versus 15 (placebo group). There was no significant difference between the drug treatment and placebo group in the percentages of patients with neurologic improvement at 24 h (rtPA 47% vs placebo 57%; relative risk (RR) 1.2, $p = 0.21$), although a post hoc analysis comparing the median NIHSS Scores at 24 h showed a median of 8 in the rtPA-treated group versus 12 in the placebo group ($p < 0.02$). Furthermore, a benefit was observed for the rtPA group at 3 months for all four outcome measures. The long-term clinical benefit of rtPA was confirmed in all single scores as well as in the global test: BI (50% vs 38%; OR 1.6 (95% CI 1.1–2.5), $p = 0.026$); mRS (39% vs 26%; OR 1.7 (95% CI 1.1–2.5), $p = 0.019$); GOS (44% vs 32%; OR 1.6 (95% CI 1.1–2.5), $p = 0.025$); NIHSS (31% vs 20%; OR 1.7 (95% CI 1.0–2.8), $p = 0.033$); and combined endpoint (OR 1.7 (95% CI 1.2–2.6), $p = 0.008$). For every 100 patients treated with rtPA, an additional 11–13 will have a favorable outcome, as compared with 100 not treated with rtPA. Outcome did not vary by stroke subtype at baseline, meaning that patients with small-vessel disease benefited as well as patients with, for instance, cardioembolic stroke. On the other hand, small-vessel disease was clinically defined and not by imaging studies. Symptomatic ICH within 36 h after the onset of stroke occurred in 6.4% of patients given rtPA, but in only 0.6% of patients given placebo ($p < 0.001$). Nevertheless, severe disability and death were higher in the nontreated group (mortality at 3 months: rtPA 17% vs placebo 21%; $p = 0.30$). After publication of the NINDS trial in 1996, rtPA received US Food and Drug Administration (FDA) approval for the treatment of acute ischemic stroke in a time window of 3 h.

ECASS I, a prospective, multicenter, randomized, double-blind, placebo-controlled trial, recruited 620 patients for treatment either with 1.1 mg/kg rtPA or placebo within 6 h after stroke symptom onset.[20] Anticoagulants, neuroprotectants, and rheologic therapy were prohibited during the first 24 h. Patients with a severe deficit (hemiplegia, forced head and eye movement, or impairment of consciousness), with only mild or improving stroke symptoms, or with CT signs of early infarction exceeding 33% of the middle cerebral artery (MCA) territory were excluded. Primary endpoints included a difference of 15 points in the BI and 1 point in the MRS at 90 days in favor of rtPA. Secondary endpoints included combined BI and MRS, Scandinavian Stroke Scale (SSS) at 90 days, and 30-day mortality. In anticipation of a substantial number of protocol violations due to the first-time early CT signs of infarction were being used as an inclusion criterion, the investigators prospectively specified a target population (TP) analysis in addition to the primary intention-to-treat (ITT) analysis, which was performed at the end of the trial. The median NIHSS Scores at baseline were 13 (rtPA patients) and 12 (placebo group), respectively. ECASS I was the first trial of thrombolysis to use CT exclusion criteria.[23–26] In spite of these predefined parameters, there were 109 protocol violations in ECASS I (17.4%), 66 (11%) of which were CT protocol violations, 52 (8.4%) of these being due to maldetection of early infarct signs. There was no difference in the primary endpoints in the ITT analysis, while the TP analysis revealed a significant difference in the mRS (but not BI) in favor of rtPA-treated patients ($p = 0.035$). Of the secondary endpoints, the combined BI and MRS showed a difference in favor of rtPA-treated patients ($p < 0.001$). Neurologic recovery at 90 days was significantly better for rtPA-treated patients in the TP ($p = 0.03$). There was a nonsignificant trend towards a higher mortality rate at 30 days ($p = 0.08$) and a significant increase in parenchymal ICH (19.8% vs 6.5%; $p < 0.001$). There was a significant inverse relationship between protocol violation in rtPA-treated patients and 7-day survival. A post hoc analysis of the ECASS I 3 h cohort (87 patients) did not reveal a significant difference between rtPA and placebo group outcomes.[27]

ECASS II randomized a total of 800 patients (409 rtPA and 391 placebo) to treatment with either 0.9 mg/kg rtPA or placebo within 6 h (stratified into a 0–3 h and a 3–6 h group) after stroke symptom onset.[21] The primary endpoint was the mRS at 90 days, dichotomized for favorable (Score 0–1) and unfavorable (Score 2–6) outcome. Analyses were by ITT, and an 8% absolute difference was aimed for in the primary endpoint. Secondary endpoints were a combined BI and MRS at day 90 and NIHSS Score at day 30. A post hoc analysis requested by the board of reviewers was performed for an alternative dichotomization into independent versus death and dependent outcome (mRS 0–2 vs 3–6). The baseline median NIHSS Score was 11 in both groups, which is 2–3 points less than in NINDS and ECASS I. The safety analysis showed a similar mortality rate in the two groups (10.5% vs 10.7%): there were substantially more fatal ICH in the rtPA group (11 vs 2 patients), whereas fewer patients died due to space-occupying brain edema (8 vs 17 patients). There was a fourfold increase in symptomatic parenchymal ICH (48 vs 12 patients) in the rtPA group, which was a far lower rate than in ECASS I. The primary endpoint was negative for rtPA (mRS 0–1: 40.3% vs 36.6%; $\Delta = 3.7\%$; $p = 0.277$). There was a trend for the combined BI/mRS endpoint ($p = 0.098$) and a significant difference in day-30 NIHSS Score ($p = 0.035$). With the alternative dichotomization, a significant advantage for patients treated with rtPA (mRS 0–2: 54.3% vs 46.0%; $\Delta = 8.3\%$; $p = 0.024$) was demonstrated. As in ECASS I, the 3 h cohort did not show any significant differences, due to the small patient numbers (80 patients per group). Symptomatic ICH occurred in 36 (8.8%) rtPA-treated patients and 13 (3.4%) placebo-treated patients. Interestingly, there was a high number of benign spontaneous disease courses in the placebo group (36.6%), which is larger than the favorable outcome rate in the ECASS I rtPA group (35.9%). Furthermore, a comparison of the 3 h cohorts of ECASS I and II and NINDS demonstrates a surprisingly high number of favorable outcomes among the placebo group patients in ECASS II (ECASS I rtPA 38.5%; NINDS rtPA 38.7%; ECASS II placebo 37.7%). Whether this is due to general improvements in the treatment of acute stroke patients, a less severe baseline deficit, or other factors is unclear. While negative for the primary endpoint, ECASS II was a clinically highly relevant study and showed that treatment of ischemic stroke with rtPA in a time window of less than 6 h may lead to an improved outcome if given to selected patients in experienced centers.

The ATLANTIS study began in 1991 and was originally designed to assess the efficacy and safety of thrombolytic therapy with rtPA within 0–6 h after stroke symptom onset.[22] In 1993, the time window was changed, due to safety concerns, to 0–5 h and restarted as part B (ITT), only to be further modified in 1996 to a 3–5 h window (TP) after rtPA had been approved by the FDA. Part A enrolled 142 patients (22 < 3 h and 46 > 5 h).[28] The primary endpoint was an improvement of 4 or more points on the NIHSS at 24 h and day 30; secondary endpoints included functional outcome (BI and mRS) at days 30 and 90. There was a significant improvement at 24 h in the rtPA group (40% vs 21%; $p = 0.02$); this effect, however, was reversed at day 30 (60% vs 75%; $p = 0.05$). rtPA significantly raised the rate of symptomatic ICH (11% vs 0%; $p < 0.01$) and mortality at 90 days (23% vs 7%; $p < 0.01$). The primary endpoint for part B was an NIHSS Score ≤ 1 at 90 days; secondary endpoints were outcome at days 30 and 90 according to BI, mRS, and GOS. An ITT population of 613 acute ischemic stroke patients was enrolled, with 547 of these being treated as assigned within 3–5 h of symptom onset (TP). There were no differences on any of the primary (34% vs 32%; $p = 0.65$) or secondary functional outcome measures; however, there was a significant difference in the rate of major neurologic recovery (complete or ≥11 NIHSS points improvement: 44.9% vs 36%; $p = 0.03$), which did not affect overall outcome. Treatment with rtPA significantly increased the rate of symptomatic ICH (7.0% vs 1.1%; $p < 0.001$). As in ECASS II (median baseline NIHSS Score 11), the median baseline NIHSS Score was substantially lower than in the NINDS trial (10 vs 14), which (as in ECASS II) may have led to a better than expected outcome in the placebo group. In contrast to ECASS II, ATLANTIS was negative for the alternate outcome measurement independence (mRS 0–2) versus dependence or death (mRS 3–6) (rtPA 54% vs placebo 56%; $p = 0.75$). The authors concluded that thrombolysis with rtPA for acute ischemic stroke later than 3 h after symptom onset cannot be recommended.

Meta-analyses

A search of the literature reveals three large meta-analyses. The first meta-analysis by Hacke et al from 1999 covered the NINDS study and both ECASS trials, with a total of 2044 patients included (1034 rtPA patients vs 1010 placebo patients). The authors assessed the benefit of rtPA, dichotomizing the outcome into dependent versus independent or dead (mRS 0–2 vs 3–6) and favorable versus unfavorable (mRS 0–1 vs mRS 2–6). Risk in these three trials can be defined as symptomatic intracerebral hemorrhage (sICH) and mortality. Differences between the trials, such as the dose of rtPA (1.1 mg/kg in ECASS I vs 0.9 mg/kg in NINDS and ECASS II), the therapeutic time window (3 h in NINDS vs 6 h in ECASS I and II), and different definitions of sICH, were taken into account. ICH occurred significantly more often in patients receiving rtPA (144 of 1034 vs 43 of 1010; OR 3.23, 95% CI 2.39–4.37), and was slightly less increased in the 3 h time window and at the lower dosage (41 of 393 vs 15 of 389; OR 2.68, 95% CI 1.56–4.62). There was no significant difference in mortality between rtPA and placebo (OR 1.07, 95% CI 0.84–1.36), but a slight trend towards a lower mortality in the 0.9 mg/kg and 3 h group (OR 0.91, 95% CI 0.63–1.32). rtPA, on the other hand, led to a 37% reduction in death and dependence, regardless of dose and time window (OR 0.63, 95% CI 0.53–0.76). If treated with the lower dose and within 3 h, the chance of an unfavorable outcome was reduced by 45% (OR 0.55, 95% CI 0.41–0.72). For every 1000 patients treated with either dose, there are 90 fewer patients who are dead or disabled but 96 hemorrhages more than expected with placebo. Conversely, for 1000 patients treated with 0.9 mg/kg and within 3 h, there are 65 additional ICH and 140 fewer patients dead or disabled. The number needed to treat (NNT) for all doses and time windows is 11; for the 3 h and 0.9 mg/kg group, it is 7. These numbers are far better than the NNT for thrombolysis in myocardial infarctions, which is 30–40.[29]

Wardlaw et al[30] included in their Cochrane Library meta-analysis all randomized trials of thrombolysis regardless of time window, dosage, administration route, and substance. Seventeen trials with a total of 5216 patients (2889 of whom were from rtPA trials) were included. The main objectives were to show that thrombolytic therapy reduces the risk of late death, that it may increase the risk of early and fatal ICH, and that the benefit at outcome (reduction of death and dependence) offsets any early hazard. Symptomatic and fatal ICH were significantly more common as a result of thrombolytic therapy (symptomatic ICH: OR 3.53, 95% CI 2.79–4.45, $p < 0.000001$; fatal ICH: OR 4.15, 95% CI 2.96–5.84). This translates into 70 additional instances of symptomatic ICH for patients receiving thrombolysis and 29 of 1000 (OR 3.2) additional instances of fatal ICH in rtPA patients but 92 of 1000 (OR 6.03) additional ICH in those patients receiving streptokinase as opposed to placebo. Despite this, thrombolytic therapy, administered up to 6 h after ischemic stroke, significantly reduced death or dependence at the end of follow-up (55.2% vs 59.7%; OR 0.83, 95% CI 0.73–0.94, $p = 0.0015$), which is equivalent to 44 fewer patients being dead or dependent per 1000 treated (95% CI 15–73). For patients treated with rtPA only, the OR was 0.79 (95% CI 0.68–0.92, $p = 0.001$) or 57 deaths or dependence prevented per 1000 patients treated (95% CI 20–93). An alternative endpoint analysis yields similar results for favorable versus unfavorable outcome (OR 0.79 for all patients and 0.76 for rtPA patients). When treatment was given within 3 h after stroke onset, there was an even better risk reduction for dependence or death (55.2% vs 68.3%; OR 0.58, 95% CI 0.46–0.74, $p = 0.00001$) or 126 fewer dead or dependent patients per 1000 treated. The difference of benefit of rtPA in the 0–3 h window or 3–6 h window was nonsignificant but showed a trend towards better improvement with early therapy (OR 0.7 vs 0.76). The authors conclude that the significant increases in early death and fatal and nonfatal symptomatic ICH are offset by the significant reduction of disability in survivors. Therapy with rtPA is associated with less risk and more benefit than treatment with other substances.

More recently, a new meta-analysis of the NINDS, ECASS I and II, and ATLANTIS studies aimed to analyze combined data for individual patients to confirm the importance of rapid treatment.[31] Common data elements from the major thrombolytic therapy trials were pooled and analyzed using multivariable logistic regression to assess the relation of the interval from stroke onset to start of treatment on favorable 3-month outcome and on the occurrence of clinically relevant parenchymal ICH. Here, 2775 patients from six trials were randomly allocated to rtPA or placebo (median age 68 years, median baseline NIHSS Score 11). The odds of a favorable 3-month outcome increased as onset to treatment time decreased ($p = 0.005$). The odds were 2.8 (95%

CI 1.8–4.5) for 0–90 min, 1.6 (1.1–2.2) for 91–180 min, 1.4 (1.1–1.9) for 181–270 min, and 1.2 (0.9–1.5) for 271–360 min in favor of the rtPA group. The hazard ratio for death adjusted for baseline NIHSS Score was not different from 1.0 for the 0–90, 91–180, and 181–270 min intervals; for 271–360 min, it was 1.45 (95% CI 1.02–2.07). ICH was seen in 82 (5.9%) rtPA-treated patients and 15 (1.1%) controls ($p < 0.0001$). ICH was not associated with onset to treatment time but was with rtPA treatment ($p = 0.0001$) and age ($p = 0.0002$). Most interestingly the significant effect in favor of rtPA was mainly on the cost of patients in the mRS range from 2–5. The authors concluded that the sooner that rtPA is given to stroke patients, the greater the benefit, especially if started within 90 min. Thus the negative correlation of time and outcome again is established ('lost time is lost brain').

Phase IV studies

After FDA approval of rtPA for intravenous thrombolytic therapy in June 1996, the rate of thrombolysis remained fairly constant until the end of 1998.[29] At most centers where thrombolysis is performed, the NINDS protocol is used; many of these centers also use the ECASS CT criteria for early infarction. Despite level I evidence in favor of thrombolysis, it is estimated that overall only 1% of all ischemic stroke patients and 2% of the time-eligible (3 h window) are treated with rtPA – a rather low rate. This has several reasons, such as persisting doubts, fear of hemorrhage, or inadequate reimbursement. The reported outcome and complication rates seem to be similar to the NINDS trial in most instances. The CASES (Canadian Alteplase for Stroke Effectiveness Study) registry in Canada has registered more than 1000 rtPA-treated patients with a median NIHSS Score of 15, a symptomatic ICH rate of 4.6%, and a rate of 46% independent patients (mRS 0–2). In Cologne, approximately 22% of the patients who arrive within 3 h after symptom onset (5% of all ischemic stroke patients) receive thrombolysis.[32] This rate was achieved after cooperation between emergency caregivers, internists, and neurologists was initiated and the referral system optimized. The average door-to-needle time in Cologne is 48 min. The rates of total, symptomatic, and fatal ICH were 11%, 5%, and 1%, respectively. Of these patients, 53% recovered to a fully independent functional state. The same group have published their data on long-term follow-up after thrombolytic therapy, where 150 patients treated within 3 hours were re-evaluated after 12 months.[33] After 12 months, 41% of the patients had an mRS ≤1 and 52% an mRS ≤2. The stroke recurrence rate (6.6%/year; transient ischemic attack (TIA) 3.3%/year) was consistent with that of population-based studies.[34] These results are nearly identical to the late follow-up outcome analysis published by Kwiatkowski et al[35] in 1999. In Houston, 30 patients were treated prospectively following the NINDS protocol.[36] Six percent of all patients hospitalized with ischemic stroke received intravenous rtPA at the university hospital and 1.1% at community hospitals. The rates of total, symptomatic, and fatal ICH were 10%, 7%, and 3%, respectively, and 37% of patients recovered to fully independent function. The average door-to-needle time was 1 h 40 min.

Two studies presented divergent results. Albers et al[37] reported the STARS (Standard Treatment with Alteplase to Reverse Stroke) study results, a phase IV trial mandated by the FDA. STARS was a prospective, multicenter study of consecutive patients, who received intravenous rtPA according to NINDS criteria. Outcome measurement was mRS at 30 days. Here, 389 patients received rtPA within 2 h 44 min, and the median baseline NIHSS Score was 13. The 30-day mortality rate was 13%, 35% of patients had very favorable outcomes (mRS ≤1), and 43% were functionally independent (mRS ≤2) at day 30. Another 3.3% of the patients experienced symptomatic ICH, which was fatal in 7. Asymptomatic ICH was seen in 8.2%. Protocol violations were reported for 32.6% of the patients, and consisted mostly of treatment after 3 h (13.4%), mainly due to a door-to-needle time of 1 h 36 min, treatment with anticoagulants within 24 h of rtPA administration (9.3%), and rtPA administration despite systolic blood pressure exceeding 185 mmHg (6.7%). The authors conclude that favorable clinical outcomes and low rates of symptomatic ICH can be achieved using rtPA for stroke treatment, while the time effort for emergency evaluation may leave room for logistic improvement. Another study by Katzan et al[38] yielded different results. Twenty-nine hospitals in the metropolitan area of Cleveland, Ohio prospectively assessed the rate of rtPA use, rate of ICH, and outcomes in 3948 stroke patients. Seventy patients (1.8%) admitted with ischemic stroke received rtPA. Sixteen patients (22%) experienced ICH; 11 of these (15.7%) had

a symptomatic ICH (of which 6 were fatal), and 50% had deviations from national treatment guidelines. In-hospital mortality was significantly higher ($p < 0.001$) in patients treated with rtPA (15.7%) than in patients not receiving rtPA (5.1%). The fact that blood pressure guidelines were followed in only 47.8% and that the baseline NIHSS was only documented in 40% of the patients illustrates that intravenous thrombolysis, although an effective therapy, should be performed at experienced centers only and may explain the substantially higher rate of mortality and ICH in this study compared with other investigations. Unpublished data from Canada and Germany confirm the impression that the efficacy and risk of thrombolytic therapy seen in the controlled trials can be matched or even improved in the clinical setting. First publications of the European SITS-MOST registry (see below) are expected; preliminary data hint towards a high safety, with a rate of symptomatic bleedings less than 2%.

The costs associated with intravenous thrombolytic therapy will be a factor in determining the extent of its utilization. Fagan et al[39] analyzed data from the NINDS study and the medical literature in order to estimate the health and economic outcomes associated with the use of rtPA in acute stroke patients. A Markov model was developed to compare the costs per 1000 patients treated with rtPA compared with the costs per 1000 untreated patients. In the NINDS trial, the average length of stay was significantly shorter in rtPA-treated patients than in placebo-treated patients (10.9 vs 12.4 days; $p = 0.02$) and more rtPA patients were discharged to home than to in-patient rehabilitation or a nursing home (48% vs 36%; $p = 0.002$). The Markov model estimated an increase in hospitalization costs of $1.7 million and decreases in rehabilitation costs of $1.4 million and nursing home costs of $4.8 million per 1000 treated patients, with a greater than 90% probability of cost savings. The estimated impact on long-term health outcomes was 564 (95% CI 3–850) quality-adjusted life-years saved over 30 years of the model per 1000 patients, which makes a net cost saving to the healthcare system likely. With growing experience and better training of emergency medicine personnel, internists, and neurologists throughout all stroke services, the efficacy of intravenous thrombolytic therapy with rtPA may even improve and the time window may be routinely extended to 6 h after symptom onset.

Where is the evidence?[40] While rtPA is approved for thrombolytic therapy in the 3 h time window, there is level I (positive meta-analyses from large, methodologically flawless randomized controlled trials), level II (positive secondary endpoints of large randomized controlled trials, i.e. ECASS I and II), and ample level III[41–44] and IV evidence that thrombolysis works in the 4.5–6 h time window. Accordingly, with the recommendations of the Cochrane Collaboration[30] and the European Stroke Initiative,[45] intravenous thrombolysis is safe and effective up to 6 h in selected patients, and likely best within 4.5 h after stroke onset.[31] The ideal selection tool may be stroke MRI.[46] The fact that an individual therapy based on advanced knowledge is offered that does not meet the criteria of drug approval institutions and therefore may be associated with a higher risk of hazardous if not fatal side-effects must be stressed when informed consent is obtained. Conversely, it should be stated that the drawback of a later onset of therapy may be outweighed by a sophisticated diagnostic imaging procedure telling the physician whether to treat or not to treat. Patients and their relatives should be informed not only about the hazards of thrombolytic therapy within or outside the 3 h time window but also about its potential benefit and thus the risk of *not* being treated.

Future prospects

Another trial of rtPA for ischemic stroke – ECASS III – which was demanded by the European authorities, started to randomize patients in Spring 2004. As many patients do not arrive in the hospital within 3 h, the aim of ECASS III is to extend the treatment window and show that rtPA is effective beyond 3 h. ECASS III is a double-blinded, randomized, placebo-controlled trial in the 3–4 h time window, with approximately 400 patients per study arm and the NINDS/ECASS II dose of rtPA. The primary endpoint will be an mRS of 0–1 at day 90, the secondary endpoint will be a global outcome (mRS 0–1, BI 95–100, GOS 0–1) at day 90. A tertiary endpoint will be an mRS of 0–1 at day 90, stratified by admission NIHSS Score. Safety parameters will include symptomatic ICH rate, survival at day 90, and also rates of brain herniation and symptomatic brain edema. Inclusion criteria will be age 18–80 years, clinical diagnosis of stroke (NIHSS Score ≤24)

without significant improvement, informed consent, and treatment possible within 3–4 h. Exclusion criteria will be similar to those of ECASS II, including early CT signs of ICH or extensive infarction. Furthermore, a European equivalent of the CASES registry to which every patient treated with rtPA within 3 h must be reported (SITS-MOST: Safe Implementation of Thrombolysis in Stroke Monitoring Study) commenced operation in late 2002, and currently more than 1000 patients have been enrolled. SITS-MOST is internet-based and located in Stockholm.

A phase I study with the thrombolytic drug tenecteplase has been concluded; the results, however, have not yet been published. A stroke MRI-based study of the efficacy of recombinant desmoteplase (DSPA, derived from saliva of the vampire bat *Desmodus rotundus*) for treatment of stroke in the 3–9 h time window has completed all dose-finding tiers (DIAS: Desmoplase In Acute Ischemic Stroke), and was positive for the surrogate endpoint of reperfusion according to perfusion-weighted MRI, paralleled by an improved clinical outcome regardless of the time from stroke onset.[47] A parallel phase II US trial (DEDAS – Dose Escalation study of Desmoteplase in Acute ischaemic Stroke) had completed randomization by the end of 2004, and DIAS phase III is planned. A potential advantage of desmoteplase is its long half-life, allowing single-bolus administration as well as low neurotoxicity.

IST (International Stroke Trial) 3 is a large thrombolysis trial planned to include 6000 patients in a randomized fashion with the uncertainty principle. This means that physicians who want to treat their patients with rtPA should do so; those who do not want to treat a specific patient should not. Only when they are not sure whether to treat or not should they randomize the patient. We believe that the Cleveland area experience has clearly demonstrated that physicians who do not know whom to treat and whom not to treat should avoid the use of rtPA, as there would be an abundance of hemorrhagic complications.[38] However, IST 3, if ever completed, may provide information about patients that is still lacking, such as on those older than 80 years and those in later time windows.

Combination of rtPA with glycoprotein (GP)IIb/IIIa antagonists such as tirofiban, abciximab, and eptifibatide may be a promising approach and could result in increased vessel patency rates in accordance with cardiological studies.[48] These trials, however, are at present only phase I and II[49] (Steven Warach, personal communication).

The benefits of arterial recanalization may be supplemented by neuronal protection (the first protocol drafts are underway), particularly when the two strategies are used simultaneously, and if they can be used very early following symptom onset. A very interesting approach is ultrasound-enhanced recanalization under treatment with rtPA. Clot lysis facilitation with transcranial ultrasound is another option. Two preliminary studies have been undertaken so far: TRUMBI (Transcranial Low-Frequency Ultrasound-Mediated Thrombolysis in Brain Ischemia) was an international trial that has recently been terminated for safety reasons; CLOTBUST was an oligocentric trial headed by the University Medical Center in Houston, Texas. Preliminary unpublished data from CLOTBUST (Combined Lysis Of Thrombus in Brain ischemia using 2MHz transcranical Ultrasound and Systemic TPA) (AV Alexandrov and JC Grotta) showed a significantly higher rate of early recanalization in patients treated with rtPA and ultrasound as opposed to rtPA alone.

At present, thrombolytic therapy is still underutilized. Among the major problems are that relatively few patients meet the clinical and time criteria. Educating the general public to regard stroke as a treatable emergency and training emergency caregivers in the use of thrombolysis can decrease these problems, but demand a continuous effort. Healthcare institutions should be made aware of the potential long-term cost savings, once stroke management has been optimized and thrombolysis becomes more widely available. As we have already pointed out above, patients and their relatives should be informed not only about the hazards of thrombolytic therapy but also about its potential benefit and thus the risk of *not* being treated.

Conclusions

Thrombolysis is an effective therapy for ischemic stroke, whether performed intravenously within 3 h or intra-arterially within 3–6 h (evidence level I). Meta-analyses are applied in other fields of medicine routinely to establish level I evidence and a rationale for governmental approval for a specific drug therapy. In that regard, there is level I evidence for an effect of intravenous thrombolysis up to 4.5 h and level II evidence for up to 9 h, especially when improved selection criteria such as modern MRI protocols are applied. Sadly, thrombolysis is still underused. Positive results from studies currently underway may encourage more centers to offer this therapy to an overall increasing number of stroke patients in Europe after the approval of the European Agency for the Evaluation of Medicinal Products (EMEA), and thereby reduce the considerable socioeconomic burden of stroke.

References

1. Astrup J, Siesjö B, Symon L. Thresholds in cerebral ischemia – the ischemic penumbra. Stroke 1981;12: 723–5.
2. Davis S, Fisher M, Warach S. Magnetic Resonance Imaging in Stroke. Cambridge: Cambridge University Press, 2003.
3. Fiebach JB, Schellinger PD. Stroke MRI. Darmstadt: Steinkopff Verlag, 2003.
4. Schellinger PD, Fiebach JB, Mohr A, et al. Thrombolytic therapy for ischemic stroke – a review. Part II – Intra-arterial thrombolysis, vertebrobasilar stroke, phase IV trials, and stroke imaging. Crit Care Med 2001;29:1819–25.
5. Schellinger PD, Fiebach JB, Mohr A, et al. Thrombolytic therapy for ischemic stroke – a review. Part I – Intravenous thrombolysis. Crit Care Med 2001;29:1812–18.
6. Meyer JS, Gilroy J, Barnhart MI, Johnson JF. Therapeutic thrombolysis in cerebral thromboembolism. Neurology 1963;13:927–37.
7. Abe T, Kazama M, Naito I. Clinical evaluation for efficacy of tissue cultured urokinase (TCUK) on cerebral thrombosis by means of multi-centre double blind study (transl from Japanese). Blood-Vessel 1981;12: 321–41.
8. Atarashi J, Ohtomo E, Araki G, et al. Clinical utility of urokinase in the treatment of acute stage cerebral thrombosis: multi-center double blind study in comparison with placebo (transl from Japanese). Clin Eval 1985;13:659–709.

9. Ohtomo E, Araki G, Itoh E, et al. Clinical efficacy of urokinase in the treatment of cerebral thrombosis. Multi-center double blind study in comparison with placebo (transl from Japanese). Clin Eval 1985;15: 711–31.

10. Haley EC Jr, Brott TG, Sheppard GL, et al. Pilot randomized trial of tissue plasminogen activator in acute ischemic stroke. The TPA Bridging Study Group. Stroke 1993;24:1000–4.

11. Mori E, Yoneda Y, Tabuchi M, et al. Intravenous recombinant tissue plasminogen activator in acute carotid artery territory stroke. Neurology 1992;42: 976–82.

12. Yamaguchi T, Hayakawa T, Kiuchi H, Japanese Thrombolysis Study Group. Intravenous tissue plasminogen activator ameliorates the outcome of hyperacute embolic stroke. Cerebrovasc Dis 1993;3:269–72.

13. Morris AD, Ritchie C, Grosset DG, et al. A pilot study of streptokinase for acute cerebral infarction. Q J Med 1995;88:727–31.

14. The Multicentre Acute Stroke Trial – Italy (MAST-I) Group. Randomised controlled trial of streptokinase, aspirin, and combination of both in treatment of acute ischaemic stroke. Lancet 1995;346:1509–14.

15. The Multicenter Acute Stroke Trial – Europe Study Group. Thrombolytic therapy with streptokinase in acute ischemic stroke. N Engl J Med 1996;335:145–50.

16. Donnan GA, Davis SM, Chambers BR, et al. Streptokinase for acute ischemic stroke with relationship to time of administration: Australian Streptokinase (ASK) Trial Study Group. JAMA 1996;276:961–6.

17. Cornu C, Boutitie F, Candelise L, et al. Streptokinase in acute ischemic stroke: an individual patient data meta-analysis: the Thrombolysis in Acute Stroke Pooling Project. Stroke 2000;31:1555–60.

18. Wardlaw JM, del Zoppo G, Yamaguchi T. Thrombolysis for acute ischaemic stroke. In: The Cochrane Library, Issue 1, 2000. Oxford: Update Software, 2000.

19. The National Institute of Neurological Disorders and Stroke rt-PA Stroke Study Group. Tissue plasminogen activator for acute ischemic stroke. N Engl J Med 1995;333:1581–7.

20. Hacke W, Kaste M, Fieschi C, et al. Intravenous thrombolysis with recombinant tissue plasminogen activator for acute hemispheric stroke. The European Cooperative Acute Stroke Study. JAMA 1995;274:1017–25.

21. Hacke W, Kaste M, Fieschi C, et al. Randomised double-blind placebo-controlled trial of thrombolytic therapy with intravenous alteplase in acute ischaemic stroke (ECASS II). Lancet 1998;352:1245–1251.

22. Clark WM, Wissman S, Albers GW, et al. Recombinant tissue-type plasminogen activator (Alteplase) for ischemic stroke 3 to 5 hours after symptom onset. The ATLANTIS study: a randomized controlled trial. Alteplase Thrombolysis for Acute Noninterventional Therapy in Ischemic Stroke. JAMA 1999;282:2019–26.

23. von Kummer R, Meyding-Lamade U, Forsting M, et al. Sensitivity and prognostic value of early CT in occlusion of the middle cerebral artery trunk. AJNR Am J Neuroradiol 1994;15:9–15.

24. von Kummer R, Nolte PN, Schnittger H, et al. Detectability of cerebral hemisphere ischaemic infarcts by CT within 6 h of stroke. Neuroradiology 1996;38:31–3.

25. von Kummer R, Allen KL, Holle R, et al. Acute stroke: usefulness of early CT findings before thrombolytic therapy. Radiology 1997;205:327–333.

26. von Kummer R. Effect of training in reading CT scans on patient selection for ECASS II. Neurology 1998;51:S50–2.

27. Steiner T, Bluhmki E, Kaste M, et al. The ECASS 3-hour cohort. Secondary analysis of ECASS data by time stratification. Cerebrovasc Dis 1998;8:198–203.

28. Clark WM, Albers GW, Madden KP, Hamilton S. The rtPA (alteplase) 0- to 6-hour acute stroke trial, part A (A0276g): results of a double-blind, placebo-controlled, multicenter study. Thrombolytic Therapy in Acute Ischemic Stroke study investigators. Stroke 2000;31:811–16.

29. Hacke W, Brott T, Caplan L, et al. Thrombolysis in acute ischemic stroke: controlled trials and clinical experience. Neurology 1999;53:S3–14.

30. Wardlaw JM, del Zoppo G, Yamaguchi T. Thrombolysis for acute ischaemic stroke. In: The Cochrane Library, Issue 1, 2002. Oxford: Update Software, 2002.

31. Hacke W, Donnan G, Fieschi C, et al. Association of outcome with early stroke treatment: pooled analysis of ATLANTIS, ECASS, and NINDS rt-PA stroke trials. Lancet 2004;363:768–74.

32. Grond M, Stenzel C, Schmulling S, et al. Early intravenous thrombolysis for acute ischemic stroke in a community-based approach. Stroke 1998;29:1544–9.

33. Schmulling S, Grond M, Rudolf J, Heiss WD. One-year follow-up in acute stroke patients treated with rtPA in clinical routine. Stroke 2000;31:1552–4.

34. Sacco RL, Shi T, Zamanillo MC, Kargman DE. Predictors of mortality and recurrence after hospitalized cerebral infarction in an urban community: the Northern Manhattan Stroke Study. Neurology 1994;44:626–34.

35. Kwiatkowski TG, Libman RB, Frankel M, et al. Effects of tissue plasminogen activator for acute ischemic stroke at one year. National Institute of Neurological Disorders and Stroke Recombinant Tissue Plasminogen

Activator Stroke Study Group. N Engl J Med 1999;340:1781–7.

36. Chiu D, Krieger D, Villar-Cordova C, et al. Intravenous tissue plasminogen activator for acute ischemic stroke – feasibility, safety and efficacy in the first year of clinical practice. Stroke 1998;29:18–22.

37. Albers GW, Bates VE, Clark WM, et al. Intravenous tissue-type plasminogen activator for treatment of acute stroke: the Standard Treatment with Alteplase to Reverse Stroke (STARS) study. JAMA 2000;283: 1145–50.

38. Katzan IL, Furlan AJ, Lloyd LE, et al. Use of tissue-type plasminogen activator for acute ischemic stroke: the Cleveland area experience. JAMA 2000;283:1151–8.

39. Fagan SC, Morgenstern LB, Petitta A, et al. Cost-effectiveness of tissue plasminogen activator for acute ischemic stroke. NINDS rt-PA Stroke Study Group. Neurology 1998;50:883–90.

40. Kaste M. Approval of alteplase in Europe: Will it change stroke management? Lancet Neurol 2003;2: 207–8.

41. Röther J, Schellinger PD, Gass A, et al. Effect of intravenous thrombolysis on MRI parameters and functional outcome in acute stroke < 6 h. Stroke 2002;33: 2438–2445.

42. Parsons MW, Barber PA, Chalk J, et al. Diffusion- and perfusion-weighted MRI response to thrombolysis in stroke. Ann Neurol 2002;51:28–37.

43. Schellinger PD, Jansen O, Fiebach JB, et al. Monitoring intravenous recombinant tissue plasminogen activator thrombolysis for acute ischemic stroke with diffusion and perfusion MRI. Stroke 2000;31:1318–28.

44. Külkens S, Schwark C, Schellinger PD, et al. Thrombolysis in ischemic stroke 3 to 6 hours after symptom onset using a MR-based algorithm. In: Proceedings of International Stroke Conference, Phoenix, AZ, USA, February 13–15th, 2003.

45. The European Stroke Initiative. Recommendations for Stroke Management. Cerebrovasc Dis 2000;10: 1–34.

46. Schellinger PD, Fiebach JB, Hacke W. Imaging-based decision making in thrombolytic therapy for ischemic stroke: present status. Stroke 2003;34:575–83.

47. Warach S. Early reperfusion related to clinical response in DIAS – phase II, randomized, placebo-controlled dose finding trial of IV desmoteplase 3–9 hours from onset in patients with diffusion–perfusion mismatch. In proceedings of ASA–International Stroke Conference, San Diego, CA, 2004.

48. Hacke W. Abciximab in Emergent Stroke Treatment Trial (ABESTT). In: Proceedings of International Stroke Conference, Phoenix, AZ, USA, February 13th–15th, 2003.

49. Seitz RJ, Hamzavi M, Junghans U, et al. Thrombolysis with recombinant tissue plasminogen activator and tirofiban in stroke: preliminary observations. Stroke 2003;34:1932–5.

14

Complications of thrombolysis

Vincent Larrue

Introduction

Complications of thrombolysis for acute ischemic stroke include intracranial hemorrhage, extracranial hemorrhage, and, rarely, orolingual angioedema and hypotension.[1] Intracerebral hemorrhage (ICH) is the most common complication. This can be fatal or associated with poor functional outcome. Therefore, the fear of causing a severe ICH has been a limiting factor to a broader use of thrombolysis in acute ischemic stroke.[2] However, recent studies have shown that careful selection of patients based on a better knowledge of risk factors for ICH improves the safety of this treatment. Postmarketing studies of alteplase in acute ischemic stroke have confirmed an acceptable safety profile in clinical routine provided the guidelines for drug prescription and administration are rigorously applied.

Classification of ICH

Several classifications have been used to describe ICH in the clinical trials of alteplase for acute ischemic stroke. In ECASS I and II (European Cooperative Acute Stroke Studies) ICH were classified according to their appearance on computed tomography (CT) without consideration of their clinical consequences. Hemorrhagic infarction type 1 (HI1) was defined as small petechiae along the margins of the infarct; hemorrhagic infarction type 2 (HI2) as confluent petechiae within the infarcted area but no space-occupying effect; parenchymal hemorrhage type 1 (PH1) as blood clots in less than 30% of the

infarcted area with some space-occupying effect; and parenchymal hemorrhage type 2 (PH2) as blood clots in more than 30% of the infarcted area with a substantial space-occupying effect. ICH that developed at a distance from the ischemic area were described as remote PH.[3,4]

In the NINDS (National Institute of Neurological Disorders and Stroke) study of recombinant tissue-type plasminogen activator (rtPA) and stroke, ICH were classified using clinical criteria into symptomatic or asymptomatic ICH whatever their appearance on brain imaging. Symptomatic ICH was defined as a CT-documented hemorrhage that was temporally related to deterioration in the patient's clinical condition. Asymptomatic ICH was defined as a CT-documented hemorrhage that was not associated with deterioration in the patient's neurological condition.[5]

Both classifications of ICH have limitations. The CT-based classification provides no information on the clinical consequences of ICH, whereas the clinical classification does not acknowledge the contribution of ischemic edema to clinical deterioration. In an attempt to overcome these issues, ECASS II used a definition of symptomatic ICH incorporating brain imaging criteria: an ICH was defined as symptomatic if the patient had clinical deterioration causing an increase in the National Institutes of Health Stroke Scale (NIHSS) Score of 4 points or more, and the hemorrhage was likely to be the cause of clinical deterioration.[4]

The correlation between the clinical classification and the CT-based classification of ICH was evaluated in secondary analyses of ECASS II and the NINDS study. In the NINDS study, most symptomatic

Table 14.1   Incidence (%) of asymptomatic and symptomatic intracerebral hemorrhage (ICH) in the randomized controlled trials of intravenous alteplase in acute ischemic stroke

Study	Placebo		Alteplase	
	Asymptomatic	Symptomatic	Asymptomatic	Symptomatic
NINDS (n = 624)	2.6	0.6	4.2	6.4
ECASS II (n = 800)	36.2	3.9	37.8	8.9
ATLANTIS (n = 613)	4.2	1.3	11.3	6.7

NINDS, National Institute of Neurological Disorders and Stroke; ECASS, European Cooperative Acute Stroke Study; ATLANTIS, Alteplase Thrombolysis for Acute Noninterventional Therapy in Ischemic Stroke.

ICH (68.2%) were classified as PH.[6] A similar proportion (73.5%) of symptomatic ICH were considered PH in ECASS II.[7] Furthermore, in ECASS II, only 6 of 24 (25%) PH1 but 30 of 36 (83%) PH2 were symptomatic.[8] These data suggest that the main determinant of clinical deterioration after ICH is the volume of the hemorrhagic component rather than associated ischemic edema.

Incidence of ICH after intravenous alteplase for acute stroke

Spontaneous ICH is a common event during the natural course of brain infarction. However, the incidence of this complication varies greatly across studies. In the placebo groups of the four large randomized controlled trials of intravenous alteplase in acute stroke, an ICH was found on the repeat CT scans in 3.2–40.1% of patients (Tables 14.1 and 14.2).[3–5,9] These large differences may be explained by differences in the timing of repeat brain imaging or in the methods used to recognize ICH. Recent studies using magnetic resonance imaging (MRI) indicate that gradient-echo imaging is far more sensitive and accurate than CT to demonstrate hemorrhagic transformation.[10] This suggests that the incidence of ICH may have been underestimated in some previous studies using only CT.

Most ICH that occurred in the placebo groups of the randomized controlled trials were clinically asymptomatic or classified as HI (Tables 14.1 and 14.2).

All randomized controlled trials have shown an increased incidence of ICH in patients treated with alteplase compared with those receiving placebo. The

Table 14.2   Incidence (%) of hemorrhagic infarction (HI) and parenchymal hemorrhage (PH) in the randomized controlled trials of intravenous alteplase in acute ischemic stroke

Study	Placebo		Alteplase	
	HI	PH	HI	PH
ECASS I (n = 620)	30.3	6.5	23.0	19.8
ECASS II (n = 800)	36.5	3.1	34.9	11.8

difference was largely explained by a much higher incidence of symptomatic ICH in patients treated with alteplase. The findings regarding asymptomatic ICH were less consistent across studies. The incidence of asymptomatic ICH was higher in the alteplase group than in the placebo group in both the ATLANTIS (Alteplase Thrombolysis for Acute Noninterventional Therapy in Ischemic Stroke) and NINDS studies but was not in ECASS II (Table 14.1).[4,5,9] In the European studies, which used the CT-based classification of ICH, PH was strongly associated with alteplase. In contrast, HI were no more frequent in patients treated with alteplase than in those receiving placebo (Table 14.2).[3,4]

A systematic review of summarized data from the trials of alteplase in acute ischemic stroke given 6 h or less after symptom onset showed an increased rate of symptomatic ICH in patients treated with alteplase (odds ratio (OR) 3.13, 95% confidence interval (CI) 2.34–4.19; $p < 0.00001$), equivalent to 62 extra symptomatic ICH per 1000 patients treated.[11]

In a systematic review of individual patient data from ECASS I and II and the NINDS and ATLANTIS studies, PH2 was seen in 82 (5.9%) patients treated with alteplase and in 15 (1.1%) patients given placebo ($p < 0.0001$).[12]

Timing of ICH

Most symptomatic ICH and PH occur in the first 24 h after thrombolysis. In the NINDS study, 8 of 22 patients with symptomatic ICH had onset of symptoms within the first 12 h, and all had onset of symptoms within the first 24 h.[6] In ECASS I, 87% of PH occurred within 24 h of initiation of treatment. In contrast, HI may occur later. Thus, in ECASS I, only 24% of HI were visible on the 24 h CT scan.[13]

Clinical significance of ICH

Symptomatic ICH is usually fatal or associated with poor functional outcome. In the NINDS study, 15 of the 20 alteplase-treated patients with a symptomatic ICH were dead at 3 months, 3 had a Rankin Score of 4 or 5, and 2 had a Rankin Score of 0 or 1. One of the 2 placebo-treated patients with a symptomatic ICH died on the second day, and the other had a Rankin Score of 4 at 3 months.[6]

Asymptomatic ICH has no negative impact on outcome. In an analysis of combined data from the NINDS and ATLANTIS studies, asymptomatic ICH were found in 9.9% of patients treated with rtPA and 4.2% of patients treated with placebo. Asymptomatic ICH did not affect outcome at 90 days in either the placebo or alteplase groups.[14]

The data from ECASS II, where more ICH occurred, have allowed a refined analysis of outcome stratified by category of ICH and treatment group. Among placebo-treated patients, bad outcome, defined as death or a modified Rankin Score of 5 at 3 months, was more common in patients with symptomatic ICH or PH than in patients with HI or without ICH. There were significant interactions for bad outcome between alteplase and PH (OR 4.8, 95% CI 1.2–24.7) and between alteplase and symptomatic ICH (OR 6.9, 95% CI 1.8–30.3), suggesting that both categories of ICH were not only more common but also more severe in patients treated with alteplase.

Table 14.3 Distribution of patients with bad outcome at 3 months stratified by category of ICH and treatment group in ECASS II. Bad outcome is considered a modified Rankin Score of 5–6. Values are number of patients in category with bad outcome/number of total patients in category, with percentages in parentheses

Category of ICH	Placebo (n = 386)	Alteplase (n = 407)
No ICH	28/233 (12.0%)	21/217 (9.7%)
HI	25/141 (17.7%)	14/142 (9.9%)[a]
PH	3/12 (25.0%)	24/48 (50.0%)[a]
Symptomatic ICH	5/13 (38.5%)	26/36 (72.2%)[a]

[a]Significant rtPA by category of ICH interaction in logistic regression analysis.

In contrast, among patients with HI, the odds for bad outcome were reduced in those treated with alteplase compared with placebo (OR 0.36, 95% CI 0.15–0.81), suggesting that alteplase may benefit some patients despite minor degrees of hemorrhagic transformation (Table 14.3).[7]

Mechanisms of ICH

Numerous experimental studies have consistently shown that two conditions are required for an ICH to occur after brain infarction. First, the vessel wall must be weakened to allow leakage of blood in the surrounding brain tissue. Second, there must be some reperfusion of the ischemic area, either by lysis of the offending thrombus or via the collateral circulation.[15]

Studies using MRI have confirmed the relationship between hemorrhagic transformation and the initial severity of ischemia. The apparent diffusion coefficient of water was lower in the regions of the ischemic area destined to hemorrhagic transformation than in the regions without subsequent hemorrhage.[16,17]

A clinical study using TCD has clarified the relationship between the duration of cerebral arterial occlusion and the development of ICH. Serial TCD examinations were performed in 32 patients with proximal middle cerebral artery (MCA) occlusion, and treated with intravenous alteplase within 3 h of symptom onset. HI were associated with early recanalization, whereas PH were associated with delayed recanalization. Moreover, the volume of infarct was reduced and the clinical outcome at 3 months was improved in patients with HI compared with patients without ICH.[18] These results suggest that HI is a marker of successful early recanalization and improved outcome, which is consistent with the above-mentioned findings in ECASS II of an improved outcome despite HI in patients treated with alteplase.[7]

Taken together, these data suggest a time-dependent model of ICH pathogenesis. Early reperfusion may be associated with a small amount of hemorrhagic transformation limited to the most severely ischemic regions within the ischemic area, whereas late reperfusion of a large area of severe ischemia may cause massive ICH.

Most ICH that occur after thrombolysis with intravenous alteplase develop within the boundaries of the ischemic area, and therefore result from hemorrhagic transformation of a cerebral infarct. However, a substantial number of ICH develop at a distance from the ischemic area. These ICH were described as remote PH in the European studies. In ECASS I, 25 of 82 PH were remote PH: 22 in the alteplase group and 3 in the placebo group.[7] In ECASS II, remote PH were noted in 14 of 60 patients with PH: 13 in the alteplase group and 1 in the placebo group.[13] Finally, in the NINDS study, 4 of the 22 symptomatic ICH among patients treated with alteplase occurred outside of the distribution of the presenting ischemic stroke.[6] Several hypotheses can be considered to explain the occurrence of remote PH. These include unrecognized brain ischemia on initial imaging, and previous weakening of the vessel wall by hypertension or cerebral amyloid angiopathy.[19,20] In a pooled analysis of pathological examination of brain from patients who died from ICH after thrombolysis for stroke, 7 of 10 patients (mean age 66 years) had cerebral amyloid angiopathy, compared with an autopsy prevalence of 22% in unselected populations in that age range (OR 8.43, 95% CI 1.8–51.9; $p = 0.0005$).[21]

Advances in the understanding of the molecular mechanisms of tissue-type plasminogen activator (tPA)-induced ICH have been accomplished recently. Interaction of tPA with the blood–brain barrier causes an increase in its permeability, with resultant passage of proteinases and other harmful substances from the blood into the brain, and degradation of the vascular matrix.[22] It seems that tPA acts through a specific signaling pathway and upregulates matrix metalloproteinase-9 (MMP-9).[23] Targeting this pathway may offer new approaches for reducing the incidence and severity of ICH associated with alteplase.

Risk factors for ICH

A better knowledge of risk factors for ICH after alteplase for acute stroke may improve the selection of patients and, consequently, the safety of this treatment. Several analyses of risk factors for ICH have been published. These were derived from secondary analyses of randomized controlled trials or cohort studies conducted after registration of the drug.

Dose of alteplase

In a pilot study including 74 patients treated within 90 min of symptom onset over seven dose tiers of alteplase, ranging from 0.35 to 1.08 mg/kg, the investigators of the NINDS study found that symptomatic ICH was related to increasing doses of alteplase ($p = 0.045$) and did not occur in any of the 58 patients treated with 0.85 mg/kg or less.[24] The greater experience of thrombolysis in myocardial infarction also supports an increased risk of ICH with higher doses. In acute stroke, the patient's weight is frequently estimated by the treating physician. Discrepancies between the actual and estimated weight may occur and result in an incorrect dose. This was evaluated in the Multicenter rt-PA Acute Stroke Survey, a survey of 1205 patients treated in routine clinical practice with intravenous rtPA for acute stroke. Data on actual weight and rtPA dose were available in 769 patients. Forty-one patients had a symptomatic ICH while 51 had an asymptomatic ICH. There was a nonsignificant trend toward an increased risk of any ICH as the degree of overdosage increased ($p = 0.09$), which became significant after adjustment for other relevant variables.[25] Thus, in clinical practice, overdosage caused by an overestimation of weight may result in an increased risk of ICH. Every effort should be made to obtain the most accurate weight.

Age

Advancing age is a major risk factor for symptomatic ICH and PH. This was found in ECASS I and II but not confirmed in the NINDS study.[6,7,13] It should be recalled, however, that only 22 symptomatic ICH occurred in the NINDS study, which limits the power of analyses derived from this study. In the pooled analysis of ECASS I and II and the ATLANTIS and NINDS studies, advancing age was strongly associated with PH2 ($p = 0.0002$).[12]

The safety of thrombolysis with alteplase in patients over 80 years of age is unknown because only 42 such patients were included in the randomized controlled trials of alteplase for acute ischemic stroke.[11] In a review of prospectively collected data on 62 patients, aged 80 years and over, and treated with intravenous alteplase at a tertiary center, the rate of symptomatic ICH was 9.7%, which is double that seen in most case series of younger patients.[26]

Time interval from stroke onset to start of treatment

The risk of PH or symptomatic ICH was not related to the time elapsed from the onset of stroke to initiation of treatment in any of the randomized controlled trials.[6,7,13] However, the number of PH or symptomatic ICH that occurred in patients treated within 3 h of symptom onset in these trials may be insufficient to assess the relationship of ICH with time to treatment within this time frame. Among patients given alteplase within 3 h of symptom onset, there were only 20 symptomatic ICH in the NINDS study, 7 PH in ECASS II, and 12 PH in ECASS I.[6,7,11] In the pooled analysis of these trials, 3% of patients treated with rtPA within 90 min of symptom onset, and 6% of those treated between 91 and 180 min, suffered a PH2. This trend was not significant after adjustment on other variables.[12] More data are needed to reliably assess the relationship of time to treatment with ICH.

Clinical severity of stroke

The clinical severity of stroke was evaluated using the Scandinavian Stroke Scale (SSS) in ECASS I and the

NIHSS in the NINDS trial, ECASS II, and ATLANTIS. The severity of the neurological deficit at baseline was associated with an increased risk of symptomatic ICH in the NINDS study but was not in ECASS II.[6,7] In ECASS I and II, the severity of the neurological deficit was associated with HI but not with PH.[7,13] In the pooled analysis of the NINDS and ATLANTIS studies and ECASS I and II, PH2 was not associated with the initial severity of the neurological deficit.[12] Hence, there is currently no firm evidence to support the notion of an increased risk of severe ICH in patients with a severe neurological deficit.

Early signs of cerebral ischemia on CT

Early signs of cerebral ischemia on CT include hypodensity (less than the white matter density), mass effect (effacement of the cortical sulci, sylvian fissure, or other basal cisterns, or compression of the ventricular system), and subtle changes. Subtle changes result from the relative attenuation of gray matter density. Thus, the affected gray matter can no longer be distinguished from the adjacent white matter: there is loss of the insular ribbon, effacement of the lenticular nucleus, loss of cortico–subcortical differentiation.[27] Subtle changes are difficult to recognize and quantify.[28] However, specific training and the use of a quantitative CT score can both improve the identification and quantification of these signs.[29]

In the NINDS study, 31% of patients with hypodensity or mass effect developed a symptomatic ICH, compared with 6% of patients without these CT findings. This association remained significant after adjustment for other variables, including the baseline NIH stroke scale score.[6] The NINDS study data were later reanalyzed to assess the impact of subtle changes. Among patients treated with rtPA, symptomatic ICH had occurred in 5 (14%) of the patients with frank or subtle signs in more than one-third of the MCA territory, 4 (8%) of the patients with signs in less than one-third of the MCA territory, and 11 (5%) of the patients without early signs. However, the association of early signs of ischemia with symptomatic ICH was not significant after adjustment for the baseline NIHSS Score.[30]

In ECASS I, early signs of cerebral ischemia (attenuation of density, or mass effect) were associated with HI but not with PH.[13] In ECASS II, the risk of PH and the risk of symptomatic ICH were both significantly increased in patients with frank or subtle attenuation of density in more than one-third of the MCA territory in multivariate analysis.[7]

An association of extended early signs with symptomatic ICH was also found in two prospective cohort studies of patients treated with intravenous rtPA within 3 h of symptom onset. The ASPECTS (Alberta Stroke Program Early CT Score) Study Group reported symptomatic ICH in 9 (13.8%) of 65 patients with attenuation of density or focal brain swelling in more than one-third of the MCA territory, and in only 1 (1.1%) of 91 patients with these signs in one-third or less the MCA territory (including patients without any signs). This association remained significant in multivariate analysis.[29]

In the STARS (Standard Treatment with Alteplase to Reverse Stroke) study, 2 (29%) of the 7 patients who had hypodensity in more than one-third of the MCA territory on the baseline CT scan had a symptomatic ICH, compared with 11 (3%) of the 382 patients who had no hypodensity or hypodensity in less than one-third of the MCA territory (p = 0.02).[31]

Similar findings were reported in a multicenter retrospective and prospective analysis comprising 1205 patients treated in routine clinical practice with intravenous rtPA within 3 h of symptom. In this sample, which includes data from the STARS and ASPECTS studies, the adjusted odds ratio for symptomatic ICH in patients with early signs in more than one-third of the MCA territory was 6.7 (95% CI 2.14–21.01).[32]

The results of a systematic review of clinical trials[7,13,29] and prospective cohort studies[28,30] that reported on ICH after intravenous alteplase for ischemic stroke and included data on the extent of early signs of ischemia on pretreatment CT scan are summarized in Figure 14.1. For the purpose of this review, a severe ICH was defined as symptomatic ICH or PH. Overall, 140 severe ICH occurred in 1561 patients. There were 29 (18.0%) severe ICH among 161 patients with early signs in more than one-third of the MCA territory, and 111 (7.9%) among 1400 patients with signs in less than one-third of the MCA territory or without any signs. The pooled odds ratio for a severe ICH in patients with extended signs was

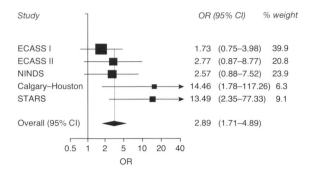

Figure 14.1
Effect of early signs of ischemia in more than one-third of middle cerebral artery territory on risk of severe intracerebral hemorrhage (ICH) (symptomatic ICH or parenchymal hemorrhage (PH)) in patients treated with intravenous alteplase for stroke: systematic review of randomized controlled trials (alteplase group only) and cohort studies. The odds ratio (OR) for each study is represented by a square, the area of which is proportional to the statistical power of the estimate. Each line represents the 95% confidence interval (CI) of the OR. An arrow at the end of the line indicates that the confidence interval extends beyond the horizontal-axis log scale (which was forced to be in the range 0–40). The diamond represents the overall pooled estimate. Test for heterogeneity among studies: $\chi^2 = 6.78$; df = 4; p = 0.15. ECASS, European Cooperative Acute Stroke Study; NINDS, National Institute of Neurological Disorders and Stroke; STARS, Standard Treatment with Alatephase or Reverse Stroke.

2.89 (95% CI 1.71–4.89). There was no significant heterogeneity among studies (p = 0.15).[33]

Currently available data indicate a high risk of symptomatic ICH or PH in patients with extended signs of ischemia on CT, and warrant the continued exclusion of these patients from thrombolytic therapy.

Cerebral microbleeds

Asymptomatic cerebral microbleeds can be identified with T2*-weighted gradient-echo MRI. Whether microbleeds on pretreatment MRI are associated with an increased risk of ICH after thrombolysis has not been determined. In two short series including 44 patients (8 with microbleeds) and 41 patients (5 with microbleeds), respectively, there were no more ICH after thrombolysis for acute stroke in patients with microbleeds than in those without.[34,35]

Blood glucose

Experimental studies in animals suggest that hyperglycemia may increase the permeability of the blood–brain barrier and promote hemorrhagic transformation of cerebral infarcts.[36] In the NINDS trial, the risk of symptomatic ICH increased as the admission blood glucose increased.[37] A similar finding was reported in a retrospective analysis of 138 patients treated in routine clinical practice with intravenous alteplase within 3 h of symptom onset.[38]

In contrast, admission blood glucose was not related to PH or symptomatic ICH in the ATLANTIS study or in ECASS I and II.[6,7,13] It should be recalled that patients with extreme hyperglycemia were excluded from the trials of intravenous alteplase in stroke. Thus, available data would not support the decision to withold thrombolytic therapy in a patient because of hyperglycemia, unless blood glucose is above 400 mg/dl (22.2 mmol/l).

High blood pressure

Acute hypertension increases the incidence and severity of hemorrhagic transformation in animal studies.[39] Also, elevated diastolic blood pressure on admission was associated with increased risk of ICH in the pilot phase of the NINDS Study.[40] Consequently, patients with baseline systolic blood pressure greater than 185 mmHg or diastolic blood pressure greater than 110 mmHg were excluded from the randomized controlled trials. Furthermore, a treatment algorithm that included aggressive measures to maintain blood pressure at less than 185/110 mmHg was applied in the NINDS study, ECASS II, and the ATLANTIS study. In spite of these precautionary measures, high systolic blood pressure at baseline was associated with PH in ECASS II.[7] In contrast, no association was found between high blood pressure and symptomatic ICH or PH in either the NINDS study or ECASS I.[6,13]

Aspirin use before stroke

In ECASS II, the risk of symptomatic ICH and the risk of PH after alteplase were strongly increased in patients taking aspirin before the occurrence of stroke.[7] These findings were not confirmed in either ECASS I or the NINDS study.[6,13] Further data are needed to assess the relationship between aspirin use before stroke and ICH.

Cardiac diseases

A history of congestive heart failure was associated with both PH and symptomatic ICH in ECASS II, whereas atrial fibrillation on admission and a history of myocardial infarction were not.[7] This finding needs confirmation.

Postmarketing studies

The safety of alteplase in acute ischemic stroke in clinical routine has been assessed in several postmarketing studies. In a meta-analysis of 15 published open-label studies, the rate of symptomatic ICH in 2639 patients was 5.2% (95% CI 4.3–6.0), which is slightly lower than the 6.4% rate in the alteplase group of the NINDS study. Comparisons across studies showed that the mortality rate correlated with the percentage of protocol violations.[41] Furthermore, implementation of a quality improvement program in centers with initially unfavorable results can reduce the rates of protocol violations and symptomatic ICH. In the nine hospitals participating in the Cleveland Clinic Health System, the rate of symptomatic ICH dropped from 13.4% to 6.4% and that of protocol violations from 33% to 17% after implementation of such a program.[42]

Conclusions

Thrombolysis with intravenous alteplase has revolutionized the care of stroke patients. This treatment is effective despite an increased risk of ICH in treated patients. The risk of ICH can be reduced by careful selection of patients based on clinical and radiological criteria. Age and the initial severity of brain ischemia are the main determinants of ICH. Increasing knowledge of the pathophysiology of tPA-induced ICH may lead to the development of drugs that might reduce the incidence and severity of this complication.

References

1. Engelter ST, Fluri F, Buitrago-Téllez C, et al. Life-threatening orolingual angioedema during thrombolysis in acute ischemic stroke. J Neurol 2005;252:1167–70.

2. Mitka M. Tensions remain over tPA for stroke. JAMA 2003;289:1363–4.

3. Hacke W, Kaste M, Fieschi C, et al. Intravenous thrombolysis with recombinant tissue plasminogen activator for acute hemispheric stroke: the European Cooperative Acute Stroke Study (ECASS). JAMA 1995;274:1017–25.

4. Hacke W, Kaste M, Fieschi C, et al. Randomised double-blind placebo-controlled trial of thrombolytic therapy with intravenous alteplase in acute ischaemic stroke (ECASS II). Lancet 1998;352:1245–51.

5. The National Institute of Neurological Disorders and Stroke rt-PA Stroke Study Group. Tissue plasminogen for acute ischemic stroke. N Engl J Med 1995;333:1581–7

6. The NINDS t-PA Stroke Study Group. Intracerebral hemorrhage after intravenous t-PA therapy for ischemic stroke. Stroke 1997;28:2109–2118.

7. Larrue V, von Kummer R, Müller A, et al. Risk factors for severe hemorrhagic transformation in ischemic stroke patients treated with recombinant tissue plasminogen activator. Stroke 2001;32:438–41.

8. Berger C, Fiorelli M, Steiner T, et al. Hemorrhagic transformation of ischemic brain tissue: asymptomatic or symptomatic? Stroke 2001;32:1330–5.

9. Clark WM, Wissman S, Albers GW. Recombinant tissue-type plasminogen activator (alteplase) for ischemic stroke 3 to 5 hours after symptom onset: the ATLANTIS study: a randomized controlled trial. JAMA 1999;282:2019–26.

10. Arnould MC, Grandin CB, Peeters A, et al. Comparison of CT and three MR sequences for detecting and categorizing early (48 hours) hemorrhagic transformation in hyperacute ischemic stroke. AJNR Am J Neuroradiol 2004;25:939–44.

11. Wardlaw J, Del Zoppo G, Yamaguchi T, et al. Thrombolysis in acute ischemic stroke, Cochrane Database Syst Rev 2003;3:CD000213.

12. Hacke W, Donnan G, Fieschi C, et al. Association of outcome with early stroke treatment: pooled analysis of ATLANTIS, ECASS, and NINDS rt-PA stroke trials. Lancet 2004;363:768–74.

13. Larrue V, von Kummer R, del Zoppo G, et al. Hemorrhagic transformation in acute ischemic stroke: potential contributing factors in the European Cooperative Acute Stroke Study. Stroke 1997;28:957–60.

14. Kent DM, Hinchey J, Price LL, et al. In acute ischemic stroke, are asymptomatic intracranial hemorrhages clinically innocuous? Stroke 2004;35:1141–6.

15. Lyden PD, Zivin JA. Hemorrhagic transformation after cerebral ischemia: mechanisms and incidence. Cerebrovasc Brain Metab Rev 1993;5:1–16.

16. Tong D, Adami A, Moseley M, et al. Relationship between apparent diffusion coefficient and subsequent hemorrhagic transformation following acute ischemic stroke. Stroke 2000;31:2378–84.

17. Selim M, Fink JN, Kumar S, et al. Predictors of hemorrhagic transformation after intravenous recombinant tissue plasminogen activator: prognostic value of initial apparent diffusion coefficient and diffusion-weighted lesion volume. Stroke 2002;33:2047–52.

18. Molina CA, Alvarez-Sabin J, Montaner J, et al. Thrombolysis-related hemorrhagic infarction: a marker of early reperfusion, reduced infarct size, and improved outcome in patients with proximal middle cerebral artery occlusion. Stroke 2002;33:1551–6.

19. Sloan MA, Price TR, Petito CK, et al. Clinical features and pathogenesis of intracerebral hemorrhages after rt-PA and heparin therapy for acute myocardial infarction in the Thrombolysis in Myocardial Infarction (TIMI) II pilot and randomized clinical trial experience. Neurology 1995;45:649–58.

20. Winkler DT, Biedermann LT, Tolnay M, et al. Thrombolysis induces cerebral hemorrhage in a mouse model of cerebral amyloid angiopathy. Ann Neurol 2002;51:790–3.

21. McCarron M, Nicoll JAR. Thrombolysis and intracerebral haemorrhage. Lancet Neurol 2004;3:484–92.

22. Yepes M, Lawrence DA. Tissue-type plasminogen activator and neuroserpin: a well-balanced act in the nervous system? Trends Cardiovasc Med 2004;14:173–80.

23. Wang X, Lee SR, Arai K, et al. Lipoprotein receptor-mediated induction of matrix metalloproteinase by tissue plasminogen activator. Nat Med 2003;9: 1313–17.

24. Brott TG, Haley EC Jr, Levy DE, et al. Urgent therapy for stroke. Part 1. Pilot study of tissue plasminogen activator administered within 90 minutes. Stroke 1992;23:632–40.

25. Messe SR, Tanne D, Demchuk AM, et al. Dosing errors may impact the risk of rt-PA for stroke: the Multicenter rt-PA Acute Stroke Survey. J Stroke Cerebrovasc Dis 2004;13:35–40.

26. Simon JE, Sandler DL, Pexman JHW, et al. Is intravenous recombinant tissue plasminogen activator (rt-PA) safe for use in patients over 80 years old with acute ischemic stroke? The Calgary experience. Age Ageing 2004;33:143–9.

27. Moulin T, Cattin F, Crepin-Leblond T, et al. Early CT signs in acute middle cerebral artery infarction: predictive value for subsequent infarct locations and outcome. Neurology 1996;47:366–75.

28. Grotta JC, Chiu D, Lu M, et al. Agreement and variability in the interpretation of early CT changes in stroke patients qualifying for intravenous rtPA therapy. Stroke 1999;30:1528–33.

29. Barber P, Demchuk AM, Zhang J, et al. Validity and reliability of a quantitative computed tomography score in predicting outcome of hyperacute stroke before thrombolytic therapy. Lancet 2000;355:1670–4.

30. Patel SC, Levine SR, Tilley BC, et al. Lack of clinical significance of early ischemic changes on computed tomography in acute stroke. JAMA 2001;286:2830–8.

31. Albers GW, Bates VE, Clark WM, et al. Intravenous tissue-type plasminogen activator for treatment of acute stroke: the Standard Treatment with Alteplase to Reverse Stroke (STARS) study. JAMA 2000;283:1145–50.

32. Tanne D, Kasner SE, Demchuk AM, et al. Markers of increased risk of intracerebral hemorrhage after intravenous recombinant tissue plasminogen activator therapy for acute ischemic stroke in clinical practice: the Multicenter rt-PA Acute Stroke Survey. Circulation 2002;105:1679–85.

33. Larrue V, Lauwers-Cances V. Risk of severe intracerebral hemorrhage after rtPA for ischemic stroke in patients with extended ischemic changes on computed tomography. Cerebrovasc Dis 2003;16(Suppl 4):110.

34. Kidwell CS, Saver JL, Villablanca JP, et al. Magnetic resonance imaging detection of microbleeds before thrombolysis: an emerging application. Stroke 2002; 33:95–8.

35. Derex L, Nighogossian N, Hermier M, et al. Thrombolysis for ischemic stroke in patients with old microbleeds on pretreatment MRI. Cerebrovasc Dis 2004;17:238–41.

36. Kawai N, Keep RF, Betz AL. Hyperglycemia and the vascular effects of cerebral ischemia. Stroke 1997;28: 149–54.

37. Bruno A, Levine SR, Frankel MR, et al. Admission glucose level and clinical outcomes in the NINDS rt-PA Stroke Trial. Neurology 2002;59: 669–74.

38. Demchuk AM, Morgernstern LB, Krieger DW, et al. Serum glucose level and diabetes predict tissue plasminogen activator-related intracerebral hemorrhage in acute ischemic stroke. Stroke 1999;30:34–9.

39. Bowes MP, Zivin JA, Thomas GR, et al. Acute hypertension but not thrombolysis increases the incidence and severity of hemorrhagic transformation following experimental stroke in rabbits. Exp Neurol 1996;141:40–6.

40. Levy DE, Brott T, Haley EC, et al. Factors related to intracranial hematoma formation in patients receiving tissue-type plasminogen activator for acute ischemic stroke. Stroke 1994;25:291–7.

41. Graham G. Tissue plasminogen activator for acute ischemic stroke in clinical practice. A meta-analysis of safety data. Stroke 2003;34:2847–50.

42. Katzan I, Hammer M, Furlan A, et al. Quality improvement and tissue-type plasminogen activator for acute ischemic stroke: a Cleveland update. Stroke 2003;34:799–800.

15

Implementation of thrombolytic therapy for stroke in routine practice

Guntram W Ickenstein, Heinrich J Audebert, and Nils Gunnar Wahlgren

Safe implementation of thrombolysis in stroke (SITS)

Intravenous treatment with alteplase, a recombinant tissue-type plasminogen activator (rtPA), was approved in the USA in 1996 and by the European Union (EU) regulatory authorities in 2002 for the treatment of acute ischemic stroke within 3 h of symptom onset. At the Karolinska Stroke Update Consensus meeting in 2000, it was concluded that intravenous rtPA within 3 h after onset of symptoms in patients with acute ischemic stroke is a highly effective evidence-based treatment (grade A evidence).[1] For the EU, Iceland and Norway, two major conditions were set for temporary approval between 2003 and 2005. The first condition was that all patients treated with alteplase during a 3-year period within the EU, Norway, and Iceland, will be registered in the Safe Implementation of Thrombolysis in Stroke (SITS) internet database in accordance with the SITS Monitoring Study (SITS-MOST) protocol. The second condition was that a randomized controlled study of alteplase versus placebo, later called ECASS III (European Cooperative Acute Stroke Study III), should be launched for patients who could be treated within a 3–4 h time interval. In a later protocol amendment, this interval has been extended to 4½ h.

Since the safety and efficacy of a treatment may be different in the setting of randomized controlled trials and during implementation into clinical routine, the benefits demonstrated in clinical studies combined with the observed potential for hemorrhagic complications call for continous quality control through clinical audit as routine clinical use of rtPA in stroke becomes established. Treatment may be in the hands of less experienced clinical centers, inclusion and exclusion criteria may be less strictly followed, and treatment outcome is generally not systematically monitored.

SITS-MOST is an observational safety monitoring study for EU countries embedded within the SITS International Stroke Thrombolysis Register (SITS-ISTR) (Figure 15.1). A similar study was launched in South Korea during 2005. The registry is available to clinicians worldwide and is driven by independent collaborators, having been established by the European Cooperative Acute Stroke Study (ECASS).[2] The International Coordinating Centre is at the Karolinska University Hospital in Stockholm.

The EU approval includes a condition that treatment should be given under the responsibility of a physician trained in neurological care. Criteria for center participation are specified in the SITS-MOST protocol. A center must have solid experience of acute stroke treatment. The physician on call at the emergency department of the hospital must have the authority to initiate thrombolysis treatment or have immediate access to a colleague with this authority.

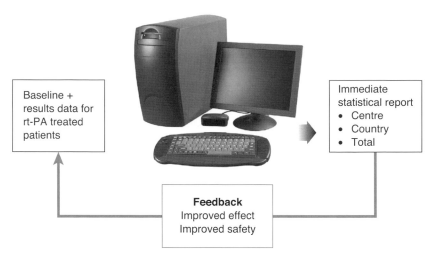

Figure 15.1
SITS registry: automatic feed back of entered data

During thrombolysis and the first day after admission, patients will be admitted to an intermediate care unit (IMC) or intensive care unit (ICU), preferably but not necessarily within the stroke unit. These units should have monitoring equipment for the management of oxygen saturation blood pressure, blood glucose, body temperature, pulse rate, and electrocardiography (ECG). Also, a nurse should be constantly present in the room during procedures, qualified to monitor level of consciousness and neurological impairment. The ward responsible for thrombolysis treatment should be specialized in stroke management, with a multidisciplinary team including a trained stroke nurse, and usually also including a physiotherapist, occupational therapist, speech therapist, social worker, and neuropsychologist. The ward should also adhere to a policy of early rehabilitation.

Now that alteplase has been provisionally licensed in Europe, SITS-MOST aims to prove that it is as safe and as beneficial in routine clinical practice in a large number of European clinical centers as it has been shown to be in randomized clinical trials such as the NINDS (National Institute of Neurological Disorders and Stroke) trial.[3] Since the risk of early fatal and symptomatic intracranial hemorrhage is increased and these hazards in randomized trials are

offset by a reduction in the proportion of patients due to death or dependency, primary and secondary aims of SITS-MOST include:

- the incidence of symptomatic intracranial hemorrhage (SICH) within 22–36 h after thrombolytic treatment, mortality at 3 months (mRS 6), and independence for activities of daily living (ADL) at 3 months (mRS 0–2) related to background variables
- independence compared with expected outcome in a prognostic model based on the placebo arm of randomized controlled trials
- a risk model for hemorrhage and death
- outcome in stroke subgroups

The central question is not a fundamental doubt about the efficacy of rtPA in acute ischemic stroke but rather that of conditions of prescription and safety in routine clinical use. There is concern that the risk of thrombolysis might be greater under routine conditions than under the optimal experimental conditions of controlled trials conducted exclusively in experienced centers and that this higher risk might outweigh the benefit. In addition, it has been shown that intravenous rtPA within 6 h after onset of ischemic stroke

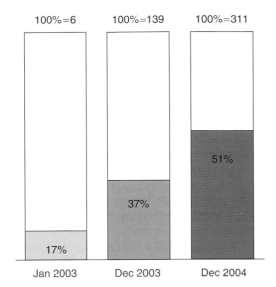

Figure 15.2
Increasing proportion of centers with more or less than five patients/year treated with rt-PA.

symptoms seems to be beneficial – although the benefit is smaller while the risks are higher.[4] Therefore, even in the 3 h time window, the question on risk and efficacy of thrombolytic treatment under routine conditions (especially outside experienced centers) needs further eludication, focusing on safety and efficacy in real medical practice. In SITS-MOST, hemorrhages on post-treatment imaging combined with clinical deterioration will be independently evaluated by a Brain Imaging Committee. Source data monitoring is performed in 10% of all patients by professional monitors. SITS has accepted a request to provide the European Medicines Evaluation Agency (EMEA) with biannual reports on the proportions of patients who experience a symptomatic intracranial hemorrhage or die following treatment or who are independent for ADL at 3-month follow-up. The outcome of the study will be compared with those of a systematic analysis of randomized controlled trails, which provides a proportion of 8.6% for symptomatic intracerebral hemorrhage, 17.3% for death and 50.1% for independence (Wardlaw JM: data from the Cochrane collaboration. Personal communication) and with the outcome of a pooled analysis of all randomized controlled trials of rtPA.[5]

Centers intending to employ intravenous thrombolysis in agreement with EU approval use an electronic application form on the SITS website (www.acutestroke.org). In this form, each center, through its local coordinator, accepts the basic conditions for participation in SITS and also confirms that they do fulfill the criteria set up by EMEA and the SITS-MOST protocol. The application is then submitted to the National Coordinator. The National Coordinator then provides the user name and password after approval of the application. Local users are appointed by a local coordinator, who is also authorized to enter user names and passwords. Data entry includes time of onset of stroke symptoms and arrival at hospital, time for brain imaging and start of treatment, age and gender, initial stroke severity (National Institutes of Health Stroke Scale: NIHSS), risk factors, stroke subtype, imaging studies before and after treatment, stroke severity after treatment, evaluation of hemorrhagic or other complications, and functional outcome with Rankin score at 3 months. Complete data entry takes a few minutes using a point-and-click design. Automatic reports, updated on a daily basis, provide statistics for the user's own center, for the user's own country, and for all registry data. This immediate feedback of results should stimulate improvement in management, which may lead to increased benefit for patients. So far, the median symptom onset-to-door time is 65 min and so is the median door-to-needle time.

The EU regulatory authorities decided that data collected through SITS and data from the randomized controlled trial within the 3–4 h time window (ECASS III) will form the basis for a final evaluation of continued licence approval after 3 years. This decision was made by the EU Commission on 29 September 2002 and was passed to the appropriate national authorities for implementation. Since this international network of stroke professionals launched the database on a secure internet connection for monitoring the safety and efficacy of rtPA in stroke, more than 6000 patients have been included in a later version started in January 2003 and over 400 patients in an earlier pilot database.

The recruitment of clinical centers with no previous experience of thrombolysis for the treatment has been increasingly successful during the period

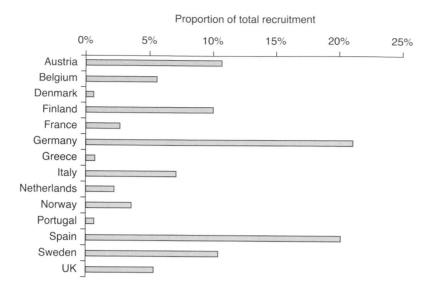

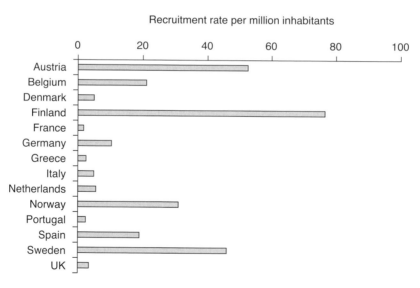

Figure 15.3
SITS-MOST recruitment.

2003–2005. The proportion of centers with more than five patients/year treated with intravenous thrombolysis before entering SITS-MOST was 17% in January 2003, 37% in December 2003, and 51% in December 2004 (Figure 15.2). Therefore SITS-MOST reaches new centers that might be reluctant to start without support from the network. The total number of centers now active to recruit patients into the SITS registry is 340 from 24 countries (Figure 15.3). About 10 new centers become active each month. The potential expansion of the treatment within the active SITS centers, following improved logistics, information to the public, and internal education, can be estimated to increase from currently about 3000 per year to about 10 000. The number of centers in Europe alone needs to be expanded several times over the next few years to fulfil the needs.

Safety of rtPA use in a telemedicine setting (TEMPIS)

The extreme sensitivity of neuronal tissue to even brief periods of ischemia mandates that ischemic stroke patients be treated as a medical emergency. For several years now, new drugs such as rtPA have offered powerful hope for people who suffer strokes, cutting the risk of death or disability. However, a decade after the US National Institutes of Health declared thrombolytic therapy to be the gold standard for stroke treatment, the vast majority of stroke patients still do not receive the medicine, because they are not treated quickly enough. Studies have found that still less than 3% of stroke patients receive thrombolytics.[6]

Published guidelines recommend that the door-to-needle time for the use of intravenous rtPA treatment in patients with stroke should be no more than 60 min.[7] Numerous communities in rural areas are medically and neurologically underserved, as demonstrated by poor utilization of proven stroke prevention therapies.[8] These same communities rely on community hospitals with limited access to neurological expertise and lesser comfort in the use of thrombolytics for stroke patients. In one study, 66% of hospitals surveyed did not have stroke protocols, and 82% did not have rapid identification for patients experiencing acute stroke.[9] Increasing the appropriate use of rtPA in acute ischemic stroke can result in an additional 12% of patients having an excellent neurological outcome at day 90 and a 48% likelihood of being discharged to home, compared with 36% of patients not receiving rtPA.[10]

The requirements for telemedicine in stroke medicine in communities without an established stroke team were first described by Levine and Gorman.[11] They listed the mandatory elements of a telestroke system: high-speed data connection to transfer imaging data and review clinical findings at a remote computer workstation. Since neurological examination and cranial computed tomography (CCT) are crucial in assessing an acute stroke patient for

possible thrombolytic intervention, the NIHSS, as an abbreviated neurological examination, has been validated for use in telemedical assessment and treatment of stroke.[12] The adequacy of neuroradiologists' reading of digitally transmitted head CT scans has been reported,[13] and the validity and reliability of stroke-trained neurologists' readings of acute stroke head CT scans via teleradiology has been evaluated, showing an excellent validity to exclude patients who have hemorrhage on the baseline non-contrast CT (NCCT).[14] Telemedicine technology has been shown to be useful and effective in the remote neurological evaluation and treatment of acute stroke patients and is now used at several hospitals in Europe and the USA as an option for stroke patients to have access to cerebrovascular expertise.[13,15,16]

In 2000, the Brain Attack Coalition (BAC) proposed a concept of a two-level stroke center that should be established in the near future: this should comprise a primary stroke center and a comprehensive stroke center.[17] Since it is unlikely that every primary stroke center would have a neurologist with expertise in vascular disease on its attending staff, a telemedicine system could be used to develop an environment in which the expertise of a stroke neurologist is available 24 h/7 days. This system could aid managed care plans in hospital selection, with a number of hospitals being linked with stroke centers as part of their telemedicine care network. By reducing complications and improving patient status at discharge, the savings to the health care system could be substantial.

In Bavaria, Germany, only half of the population has the chance to be admitted to one of the existing 19 stroke units within the critical time window of less than 3 h, and the majority of stroke patients are treated in local general hospitals in rural areas. In 2002, the Telemedicine Pilot Project for Integrated Stroke Care (TEMPIS) was established to increase the safe and proper use of tPA thrombolysis through a telemedicine 24 h/7 day stroke expert consultation service, accelerating treatment via telemedicine technology in the precious first hours when a stroke patient's brain is being damaged beyond repair.

In TEMPIS, cooperation was established between two comprehensive stroke centers (the Department of Neurology at the Munich Harlaching Hospital and the Department of Neurology at the University of

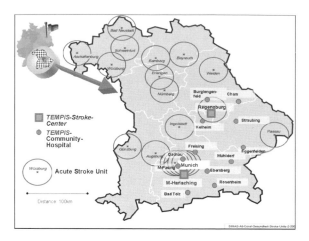

Figure 15.4
Institutions for specialized stroke care in Bavaria.
(See also color plate)

Regensburg) and 12 regional hospitals as primary stroke centers in the southeast of Bavaria. None of the 12 regional hospitals has previously had a stroke unit, 2 hospitals have small neurology departments, and in the other 10 hospitals, the internal medicine departments are responsible for acute stroke care. The locations of the two stroke centers and the distances to the regional hospitals are shown in Figure 15.4.

The initial steps for the implementation of the TEMPIS project in 2002 were:

1. Establishment of specialized stroke wards in all participating local hospitals.
2. Comprehensive stroke training for all staff members of the new stroke team.
3. Introduction of a high-speed conferencing system allowing simultaneous clinical examination and transmission of the DICOM data of brain imaging based on a 24 h/7 day service of stroke experts for teleconsultation.
4. Introduction of a newly designed and patented Stroke Lysis Box for rtPA thrombolysis for the staff of the participating local hospitals.

Each of the 14 participating hospitals was equipped with a high-speed video conferencing system (up to 30 ISDN lines). The telemedicine workstation consists of a videoconference system (Vicon ViGO Professional) and a remote-control video camera

(Sony Camera EviD100P). The DICOM interface of the local CT scanners and MRI scanners (if present) is connected to the workstation, and assessment of images is carried out using an Efilm workstation. The two stroke centers provide a 24 h telemedicine service with five full-time stroke experts on a week-by-week rotation. Predefined indications and rules to contact the stroke centers have been established. The medical staff of the community-based hospitals have completed a training program in state-of-the-art stroke treatment, which included:

- standardized optimized procedures (SOP) for diagnosis and treatment of stroke syndromes
- video training and certification in NIHSS evaluation
- rotations in the stroke units of the two comprehensive stroke centers
- update courses in extra/intracranial Doppler ultrasound studies
- day courses in swallowing disorders and dysphagia management
- stroke rehabilitation courses, including physical therapy, Bobath training, occupational therapy, and speech and language pathology

A special designed Stroke Lysis Box was introduced as a practical aid for rtPA thrombolysis to all participating telestroke hospitals, and in the following months the data on all rtPA thrombolyses were collected.[18] The Stroke Lysis Box is designed as a portable information and action box to manage patients who qualify for thrombolysis. It contains all information and medication for rtPA management and for the management of oxygen saturation, blood pressure, blood glucose, and temperature, injection materials, and infusion sets. Thus the information and material needed for thrombolytic therapy are readily available and also protected from dust and liquids in this disposable and portable box (Figure 15.5). Preprinted diagnostic/treatment orders in the Stroke-Lysis-Box, a checklist of treatment inclusion/exclusion criteria, and printed information for patients and families help to focus on the patient and to explain the rationale and risks of the proposed treatment.

A log sheet that documents call time, response times, CT times, and rtPA treatment times has to be completed by the attending physicians and faxed to the comprehensive stroke center for quality improvement monitoring. Also, initial training and ongoing

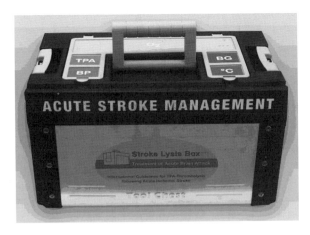

Figure 15.5
Stroke Lysis Box for rtPA thrombolysis.

mentoring on management of acute stroke patients enhances the care provided to this population by increasing staff awareness and confidence of the disease process. For analysis of intracranial hemorrhages, CT scans are required post thrombolysis and when any clinical deterioration occurs, and are evaluated by a radiologist blinded to the clinical course of all patients. Bleeds are categorized according to the criteria published by Fiorelli et al[19] for the ECASS I cohort. According to the NINDS definition, hemorrhage is considered symptomatic 'if it was not seen on a previous CT scan and there had subsequently been either a suspicion of hemorrhage and any decline of neurologic status' within 36 h after rtPA treatment.[3]

In the first year of the TEMPIS project 2182 teleconferences were performed (Figure 15.6). The mean number of teleconsultations initiated by the 12 remote hospitals was around 200 per month, with up to 20 per day. A high number (11.7%) of nonstroke diagnoses was found in the teleconsultations. Interhospital transfer to stroke centers or neurosurgical departments was indicated in 12.1% of all presented patients.

In a 12-month period before the introduction of the telemedicine network, the community hospitals in the TEMPIS project reported only 10 patients who received thrombolytic therapy. While 5 out of 12 community hospitals had experience with rtPA, 7 hospitals did not treat stroke patients with rtPA prior to the start of the TEMPIS project. In the

first 12 months of the project, 396 stroke patients were presented in the 3 h time window to clarify the indication for systemic rtPA thrombolysis. Out of 4179 stroke and transient ischemic attack (TIA) patients, 86 (2.1%) received rtPA according to TEMPIS protocol standards. During the following 18 months, 206 additional patients received systemic thrombolysis. The results of the first safety analysis were published after 106 rtPA treatments.[20]

The mean door-to-CT completion time was 20 min and the mean time between CT completion and rtPA treatment was 56 min, which still leaves possibilities for improvement, since the NINDS Consensus Conference recommended stroke evaluation targets for potential thrombolytic candidates of 45 min door to CT read, 60 min door to treatment, 15 min access to neurological expertise, and 2 h access to neurosurgical expertise.[21] Since all stroke experts in the comprehensive stroke centers are experienced in interpreting CCT and MRI studies and are available 24 h/7 days to read these scans, they could interpret the images within 15–20 min of their completion.[22] TEMPIS protocol violations occurred in 18 cases. Four patients had either 3 points (4×) or 4 points (3×) in the NIH Stroke Scale, and six patients had more than 20 NIHSS points (2×21, 1×22 and 3×23). In five cases, administration of rtPA was started later than 3h from onset (all within 15min after the 3 h time window). Symptomatic intracerebral hemorrhage occurred in 8.5% in the 14-month study period – including three patients with microbleeds and no mass effect.

Discussion and conclusions regarding rtPA use in routine clinical practice

Many physicians, especially those who are not neurologists, remain hesitant to use rtPA in acute stroke patients, suggesting that additional training methods and tools are desperately needed in many communities.[17] Since the NINDS-sponsored trial of rtPA in acute stroke was conducted at a relatively small number of experienced stroke centers, one commonly expressed concern is that similar results might not be obtained when rtPA is used in a variety of clinical settings. After publication of the NINDS

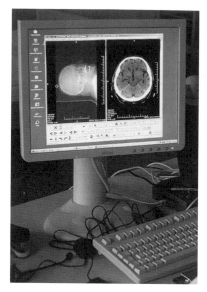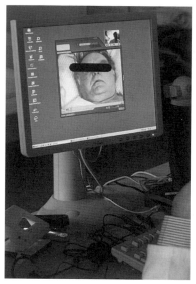

Figure 15.6
Screenshots of a telestroke conference in the TEMPIS project. (See also color plate)

trial results, more than a dozen reports of experience with rtPA in open-label, routine clinical use have been published. In 2639 treated patients, the symptomatic intracerebral hemorrhage rate was 5.2% (95% confidence interval 4.3–6.0),[23] which is slightly lower than the 6.4% rate of the NINDS trial.[3] The mean total death rate (13.4%) and proportion of subjects achieving a very favorable outcome (37.1%) were comparable to the NINDS trial results.[23] During 2006, the proportions of symptomatic hemorrhage, mortality, and independence for ADL in over 4500 patients included in SITS-MOST will be published. As public awareness of the availability of treatment for acute stroke increases, public expectations of stroke treatment rise. However, a confident, well-equipped staff is one of the most important components in the successful delivery of thrombolytic therapy, since the risk of symptomatic intracerebral hemorrhage is a major limitation to the use of thrombolytic medication, and can be as high as 15.7%.[24] Therefore, patient selection is crucial and it is important to establish a stroke team in the stroke centers that has the experience to monitor patients after rtPA treatment. As a result, community hospitals will increasingly face medicolegal risks both for treating and for not treating patients with newly available

agents. With a backup of stroke experts in professional networks such as SITS and in the telestroke setting, patients and family members can be assured that they speak with the expert face to face or online in the emergency unit and that all treatment options are standardized and discussed. This will lift a huge burden from the less stroke-experienced doctors in local hospitals in rural areas.

Another major problem confronting all community hospital stroke programs is one that has been called the 'frequency factor'. Since a small number of stroke patients will qualify for acute interventions such as rtPA thrombolysis, a stroke team could have difficulties in running effectively. A recent study investigating the routine use of systemic rtPA thrombolysis has reported an increase in in-hospital mortality after administration of rtPA in hospitals with fewer than five thrombolytic therapies within 1 year.[25] These findings underline the need to have an experienced stroke expert involved in the management of acute stroke patients, since urgent therapeutic decisions in emergency stroke care have to be made on the basis of brain imaging and a structured clinical examination. With a good knowledge of functional and vascular cerebral anatomy, the stroke expert can quickly determine the neuroanatomical localization of the brain lesion and can guide special treatment options. Since such experience and resources are available mainly in stroke centers of teaching hospitals, a networking system such as SITS and TEMPIS can allow each hospital to have access to the experience of all programs in the network. In a recent study, remote examination in the emergency room was found to be equivalent to bedside testing by an expert with the same level of experience, showing the good quality of telemedicine technology nowadays.[15]

One important aim for the SITS professional network and for the telemedicine concept is to encourage broad implementation of the treatment, and specifically to provide educational and statistical support. In Europe, where regulatory authorities require that treatment should be restricted to stroke units (or corresponding levels of stroke specialization), implementation of thrombolysis treatment has been paralleled by a systematic buildup of stroke units in some countries (e.g. Italy). In a meta-analysis, rtPA protocol deviations were reported in 19.8%, and comparison across studies showed that the mortality rate was correlated with the percentage of protocol violations ($r = 0.67$, $p = 0.018$).[23] In the Cleveland experience, where a 50% protocol deviation rate was initially reported,[24] implementation of additional training and quality improvement measures decreased the frequency of protocol violations and reduced the symptomatic intracerebral hemorrhage rates to levels close to the NINDS results.[26]

As described in several publications, telemedicine in acute stroke treatment is feasible and offers a new opportunity to improve stroke care in nonurban areas.[15,16,27–29] Due to the rapid evaluation of telestroke presentations and teleradiology consultation, this new technology may be timesaving in emergency stroke care, especially when rtPA thrombolysis is considered. In a telestroke setting, thrombolytic treatment options could be delivered to more stroke patients. In the last decade, hospital networks have been created and helicopter transport systems initiated to accelerate admission. But, even with helicopter transport, it took an average of 135 minutes from symptom onset to arrival at the designated stroke center.[30] In the TEMPIS project, which included a high involvement of the local emergency departments with continuous stroke education as well as public information to streamline local stroke

management, a mean time from symptom onset to hospital arrival of 65 min could be achieved. In addition, telestroke gives the possibilities of a first neurology expert consultation without losing time, and therefore enhances the options for rtPA treatment in the first 3 h time window. According to the protocol, the mean door-to-needle time for rtPA treatment was 76 min, which is still longer than the 60 min recommendation of the published guidelines.[7] Whereas the time needed for teleconsultation in the TEMPIS project appears to be adequate, the latencies between admission and CT diagnostics and between teleconsultation and the start of rtPA infusion still need to be reduced. Putting these measurements into practice, more patients could receive rtPA. In addition, earlier administration would provide an even higher benefit, as shown in the recently published analysis of the pooled data of the rtPA stroke trials.[5]

The TEMPIS data clearly support the necessity for adequate provider education and adherence to approved indications in institutions treating acute stroke patients with rtPA. While there is considerable information about how to carry out thrombolytic therapy in acute ischemic stroke (books, publications, and study protocols), that information is often unavailable in emergency situations. This is a critical problem for less experienced doctors who first encounter stroke patients in the emergency room. To reach the standard of rtPA thrombolysis of specialized stroke centers with a specialized stroke team, we designed and introduced a Stroke Lysis Box for rtPA thrombolysis, which has all the treatment information, medication, equipment, and screening forms for the quick and safe application of rtPA. We intended that the Stroke Lysis Box, placed in the emergency room where the telestroke connection is located, should enhance physicians' confidence in rtPA treatment, in addition to the telestroke conference, and should make the physicians' job easier by reducing the time required to find the necessary information. Our safety results show that the symptomatic intracerebral hemorrhage rate in the TEMPIS project is comparable to the NINDS data and lower than reported in inexperienced local hospitals.[24,25,31] The percentage of all types of intracranial hemorrhage is between the rates reported in the NINDS study (11%) and in ECASS II (43% in patients with rtPA treatment within 3 h).[32]

However, this safe and effective telestroke and tele-thrombolysis service with experienced stroke experts for stroke management requires a 24h on-demand teleconsultation service that needs to be reimbursed. In TEMPIS, the expenses for this service account for 300 000€ per year. Based on the calculated savings of subsequent costs by each thrombolysis of between 3300 and 4200 €,[33] the absolute increase in systemic thrombolysis of 76 rtPA treatments within one year would result in a total saving of between 250 800 and 319 200 €. Therefore, the teleconsultation service turns out to be cost-efficient regarding only the consultations for possible thrombolyses. Since a European consensus statement set the goal of having all persons with acute stroke admitted to specialized treatment facilities by the year 2005,[34] using the TEMPIS model with a development of local stroke teams in nonurban areas might be the solution to the difficult reimbursement situation of insurance companies and the problems in finding enough stroke neurologists.

In summary, the wide implementation of thrombolysis in stroke is supported by the expanding SITS network and registry. Our data from the SITS-MOST trial and the TEMPIS project show that the use of rtPA treatment in acute stroke can be extended with a rtPA thrombolysis protocol and a telemedicine stroke concept. In addition, a Stroke Lysis Box for rtPA thrombolysis can enhance confidence with thrombolysis and may lead to more frequent use of rtPA. Telestroke and telethrombolysis are practicable and can contribute to the improvement of stroke care in rural hospitals that are too distant from a specialized stroke unit. In the absence of alternatives, telemedicine should be used to extend the utilization of systemic thrombolysis in acute stroke to more remote and underserved areas in the future.

References

1. Consensus Statement on Thrombolysis, Karolinska Stroke Update 2000. In: Wahlgren NG (ed). Karolinska Stroke Update. Stockholm, 2001:28–30.
2. Hacke W, Kaste M, Fieschi C, et al, for the Second European–Australasian Acute Stroke Study Investigators. Randomised double-blind placebo-controlled trial of thrombolytic therapy with intravenous alteplase in acute ischemic stroke (ECASS II). Lancet 1998;352:1245–51.
3. The National Institute of Neurological Disorders and Stroke rt-PA Stroke Study Group. Tissue plasminogen activator for acute ischemic stroke. N Engl J Med 1995; 333:1581–7.
4. Clark WM, Wissman S, Albers GW, for the ATLANTIS Study Investigators. Recombinant tissue-type plasminogen activator (alteplase) for ischemic stroke 3 to 5 hours after symptom onset. The ATLANTIS Study: a randomized controlled trial. JAMA 1999;282:2019–26.
5. Hacke W, Donna G, Fieschi C, et al. Association of outcome with early stroke treatment pooled analysis of ATLANTIS, ECASS, and NINDS rt-PA stroke trials. Lancet 2004;363:768–74.
6. Albers GW. Advances in intravenous thrombolytic therapy for treatment of acute stroke. Neurology 2001;57:77–81.
7. Adams H, Brott T, Furlan A. Guidelines for thrombolytic therapy for acute stroke: a supplement to the guidelines for the management of patients with acute ischemic stroke. Stroke 1996;27:1711–18.
8. Gage BF. Adverse outcomes and predictors of under use of antithrombotic therapy in medicare beneficiaries with chronic atrial fibrillation. Stroke 2000;31: 822–7.
9. Goldstein L. North Carolina Stroke Prevention and Treatment Facilities Survey. Stroke 2000;31:66–70.
10. Fagan SC, Morgenstern LB, Petitta A, for the NINDS rt-PA Stroke Study Group. Cost-effectiveness of tissue plasminogen activator for acute ischemic stroke. Neurology 1998;50:883–90.
11. Levine SR, Gorman M. Telestroke: the application of telemedicine for stroke. Stroke 1999;30:464–9.
12. Wang S, Lee SB, Pardue C, et al. Remote evaluation of acute ischemic stroke; Reliability of National Institutes of Health Stroke Scale via Telestroke. Stroke 2003;34:188–92.
13. Reponen J. Initial experience with a wireless personal digital assistant as a teleradiology terminal for reporting emergency computerized tomography scans. J Telemed Telecare 2000;6:45–9.

14. Johnston KC, Worrall BB. Teleradiology assessment of computerized tomographs online reliability study (TRACTORS) for acute stroke evaluation. Telemedicine J e-Health 2003;9:227–33.

15. Handschu R, Littmann R, Reulbach U, et al. Telemedicine in emergency evaluation of acute stroke. Interrater agreement in remote video examination with a novel multimedia system. Stroke 2003;34: 2842–6.

16. Wiborg A, Widder B, for the TESS Study Group. Teleneurology to improve stroke care in rural areas. The Telemedicine in Stroke in Swabia (TESS) project. Stroke 2003;34:2957–63.

17. Alberts MJ, Hademenos G, Latchaw RE, et al, for the Brain Attack Coalition. Recommendations for the establishment of primary stroke centers. JAMA 2000; 283:3102–9.

18. Ickenstein GW, Horn M, Schenkel J, et al, for the TEMPiS Study Group. The use of telemedicine in combination with a new Stroke Lysis Box significantly increases t-PA utilization in rural communities. Neurocrit Care 2005;3:27–32.

19. Fiorelli M, Bastianello S, von Kummer R, et al. Hemorrhagic transformation within 36 hours of a cerebral infarct: relationships with early clinical deterioration and 3-month outcome in the European Cooperative Acute Stroke Study I (ECASS I) cohort. Stroke 1999;30:2280–4.

20. Audebert HJ, Kukla C, von Clarenan C, et al. Telemedicine for safe and extended thrombolysis in stroke. Stroke 2005;36:287–91.

21. NINDS Symposium. Setting New Directions for Stroke Care: Rapid Identification and Treatment of Stroke. Washington, DC, December 12–13, 1996.

22. Grotta J. Acute hospital care: resource utilisation. In: Marler J, Jones P, Emr M (eds). Proceedings of a National Symposium on Rapid Identification and Treatment of Acute Stroke. Arlington, VA: National Institute of Neurological Disorders and Stroke, 1997:87–9.

23. Graham GD. Tissue plasminogen activator for acute ischemic stroke in clinical practice. A meta-analysis of safety data. Stroke 2003;34:2847–50.

24. Katzan IL, Furlan AJ, Lloyd LE, et al. Use of tissue-type plasminogen activator for acute ischemic stroke: the Cleveland area experience. JAMA 2000; 283:1151–8.

25. Heuschmann PU, Kolominsky-Rabas PL, Roether J, et al. German Stroke Registers Study Group. Predictors of in-hospital mortality in patients with acute ischemic stroke treated with thrombolytic therapy. JAMA 2004;292:1831–8.

26. Katzan IL, Hammer MD, Furlan AJ, for the Cleveland Clinic Health System Stroke Quality Improvement Team. Quality improvement and tissue-type plasminogen activator for acute ischemic stroke: a Cleveland update. Stroke 2003;34:799–800.

27. Chodroff PH. A three-year review of telemedicine at the community level clinical and fiscal results. J Telemed Telecare 1999;5:28–30.

28. LaMonte MP, Bahouth M, Hu P, et al. Telemedicine for acute stroke. Triumphs and Pitfalls. Stroke 2003; 34.725–8.

29. Shafqat S, Kvedar JC, Guanci MM, et al. Role for telemedicine in acute stroke. Feasibility and reliability of remote administration of the NIH Stroke Scale. Stroke 1999;30:2141–5.

30. Sillimann SL, Quinn B, Huggett V, Merino JG. Use of a field-to stroke center helicopter transport program to extend thrombolytic therapy to rural residents. Stroke 2003;34:729–33.

31. Heuschmann PU, Berger K, Misselwitz B, et al. Frequency of thrombolytic therapy in patients with acute ischemic stroke and the risk of in-hospital mortality: the German Stroke Registers Study Group. Stroke. 2003;34:1106–13.

32. Fieschi C, Hacke W, Kaste M, et al. Thrombolytic therapy for acute ischaemic stroke. ECASS Study Group. Lancet 1997;350:1476.

33. Wein TH, Hickenbottom SL, Alexandrov AV. Thrombolysis, stroke units and other strategies for reducing acute stroke costs. Pharmacoeconomics 1998;14:603–11.

34. Aboderin I, Venables G. Stroke management in Europe. Pan European Consensus Meeting on Stroke Management. J Intern Med 1996;240:173–80.

16
Imaging of the ischemic penumbra

Magdy Selim, Max Wintermark, and Marc Fisher

Introduction

Several definitions of the ischemic penumbra have been proposed.[1–3] Fundamental to any definition is that the penumbra is a region of reduced blood supply that has spatial characteristics (i.e. it is situated within the vicinity of irreversibly damaged ischemic tissue) and temporal characteristics (i.e. it is progressively recruited into the infarcted tissue with time).[4] However, the penumbral tissue is potentially salvageable, if reperfusion occurs or tissue salvage therapy is initiated within a certain time period.[4] Imaging of the penumbra, therefore, requires detection of ischemic tissue and measuring reduced regional blood flow below a certain functional threshold. Multimodal magnetic resonance imaging (MRI) techniques that combine diffusion- and perfusion-weighted imaging and perfusion computed tomography (CT) have the potential capability to identify and separate brain tissue that is irreversibly injured (ischemic core), severely hypoperfused and at risk of infarction (the penumbra), mildly hypoperfused but not at risk (oligemia), and unaffected (normal).

Theoretical models underlying perfusion MRI and CT studies

Perfusion MRI and CT data relate to contrast enhancement curves evaluated in each pixel of the imaged slices. Contrast enhancement in each of these curves is directly related to the plasma concentration of contrast bolus. The central volume principle allows extraction of quantitative blood flow values from these data. The key to the central volume principle lies in solving a mathematical operation called deconvolution, which leads to a parameter called the mean transit time (MTT). The MTT designates the average time delay necessary for an instantaneous bolus of iodinated contrast material to cross the cerebral capillary network.[5–8] The regional cerebral blood volume (rCBV) relates to the relative volume occupied by blood in a pixel. It is inferred from a quantitative evaluation of a partial volume averaging effect (PVAE).[9–11] Indeed, time–concentration curves measured during perfusion studies do not all have the same areas: the latter are more extensive in pure vascular pixels than in parenchymal pixels – including blood within capillaries, but also neurons, axonal tubes, and myelin sheaths. In these parenchymal pixels, the vascular volume only represents a few percent of the total tissue volume, thus leading to a PVAE. As such, a PVAE is completely absent in a reference pixel in the center of the large superior longitudinal sinus, and the following equation ensues:

$$rCBV = \frac{\text{area under the curve in a parenthymal pixel}}{\text{area under the curve in the reference pixel}}$$

Normal values of rCBV amount to 6 ml/100 g in the gray matter and 2 ml/100 g in the white matter.[12] Finally, since the rCBV designates a blood volume and the MTT the time delay necessary for the blood to cross the local capillary network, their combination leads to the regional cerebral blood flow (rCBF):

$$rCBF = \frac{rCBV}{MTT}$$

Normal values of rCBF range around 80 ml/100 g/min in the gray matter and 20 ml/100 g/min in the white matter – of course with variations relating to local cerebral activity changes.[12]

Imaging of the ischemic penumbra with diffusion- and perfusion-weighted MRI

Diffusion- and perfusion-weighted MRI techniques assess different, but complementary, aspects of cerebral ischemia. Diffusion-weighted imaging (DWI) is highly sensitive to the shifts (diffusion) of water molecules and can detect ischemia-induced alterations in static water protons within minutes.[13–15] This diffusion slowing (i.e. cytotoxic edema) results in signal hyperintensity on DWI that can be seen as early as 2 min after the onset of cerebral ischemia,[13–15] thus making DWI an ideal imaging modality to detect and qualitatively identify ischemic brain tissue during the hyperacute phase of stroke.

The time and amplitude of the magnetic field gradient pulses influence the sensitivity of DWI to water shifts. Measurements of water diffusion at different gradient pulses (*b*-values) can be used to calculate a quantitative value for the degree of water diffusion, i.e. the apparent diffusion coefficient (ADC). The ADC of water is dependent upon the ionic membrane gradients, which derive their energy from high-energy compounds. Therefore, the ADC rapidly declines following ischemia-induced depletion of high-energy compounds.[16,17] This acute ADC decline thus allows the identification of tissue with energy failure that is indicative of the ischemic core.

Perfusion-weighted imaging (PWI) utilizes rapid acquisition of $T2^*$-weighted gradient-echo sequences following a bolus injection of a paramagnetic contrast. This results in a transient signal loss (i.e. darkening ($T2^*$ shortening)) in the perfused tissue and variable degrees of 'relative brightening' in the hypoperfused tissue.[18] Thus, PWI can be used to assess regional blood supply and to qualitatively delineate regions of decreased perfusion that may or may not proceed to infarction. Furthermore, the signal intensity (concentration)-versus-time curves from the PWI during bolus transit can be used to calculate physiological parameters of rCBV, rCBF, and mean transit time (rMTT).[19]

Therefore, combining the results of DWI and PWI can provide an estimate of the ischemic penumbra within a few minutes after the onset of cerebral ischemia, where the initial region of DWI abnormality and ADC decline (i.e. the zone of energy failure) is believed to represent the ischemic core within a larger region of reduced rCBF as defined by PWI.

The spatial and temporal components of the ischemic penumbra have been demonstrated in experimental[20–22] and human strokes[23–26] by using DWI and PWI. A mismatch in lesion size between DWI and PWI, with a core of restricted diffusion, low ADC, and absent perfusion that is surrounded by a zone of variable perfusion deficit, is often seen during the acute phase of cerebral ischemia (Figure 16.1).[20–26] This perfusion–diffusion mismatch is believed to represent penumbral ischemic tissue that is at risk of infarction if reperfusion is not restored in a timely fashion. Support is provided by results from serial DWI MRI studies showing that the initial DWI/ADC abnormality (i.e. the ischemic core) gradually expands into the hypoperfused region on initial PWI within a few hours after the ischemic insult in animal models[21,27] and 24–48 h in acute stroke patients;[23,26,28,29] and also showing chronic T2-weighted MRI lesions extending beyond the initial DWI ischemic regions into the surrounding PWI lesion regions.[30–33] Further support is provided by reports of patients with large PWI > DWI lesion mismatches who have a favorable clinical and radiological response to thrombolytic therapy and successful recanalization.[29,31,33] Such patients exhibit substantial improvement in their neurological function and smaller final infarct volumes after thrombolysis, even beyond 3 h from stroke onset.[29] Several studies have also shown a correlation between acute PWI (but not DWI) lesion size and baseline severity of neurological deficits, and that long-term neurological recovery is proportional to the volume of the mismatch that eventually escapes infarction.[28,34,35] Taken together, these findings indicate that PWI–DWI lesion mismatch serves as an approximate MRI marker for the ischemic penumbra.

However, the use of PWI–DWI mismatch pattern alone to identify the ischemic penumbra is too simplistic. It is estimated that more than 70% of stroke patients, evaluated within 6 h of stroke onset, have a mismatch between a smaller diffusion and a larger perfusion abnormality. The ischemic lesion on initial

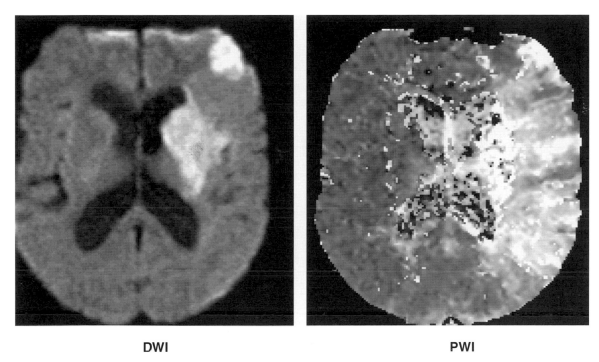

DWI   PWI

Figure 16.1
Diffusion-weighted imaging (DWI) shows a small hyperintensity in the left basal ganglia. Perfusion-weighted imaging (PWI) shows a larger area of prolonged mean transit time (MTT), indicative of a large diffusion–perfusion mismatch.

DWI often expands into the larger and surrounding hypoperfused lesion on PWI, but seldom reaches its full size.[32,34,36] Therefore, using the mismatch between PWI and DWI lesions alone may mix two sub-regions that are different: one that is at risk for infarction and may do so over time and another region of moderately reduced rCBF that does not go on to infarction. Animal and human studies have also demonstrated that there may be small areas within the DWI abnormality that possess biochemical characteristics of penumbral tissue.[17,37,38] This implies that the ischemic penumbra includes not only the perfusion–diffusion mismatch region but also portions of the diffusion abnormality, and that the use of DWI abnormality alone to estimate the ischemic core may be misleading. Calculating ADC values of the ischemic subregions is necessary for objective and quantitative interpretation of the DWI abnormality.[36]

A plethora of experimental and clinical data indicate that ADC values are decreased in regions with hypoperfusion within a few minutes of stroke onset. The severity of ADC decline within the ischemic tissue is heterogeneous, and correlates with the severity of regional perfusion deficit.[39] Ischemic regions with mild perfusion deficits and minimal decline in ADC values are potentially salvageable.[40] However, regions with low ADC will rapidly become permanently damaged if reperfusion is not restored. Desmond et al[40] studied 19 acute stroke patients with DWI and PWI within 6 h from stroke onset and showed that the mean ADC ratios in regions of the penumbra that progressed to infarction on 90-day follow-up MRI were 0.75–0.90, in comparison with contralateral homologous regions. The ADC ratios were less reduced in regions of the penumbra that escaped infarction.

The ADC decline can recover to normal values with successful reperfusion.[38,41,42] Reversal of DWI lesions, with mildly reduced ADC values, has been reported in animal models after brief temporary occlusion of the middle cerebral artery.[41] Recovery of ADC abnormalities has also been reported in experimental neuroprotective therapeutic studies in animals[43] and in stroke patients treated with intra-arterial thrombolysis up to 6 h from onset.[38] However, this reversal of DWI/ADC abnormalities appears in part to be short-lasting. Recurrent diffusion/ADC changes, after successful reperfusion, have been reported on subsequent follow-up DWI in both animal and human studies.[38,41,44] Histopathological studies demonstrate variable degrees of neuronal damage and necrosis within the regions of recurrent diffusion/ADC abnormalities that correlate with the severity of baseline CBF decline.[45] This indicates that early recovery of DWI/ADC abnormalities does not always correlate with penumbral salvage.

Determining physiological thresholds of blood volume and flow for the ischemic subregions may help refine characterization of the penumbral tissue. Schlaug et al[30] developed an operational definition for the penumbra using a retrospective analysis of admission and 2- to 3-day post-stroke DWI and PWI indices of rCBV, rCBF, and rMTT in 25 patients with acute stroke. Using PWI–DWI mismatch, they quantitatively characterized the penumbral tissue as having a 53% reduction in initial rCBV and 63% reduction in rCBF, in comparison with a contralateral control region. The ischemic core had a more severe reduction in initial rCBV (81%) and rCBF (88%). This corresponds to a CBF threshold of 18.5 ml/100 g/min in the penumbra and 6 ml/100 g/min in the core. These thresholds are in agreement with studies using positron emission tomography (PET) showing that CBF threshold in the ischemic core regions is less than 8 ml/100 g/min versus 17–45 ml/100 g/min in the penumbral tissue.[37,46–49] The study by Schlaug et al[30] showed that the initial rCBV was the best predictor of the penumbral tissue, and that the initial rCBF was slightly better than the initial rCBV in differentiating the ischemic penumbra from the core. rMTT was prolonged in both the penumbra and the core and was not good in differentiating them. However, it was excellent in differentiating abnormal (i.e. core and penumbra) from normal perfusion. A study aimed at determining the viability thresholds in the ischemic penumbra showed that the penumbral tissue on initial DWI–PWI, obtained within 6 h of stroke onset, progressed to infarction on follow-up scans at rCBF < 0.59 and rMTT > 1.63 cutoff values, calculated as ratios relative to contralateral mirror control

regions.[50] The penumbral tissue that recovered had higher rCBF and MTT values. In this study, the initial rCBV and ADC ratios did not differentiate the part of the penumbra that recovered from that which progressed into infarction, and the rCBF ratio was the best predictor of the fate of the penumbral tissue.[50] Clearly, more work is needed to validate these thresholds and to define more precise and applicable parameters for the penumbral and core regions.

It is noteworthy that there is a broad overlap between these threshold flow values in the ischemic tissue. This overlap is time-dependent; being less severe if PWI is performed within 6 h after stroke onset and greater if PWI is performed longer than 6 h after symptom onset. Therefore, determination of perfusion deficits alone provides a poor estimate of the tissue status as long as the time course of changes is not known in the individual patient. The duration of reduced perfusion parameters, such as CBF, that might lead to irreversible damage and infarction of the penumbral tissue is variable. There is evidence to suggest that viable tissue in the penumbra can be found up to 48 h after stroke onset[47,48] and that CBF thresholds increase with increasing duration of ischemia.[46] A study using in vivo proton magnetic resonance spectroscopy (^{1}H-MRS) to investigate the metabolic changes in the ischemic penumbra of patients with strokes attributed to internal carotid artery occlusive lesions suggests that chronic penumbral tissue lasting longer than previously thought may exist.[51]

The ability to determine the existence and extent of potentially salvageable penumbral tissue has important therapeutic implications. The PROACT (Prolyse [prourokinase] in Acute Cerebral Thrombolism) study showed that intra-arterial thrombolysis in stroke patients with angiographically documented middle cerebral artery occlusion resulted in significant clinical benefits, even when prourokinase was given as late as 6 h after stroke onset.[52] This implies that a portion of the penumbra was still viable in such patients, long after the current recommended 3 h window for thrombolysis. Studies using multimodal MRI with DWI, PWI, and magnetic resonance angiography (MRA) showed that the finding of a proximal vessel occlusion on MRA is almost always associated with a significant perfusion > diffusion mismatch.[23,31,53] However, not all patients with perfusion > diffusion mismatch have an identifiable arterial lesion on MRA.[29] Studies have consistently shown that patients with a perfusion > diffusion mismatch pattern and an observable lesion on MRA had a worse clinical outcome and enlargement of their initial DWI ischemic lesion volume on follow-up.[24,28,34,53] However, this natural evolution of acute perfusion > diffusion mismatch can be altered by thrombolysis.[29,33] Most recently, Parsons et al[29] studied 19 stroke patients treated with intravenous recombinant tissue-type plasminogen activator (rtPA) within 6 h from stroke onset (13 were treated between 3 and 6 h and 16 had perfusion > diffusion mismatch) and 21 untreated stroke patients (16 had perfusion > diffusion mismatch) with serial DWI, PWI, and MRA within 6 h from symptom onset, 2–3 days later and at 3-month follow-up. Patients with mismatch who were treated with rtPA had higher recanalization rates, enhanced reperfusion, greater salvage of penumbral tissue, less DWI lesion expansion, and improved clinical outcome. Of particular interest were 8 patients (4 treated with rtPA and 4 in the control group) in whom acute MRI showed perfusion > diffusion mismatch without a corresponding arterial lesion on MRA. Three of the rtPA-treated patients achieved complete penumbral salvage with no infarct expansion, in contrast to infarct expansion in all untreated patients. This study provides evidence that those patients with perfusion > diffusion mismatch can benefit from thrombolysis, even if MRA does not show a visible lesion, after 3 h from stroke onset. It also suggests that selection of patients for thrombolysis based on their PWI–DWI lesion mismatch pattern, rather than a clock-determined therapeutic window, is associated with an overall clinical and radiological improvement.

MRI with DWI and PWI has become an increasingly appealing imaging modality in evaluating acute stroke patients. It can provide rapid and noninvasive angiographic, perfusion, and lesion volume information. The ability and feasibility to use this information to acutely estimate the ischemic penumbra and to make treatment decisions has been demonstrated. Accurate definition of the ischemic penumbra, using DWI and PWI, requires identification of initial perfusion–diffusion mismatch in conjunction with ADC thresholds for tissue viability and baseline parameters of regional blood flow and volume thresholds. We can expect that future advances in MRI technology and data processing will ultimately optimize identification of the ischemic

penumbra. However, the PWI–DWI mismatch, if used in isolation, provides a practical and rapid means to roughly estimate the tissue at risk.

Imaging of cerebral hemodynamics by perfusion-CT

Perfusion-CT is a simple and accurate imaging technique affording quantitative assessment of brain perfusion. It involves dynamic acquisition of sequential CT slices on a cine mode during intravenous administration of nonionic iodinated contrast material. Data acquisition should take less than 5 min. Perfusion-CT studies are well tolerated even in acute patients, and can therefore be easily and quickly obtained in the emergency setting, as part of the admission cerebral imaging survey. Perfusion-CT can be performed in all hospitals equipped with ultrafast CT units and does not require specialized technologists or extra equipment – only postprocessing software.

The fundamentals of perfusion-CT were developed some two decades ago.[9–11,54–56] However, its implementation at that time was limited by the slowness of CT data acquisition and by the limited brain coverage by single-slice CT units. Today, CT is more technologically advanced with the introduction and spread of subsecond slice acquisition and multislice CT (MSCT) units. Indeed, with two successive acquisitions accompanied by acceptable patient radiation exposure, MSCT can assess for a depth of 40 mm of cerebral parenchyma.

Practically, perfusion-CT studies consist of two series of two slices obtained within a 5 min time interval. Each series involves 40 successive CT slices obtained every second on a stationary mode, with acquisition parameters of 80 kVp and 100 mA.[57] For each series, acquisition begins 7 s after starting the intravenous administration of a 40 ml infusion of nonionic iodinated contrast material. This intravenous administration is performed through an antecubital vein with a power injector at a rate of 5 ml/s. This protocol, combined with MSCT technology, can evaluate four 10 mm CT slices. These slices are chosen immediately above the orbits to protect the lenses, going through the basal ganglia and

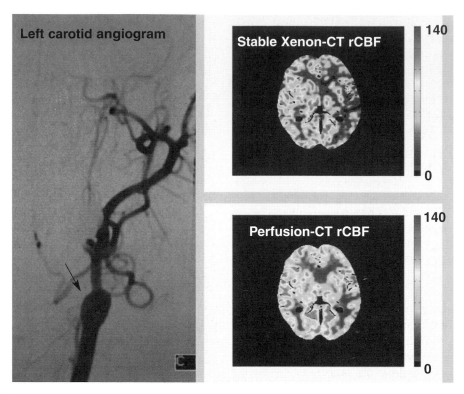

Figure 16.2
A 58-year-old male patient admitted for repeated transitory ischemic accidents. The postero-anterior angiographic view demonstrates a complete chronic occlusion of the left internal carotid artery (arrow), whereas both stable xenon-CT and perfusion-CT display a lowered regional cerebral blood flow (rCBF) in the left middle cerebral artery (MCA) territory. This area with lowered rCBF relates to an ischemic area, superimposed on a context of chronic arterial occlusion, and explains the patient's symptomatology. The perfusion-CT rCBF map (ml/100 g/min) relates closely to the corresponding reference stable xenon-CT map (ml/100 g/min), in both the gray and the white matter, as well as in the pathological ischemic area. (See also color plate)

towards the vertex. Perfusion CT series are performed after a standard cerebral CT examination of the brain parenchyma, and may be accompanied by extra- and intracranial CT angiography, the latter involving an additional dose of 70 ml of nonionic iodinated contrast material.

Quantitative validation of the accuracy of perfusion-CT results

Perfusion-CT results have been quantitatively validated against those of stable xenon-CT (Figure 16.2).[57]

Stable xenon-CT is a cerebral perfusion imaging technique requiring specialized and expensive equipment, as well as cooperation from acutely ill patients. Side-effects, such as decrease in respiratory rate, headaches, nausea and vomiting, as well as convulsions, are observed in 4.4% of patients.[58] Stable xenon-CT results have been proven to be as quantitatively accurate by comparison with radiolabelled microsphere studies, and thus stable xenon-CT constitutes an adequate gold standard for quantitative assessment of rCBF.[59–61] A strong correlation has been demonstrated between perfusion-CT and stable xenon-CT in both healthy cerebral regions and pathological cerebral regions with low rCBF, with slopes close to unity in linear regression analysis (Figure. 16.2). This accurate correlation in cerebral areas with reduced blood flows confers an adequate reliability to perfusion-CT studies in the evaluation of ischemic cerebral parenchyma.[57]

Perfusion-CT as a selection criterion in hyperacute stroke patients eligible for thrombolysis

Lowering of rCBF induces progressive inhibition of the various metabolic and electrical activities of the neurons, relating to many hemodynamic thresholds. This inhibition is first reversible, i.e. penumbra. Below 10–15 ml/100 g/min, alteration of adenosine triphosphate (ATP) synthesis results in a disturbance of membrane ion pumping. If the latter persists, irretrievable cerebral infarction occurs. Early after occlusion of a cerebral artery, an ischemic penumbra develops in the territory of cerebral parenchyma fed by this artery. With time, the infarct progressively replaces the penumbra from the center to the periphery of the ischemic arterial territory, the rate depending upon the collateral circulation and other factors.[62–64]

The purpose of thrombolysis is to rescue the penumbra.[65] However, it is associated with a significant risk of cerebral bleeding – up to 15%.[66] This explains why very strict criteria have been defined for the inclusion of acute stroke patients in intravenous thrombolysis protocols.[67–69] Assessment of brain perfusion prior to thrombolysis has been advocated as a possible selection criterion for treatment,[70–72] because extensive oligemia in the territory of an occluded MCA is related to an unfavorable risk–benefit ratio. Indeed, thrombolysis achieved in extended cerebral infarcts with limited penumbra would have little benefit and would increase the risk of intracranial bleeding.[68,73] Perfusion-CT, as described above, can easily be performed in acute stroke patients in an emergency setting. Nonionic iodinated contrast material is not toxic for ischemic neurons.[74]

Perfusion-CT can generate rCBF and rCBV maps. Penumbra and infarct can be assessed from these parameters and represented as a prognostic map (Figures 16.3–16.5). Infarct and penumbra can indeed be differentiated from each other through

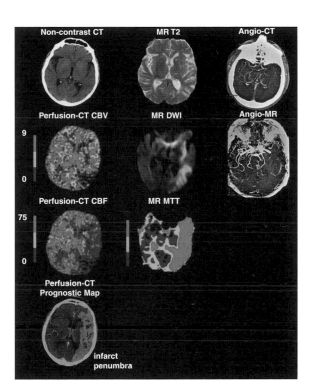

Figure 16.3

A 71-year-old male patient admitted for sudden onset of a right hemisyndrome, associated with nonfluent aphasia. Non-enhanced cerebral CT/perfusion-CT and DWI/PWI were performed 2 and 2.3 h after symptomatology onset, respectively. Non-enhanced cerebral CT demonstrates a left insula ribbon sign and left parietal hypodensity. The more sensitive perfusion-CT prognostic map clearly identifies a posterior and deep left MCA infarct (red), with penumbra (green) involving the remaining left MCA territory. Regional cerebral blood flow (rCBF) (ml/100 g/min) is lowered in both the infarct and the penumbra, whereas regional cerebral blood volume (rCBV) (ml/100 g) is lowered in the infarct, and preserved or increased in the penumbra, because of the autoregulation processes. The cerebral infarct on perfusion-CT shows a similar size to the DWI abnormality, and the cerebral ischemic lesion (infarct plus penumbra) on perfusion-CT shows a similar size to the MRI MTT abnormality. Stroke in this patient was related to an M1 occlusion, demonstrated on both CT angiography and MRA. The patient underwent unsuccessful thrombolysis. (See also color plate)

absence or persistence of vascular autoregulatory reflexes. In both penumbra and infarct, rCBF is lowered below 15–20 ml/100 g/min. However, in

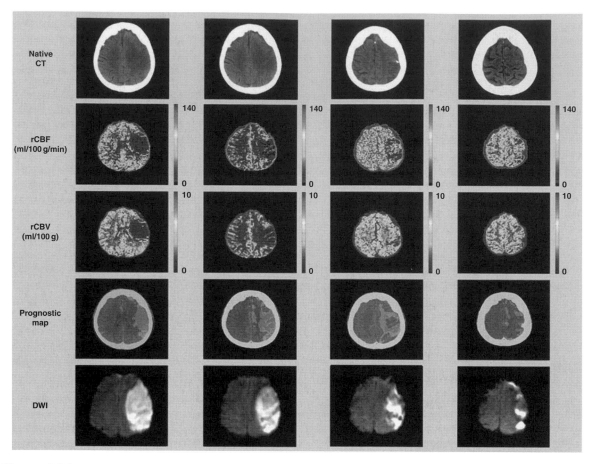

Figure 16.4

A hypertensive 43-year-old female patient was admitted at our institution 3.5 h after sudden onset of a right hemisyndrome, associated with right homonymous hemianopsia and global aphasia. Since it was contra-indicated, thrombolysis was not performed. The non-enhanced cerebral CT scan obtained 30 min after admission (top row) displays a subtle loss of the cortical ribbon in the left sylvian territory, whereas the more sensitive perfusion-CT prognostic map (fourth row) clearly identifies a posterior left MCA infarct (red), with a limited rim of penumbra (green). Due to the persistent occlusion of the left MCA (demonstrated by admission CT-angiography and delayed MRA obtained 2 days after admission), the penumbra described on the admission perfusion-CT evolved towards infarct and was completely replaced by it, as demonstrated by a close correlation of the whole ischemic area (penumbra plus infarct) as seen on the perfusion-CT with the infarct displayed on the delayed DWI (fifth row). (See also color plate)

penumbra, rCBV is increased as a result of a local vasodilatation, in an attempt to maintain autoregulation to compensate for rCBF lowering. In infarct, auto-regulatory reflexes are compromised and rCBV is lowered.[75–76] Perfusion-CT is potentially able to demonstrate the exact extent and location of infarct and penumbra in hyperacute stroke patients, within the first few minutes of cerebral ischemia.

The accuracy of such determined prognostic maps extracted from admission perfusion-CT results was demonstrated through comparison with acute and delayed MRI.[75,76] Perfusion-CT-defined infarct and penumbra were closely correlated with DWI demonstration of infarction and the DWI–PWI mismatch, respectively (Figure 16.3).[75] In the case of persistent arterial occlusion (Figure 16.4), the ischemic area

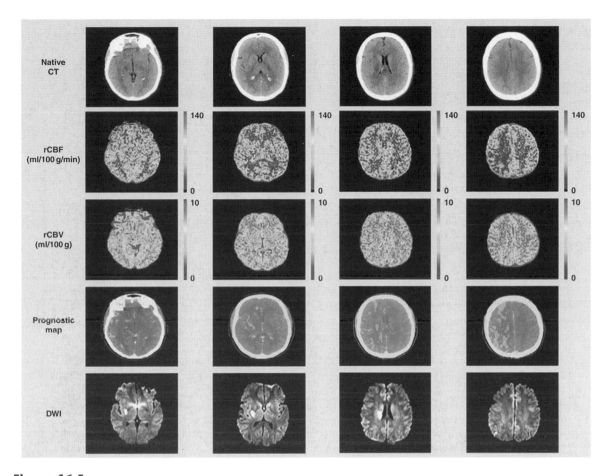

Figure 16.5
A 46-year-old female patient with suspected deep right sylvian artery stroke. The non-enhanced cerebral CT (top row) obtained on admission, 4 h after symptomatology onset, features a hypodensity and a gray matter–white matter dedifferentiation in the right internal capsula. The more sensitive perfusion-CT prognostic map (fourth row) identifies a more extensive deep left MCA penumbra (green), with a very limited infarct (red) located on the right internal capsula. No thrombolysis was performed due to time delay. Six days after admission, DWI (fifth row) demonstrates the residual irretrievable infarct, which closely correlates with the one described on the perfusion-CT prognostic map. Recanalization of the right MCA, demonstrated by delayed MRA, afforded recovery of the penumbra described on the admission perfusion-CT. (See also color plate)

(penumbra plus infarct) on the admission perfusion-CT gradually evolves towards infarct, due to the persistence of the arterial occlusion. In the case of arterial recanalization (Figure 16.5) – either spontaneous or as a result of thrombolysis most of the penumbra recovers, as demonstrated by delayed DWI.[76] The initial severity of the patient's clinical status was proportional to the admission size of the ischemic area (penumbra plus infarct) on perfusion-CT. In cases of arterial recanalization, the observed clinical improvement correlated linearly with the Lausanne Stroke Index, defined as the relative extent of penumbra compared with the whole ischemic area (penumbra plus infarct) on the admission perfusion-CT. This means that the clinical prognosis is better with a high PRR (potential recuperation ratio), i.e. when the penumbra predominates over the infarct with regard to size.[76]

Conclusions and future prospects

Developing and implementing additional acute stroke therapies will likely be aided by the availability of imaging techniques such as diffusion/perfusion-weighted MRI and perfusion-CT. These imaging techniques will provide important information about the presence of the ischemic penumbra to allow designers of clinical trials and clinicians caring for stroke patients to better choose patients eligible for treatment. This information will revolutionize how acute stroke patients are managed, because treatment decisions will be made based upon the status of the individual patient and not rigid time windows. Much additional work needs to be performed to validate and refine how these MRI and CT techniques can best be used in acute ischemic stroke, but the future appears very promising for their use in acute stroke diagnosis and management.

References

1. Astrup J, Siesjo BK, Simon L. Thresholds in cerebral ischemia: the ischemic penumbra. Stroke 1981;12:723–5.
2. Hakim AM. The cerebral ischemic penumbra. Can J Neurol Sci 1987;14:557–9.
3. Lassen NA, Fieschi C, Lenzi GL. Ischemic penumbra and neuronal death: comments on the therapeutic window in acute stroke with particular reference to thrombolytic therapy. Cerebrovasc Dis 1991;1:32–5.
4. Touzani O, Roussel S, MacKenzie ET. The ischemic penumbra. Curr Opin Neurol 2001;14:83–8.
5. Wintermark M, Maeder P, Verdun FR, et al. Using 80 kVp versus 120 kVp in perfusion CT measurement of regional cerebral blood flows. AJNR Am J Neuoradiol 2000;21:1881–4.
6. Meier P, Zierler KL. On the theory of the indicator-dilution method for measurement of blood flow and volume. J Appl Physiol 1954;12:731–44.
7. Zierler KL. Theoretical basis of indicator-dilution methods for measuring flow and volume. Circ Res 1962;10:393–407.
8. Zierler KL. Equations for measuring blood flow by external monitoring of radioisotopes. Circ Res 1965;16:309–21.
9. Axel L. Cerebral blood flow determination by rapid-sequence computed tomography. Radiology 1980;137:679–86.
10. Axel L. A method of calculating brain blood flow with a CT dynamic scanner. Adv Neurol 1981;30:67–71.
11. Axel L. Tissue mean transit time from dynamic computed tomography by a simple deconvolution technique. Invest Radiol 1983;18:94–9.
12. Lassen NA. Cerebral blood flow and oxygen consumption in man. Physiol Rev 1959;39:183–238.
13. Davis D, Ulatowski J, Eleff S, et al. Rapid monitoring of changes in water diffusion coefficients during reversible ischemia in cat and rat brain. Magn Reson Med 1994;31:454–60.
14. Röther J, De Crespigny AJ, D'Arceuil H, Mosley ME. MR detection of cortical spreading depression immediately after focal ischemia in the rat. J Cereb Blood Flow Metab 1996;16:214–20.
15. Schlaug G, Siewert B, Benfield A, et al. Time course of the apparent diffusion coefficient abnormality in human stroke. Neurology 1997;49:113–19.
16. Mintorovitch J, Yang GY, Shimizu H, et al. Diffusion-weighted magnetic resonance imaging of acute focal cerebral ischemia: comparison of signal intensity with changes in brain water and Na$^+$,K$^+$-ATPase activity. J Cereb Blood Flow Metab 1994;14:332–6.
17. Kohno K, Hoehn-Berlage M, Mies G, et al. Relationship between diffusion-weighted magnetic resonance images, cerebral blood flow and energy state in experimental brain infarction. Magn Reson Imaging 1995;13:73–80.
18. Rosen BR, Belliveau JM, Vevea JM, Brady TJ. Perfusion imaging with NMR contrast agent. Magn Reson Med 1990;14:249–65.
19. Röther J. CT and MRI in the diagnosis of acute stroke and their role in thrombolysis. Thrombolysis Res 2001;103:S125–33.
20. Hoehn-Berlage M, Eis M, Back T, et al. Changes of relaxation times (T1 and T2) and ADC after permanent middle cerebral artery occlusion in the rat: temporal evolution, regional extent, and comparison with histology. Magn Reson Med 1995;34:824–34.
21. Quast MJ, Huang NC, Hillman GR, Kent TA. The evolution of acute stroke recorded by multi-modal MRI. Magn Reson Imaging 1993;11:465–71.
22. Roussel SA, Van Bruggen N, King MD, Gadian DG. Identification of collaterally perfused areas following

focal cerebral ischemia in the rat by comparison of gradient echo and diffusion-weighted MRI. J Cereb Blood Flow Metab 1995;15:578–86.

23. Schellinger PD, Jansen O, Fiebach JB, et al. Monitoring intravenous recombinant tissue plasminogen activator thrombolysis for acute ischemic stroke with diffusion and perfusion MRI. Stroke 2000;31:1318–28.

24. Beaulieu C, De Crespigny A, Tong DC, et al. Longitudinal magnetic resonance imaging study of perfusion and diffusion in stroke: evolution of lesion volume and correlation with clinical outcome. Ann Neurol 1999;46:568–78.

25. Darby DG, Barber PA, Gerraty RP, et al. Pathophysiological topography of acute ischemia by combined diffusion-weighted and perfusion MRI. Stroke 1999;30:2043–52.

26. Baird AE, Lovblad KO, Dashe JF, et al. Clinical correlations of diffusion and perfusion lesion volumes in acute ischemic stroke. Cerebrovasc Dis 2000;10:441–8.

27. Memezawa H, Smith ML, Siesjö BK. Penumbral tissue salvaged by reperfusion following middle cerebral artery occlusion in rats. Stroke 1992;23:552–9.

28. Warach S, Dashe JF, Edelman RR. Clinical outcome in ischemic stroke predicted by early diffusion-weighted and perfusion magnetic resonance imaging: a preliminary analysis. J Cereb Blood Flow Metab 1996;16:53–9.

29. Parsons MW, Barber PA, Chalk J, et al. Diffusion- and perfusion-weighted MRI response to thrombolysis in stroke. Ann Neurol 2002;51:28–37.

30. Schlaug G, Benfield BS, Baird AE, et al. The ischemic penumbra: operationally defined by diffusion and perfusion MRI. Neurology 1999;53:1528–37.

31. Schelinger PD, Fiebach JB, Jansen O, et al. Stroke magnetic resonance imaging within 6 hours after onset of hyperacute cerebral ischemia. Ann Neurol 2001;49:460–9.

32. Baird AE, Benfield A, Schlaug G, et al. Enlargement of human cerebral ischemic lesions measured by diffusion-weighted magnetic resonance imaging. Ann Neurol 1997;41:581–9.

33. Jansen O, Schellinger P, Fiebach J, et al. Early recanalization in acute ischemic stroke saves tissue at risk defined by MRI. Lancet 1999;2036–7.

34. Barber PA, Darby DG, Desmond PM, et al. Prediction of stroke outcome with echoplanar perfusion- and diffusion-weighted MRI. Neurology 1998;51:418–26.

35. Tong DC, Yenari MA, Albers GW, et al. Correlation of perfusion- and diffusion-weighted MRI with NIHSS Score in acute (<6.5 hour) ischemic stroke. Neurology 1998;50:864–70.

36. Schwamm LH, Koroshetz WJ, Sorensen AG, et al. Time course of lesion development in patients with acute stroke: serial diffusion and hemodynamic-weighted magnetic resonance imaging. Stroke 1998;29:2268–76.

37. Back T, Hoehn-Berlage M, Kohno K, Hossmann KA. Diffusion nuclear magnetic resonance imaging in experimental stroke: correlation with cerebral metabolites. Stroke 1994;25:494–500.

38. Kidwell CS, Saver JL, Mattiello J, et al. Thrombolytic reversal of acute human cerebral ischemic injury shown by diffusion/perfusion magnetic resonance imaging. Ann Neurol 2000;47:462–9.

39. Pierce AP, Lo EH, Mandeville JB, et al. MRI measurements of water diffusion and cerebral perfusion: their relationship in a rat model of cerebral ischemia. J Cereb Blood Flow Metab 1997;17:183–90.

40. Desmond PM, Lovell AC, Rawlinson AA, et al. The value of apparent diffusion coefficient maps in early cerebral ischemia. AJNR Am J Neuroradiol 2001;22:1260–7.

41. Li F, Liu KF, Silva MD, et al. Transient and permanent resolution of ischemic lesions on diffusion-weighted imaging after brief periods of focal ischemia in rats: correlation with histopathology. Stroke 2000;31:946–54.

42. Neumann-Haefelin T, Kastrup A, De Crespigny A, et al. Serial MRI after transient focal cerebral ischemia in rats: dynamics of tissue injury, blood–brain barrier damage, and edema formation. Stroke 2000;31:1965–72.

43. Lo EH, Matsumoto K, Pierce AR, et al. Pharmacological reversal of acute changes in diffusion-weighted MRI in focal cerebral ischemia. J Cereb Blood Flow Metab 1994;14:597–603.

44. Li F, Silva MD, Liu KF, et al. Secondary decline in apparent diffusion coefficient and neurological outcome after a short period of focal brain ischemia in rats. Ann Neurol 2000;48:236–44.

45. Li F, Liu KF, Silva MD, et al. Acute post-ischemic renormalization of the apparent diffusion coefficient of water is not associated with reversal of astrocytic swelling and neuronal shrinkage in rats. AJNR Am J Neuroradiol 2002;23:180–8.

46. Hossmann KA. Viability thresholds and the penumbra of focal ischemia. Ann Neurol 1995;36:557–65.

47. Furlan M, Marchal G, Viader F, et al. Spontaneous neurological recovery after stroke and the fate of the ischemic penumbra. Ann Neurol 1996;40:216–26.

48. Marchal G, Benali K, Iglesias S, et al. Voxel-based mapping of irreversible ischemic damage with PET in acute stroke. Brain 1999;122:2387–400.

49. Heiss WD, Kracht LW, Thiel A, et al. Penumbral probability thresholds of cortical flumazenil binding and

blood flow predicting tissue outcome in patients with cerebral ischemia. Brain 2001;124:20–9.

50. Rohl L, Ostergaard L, Simonsen CZ, et al. Viability thresholds of ischemic penumbra of hyperacute stroke defined by perfusion-weighted MRI and apparent diffusion coefficient. Stroke 2001;32:1140–6.

51. Kim GE, Lee JH, Cho YP, Kim ST. Metabolic changes in the ischemic penumbra after carotid endarterectomy in stroke patients by localized in vivo proton magnetic resonance spectroscopy (^{1}H-MRS). Cardiovasc Surg 2001;9:345–55.

52. Furlan A, Higashida R, Wechsler L, et al. Intra-arterial prourokinase for acute ischemic stroke. The PROACT II study: a randomized controlled trial. JAMA 1999;282:2003–11.

53. Barber PA, Davis SM, Darby DG, et al. Absent middle cerebral artery flow predicts the presence and evolution of the ischemic penumbra. Neurology 1999;52:1125–32.

54. Ladurner G, Zilkha E, Iliff LD, et al. Measurement of regional cerebral blood volume by computerized axial tomography. J Neurol Neurosurg Psychiatry 1976;39:152–5.

55. Ladurner G, Zikha E, Sager WD, et al. Measurement of regional cerebral blood volume using the EMI 1010 scanner. Br J Radiol 1979;52:371–4.

56. Zilkha E, Ladurner G, Linette D, et al. Computer subtraction in regional cerebral blood-volume measurements using the EMI-scanner. Br J Radiol 1976;49:330–4.

57. Wintermark M, Maeder P, Thiran J-Ph, et al. Quantitative assessment of regional cerebral blood flows by perfusion CT studies at low injection rates: a critical review of the underlying theoretical models. Eur Radiol 2001;11:1220–30.

58. Wintermark M, Maeder P, Thiran J-Ph, et al. Simultaneous measurements of regional cerebral blood flows by perfusion-CT and stable xenon-CT: a validation study. AJNR Am J Neuroradiol 2001;22:905–14.

59. Latchaw RE, Yonas H, Pentheny SL, Gur D. Adverse reactions to xenon-enhanced CT cerebral blood flow determination. Radiology 1987;163:251–4.

60. Kety SS. The theory and applications of the exchange of inert gas at the lungs and tissues. Pharmacol Rev 1951;3:1–41.

61. Kelcz F, Hilal SK, Hartwell P, Joseph PM. Computed tomographic measurement of the xenon brain–blood partition coefficient and implications for regional cerebral blood flow: a preliminary report. Radiology 1978;127:385–92.

62. Yonas H, Darby JM, Marks EC, et al. CBF measured by Xe-CT: approach to analysis and normal values. J Cereb Blood Flow Metab 1991;17:716–25.

63. Symon L, Branston NM, Strong AJ, Hope TD. The concepts of thresholds of ischaemia in relation to brain structure and function. J Clin Pathol 1977;30(Suppl):149–54.

64. Hossmann KA. Viability thresholds and the penumbra of focal ischemi. Ann Neurol 1994;36:557–65.

65. Heiss WD. Ischemic penumbra: evidence from functional imaging in man. J Cereb Blood Flow Metab 2000;20:1276–93.

66. Heiss WD, Grond M, Thiel A, et al. Ischemic brain tissue salvaged from infarction with alteplase. Lancet 1997;349:1599–600.

67. Katzan IL, Furlan AJ, Lloyd LE, et al. Use of tissue-type plasminogen activator for acute ischemic stroke: the Cleveland area experience. JAMA 2000;283:1151–8.

68. National Institute of Neurological Disorders and Stroke (NINDS) rt-PA Stroke Study Group. Tissue plasminogen activator for acute ischaemic stroke. N Engl J Med 1995;33:1581–7.

69. Hacke W, Kaste M, Fieschi C. Randomised double-blind trial placebo-controlled trial of thrombolytic therapy with intravenous therapy with intravenous alteplase in acute ischaemic stroke (ECASS II). Lancet 1998;352:1245–51.

70. Hennerici M. Improving the outcome of acute stroke management. Hosp Med 1999;60:44–9.

71. Rubin G, Firlik AD, Levy EI, et al. Relationship between cerebral blood flow and clinical outcome in acute stroke. Cerebrovasc Dis 2000;10:298–306.

72. Ezura M, Takahashi A, Yoshimoto T. Evaluation of regional cerebral blood flow using single photon emission tomography for the selection of patients for local fibrinolytic therapy of acute cerebral embolism. Neurosurg Rev 1996;19:231–6.

73. Oppenheim C, Samson Y, Manai R, et al. Prediction of malignant middle cerebral artery infarction by diffusion-weighted imaging. Stroke 2000;31:2175–85.

74. Doerfler A, Engelhorn T, von Kummer R, et al. Are iodinated contrast agents detrimental in acute cerebral ischemia? An experimental study in rats. Radiology 1998;206:211–17.

75. Wintermark M, Reichhart M, Cuisenaire O, et al. Comparison of admission perfusion computed tomography and qualitative diffusion- and perfusion-weighted magnetic resonance imaging in acute stroke patients. Stroke 2002;33(8):2025–31.

76. Wintermark M, Reichhart M, Thiran JP, et al. Prognostic accuracy of cerebral blood flow measurement by perfusion computed tomography, at the time of emergency room admission, in acute stroke patients. Ann Neurol 2002;51(4):417–32.

17

Thrombolytic therapy for ischemic stroke: to select or not to select

Peter D Schellinger, Jochen B Fiebach, and Antoni Dávalos

Introduction

Since the publication of the NINDS (National Institute of Neurological Disorders and Stroke) study in 1995,[1] thrombolytic therapy with recombinant tissue-type plasminogen activator (rtPA) has been approved for treatment of acute stroke within a 3 h time window after exclusion of intracerebral hemorrhage (ICH) by noncontrast computed tomography (CT). No single phase III trial has proven the efficacy of intravenous thrombolytic therapy beyond a 3 h time window, and one small trial only the efficacy of intra- arterial thrombolysis with prourokinase between 3 and 6 h after stroke onset.[2] Currently, in Europe and the USA, this effective therapy is given to approximately 1–2% of ischemic stroke patients.[3] There are several reasons for this, including persisting doubts, fear of ICH, poorly organized services, and inadequate reimbursement, but most of all it is due to late arrival of the majority of patients. With implementation of an effective stroke care system, thrombolytic therapy can be administered in accordance with American Heart Association (AHA) guidelines in community hospitals in up to 10%[4] and in urban major stroke centers in up to 22%[5] of all ischemic stroke patients. In order to extend the therapeutic time frame for thrombolytic therapy, one must analyze the available evidence with regard to effectivity beyond 3 h[6–8] and improve the diagnostic yield of current imaging techniques to identify those patients who will benefit most likely from thrombolytic therapy while differentiating them from those who have a high therapy- associated risk of ICH beyond the established time windows. Overall, the time interval between symptom onset and induction of therapy is of essence in the first hours and progressively less important in later time windows, where selection becomes more important.[9] Therefore, an adequate treatment algorithm should take into account improved selection criteria that allow one to differentiate the ideal patients to whom therapy should be given from those who most likely will not profit from (or may even be harmed by) thrombolytic treatment, rather than utilizing only a rigid time window, CT-based ICH exclusion, and general thrombolytic therapy guidelines (e.g. arterial hypertension).

Stroke MRI: background

The target for most therapeutic interventions for focal ischemia should be ischemic tissue that can respond to treatment and is not irreversibly injured. The characterization of potentially reversible loss of function versus irreversible tissue damage is based on the concept of the ischemic penumbra.[10,11] Until recently, only xenon-CT, positron emission tomography (PET), and single photon emission CT (SPECT) imaging could approximately define ischemia and penumbra thresholds. This is, however, not feasible for caregivers in a broad population, where imaging in an acute setting is confined to CT and also increasingly MRI.[12] Only the advent of new imaging techniques such as novel MRI sequences and continuing improvement of imaging software and hardware has allowed improvements in diagnostic yield. Novel MRI techniques such as perfusion- and diffusion-weighted imaging (PWI and DWI) in the early 1990s have added another dimension to diagnostic imaging in stroke.[13–15] Warach et al[16] predicted in 1995 'that the impact of advanced echoplanar MR techniques in stroke may come to be viewed as analogous to the introduction of electrocardiography for the diagnosis of myocardial infarction, i.e. a rapid, reliable, objective, accurate, and essential emergency diagnostic test that will guide the development and application of acute therapeutic intervention'.[17]

The basics of stroke MRI will only be dealt with briefly here. The interested reader is referred to two recent textbooks in which the pathophysiological basis of DWI and PWI is covered extensively.[18,19] Aside from the new MRI techniques, a stroke MRI protocol consists at least in part of conventional or standard MRI sequences such as T2-weighted imaging (T2-WI), FLAIR (Fluid Attenuated Inversion Recovery) and MR angiography (MRA). On T2-WI, ischemic infarction appears as a hyperintense lesion. Definite signal changes, however, are seen at the earliest 2 h after stroke onset in animal experiments and 6–8 h after stroke onset in humans.[20] Neither a diagnosis of parenchymal ischemia nor the differentiation of ischemic core from penumbral tissue is possible with T2-WI. DWI allows in vitro and in vivo measurement of Brownian molecular motion of water, a phenomenon first described in 1965 that can be measured quantitatively in the form of the apparent diffusion coefficient (ADC).[21] DWI, earlier than any other imaging modality, allows one to demonstrate ischemic tissue changes within minutes after vessel occlusion with a reduction of the ADC.[22] A net shift of extracellular water into the intracellular compartment (cytotoxic edema), with a consecutive reduction of free water diffusion, is the main underlying mechanism for the ADC change.[23] In order to interpret changes on DWI correctly, a variety of artifacts must be known (anisotropy and T2 shine-through) and identified as such. In the clinical setting of a hyperacute stroke, a lesion on strongly isotropic DWI and a normal T2-WI favor an acute lesion; the maximum information can be obtained when isotropic ADC parameter maps are calculated in addition to DWI and T2-WI. Newer DWI techniques, such as FLAIR-DWI to reduce CSF contamination,[24] diffusion tensor imaging, and high-field (3 T) imaging will further improve the diagnostic reach of DWI.

PWI allows the measurement of capillary perfusion with the dynamic susceptibility contrast-enhanced (DSC) technique. Paramagnetic contrast agent is injected as an intravenous bolus and the signal change is tracked by ultrafast MRI sequences in the area of interest.[25] In analogy to concentration–time curves obtained with pulmonary artery catheters after injection of ice water (temperature probe) or indocyanine green (infrared probe), cerebrovascular hemodynamic parameters can be calculated from the MRI-derived contrast bolus–time curve. Passage of the contrast bolus causes a signal loss that increases with the perfused cerebral blood volume (CBV). In ischemic brain tissue with reduced perfusion or zero perfusion, less (or no) contrast agent is present and T2*-W images thus do remain hyperintense or keep their high signal, respectively.[26] It is not yet clear which PWI parameter gives the optimum approximation to critical hypoperfusion and allows one to differentiate infarct core from penumbra and penumbra from oligemia. Most authors, however, agree that in clinical practice, mean transit time (MTT) or time to peak enhancement (TTP) give the best prognostic information.[27,28] Calculation of the quantitative cerebral blood flow (CBF) requires knowledge of the arterial input function, which in clinical practice is estimated from a major artery such as the middle or internal carotid artery (MCA or ICA). PWI has to meet the critique that it renders only a qualitative (at best semiquantitative) index of tissue perfusion, whereas other methods such as SPECT and PET, neither of which has become a standard for patient management, offer accurate quantitative regional CBF (rCBF) measurements.[29] Evaluation of perfusion status and identification of a tissue at risk by xenon-CT, SPECT, or PET, however, are not practical for routine use.[15] While it is not yet clinically feasible to obtain quantitative PWI parameters that differentiate oligemia from relevant hypoperfusion and infarct core, relative MTT (or TTP) parameter maps may be used to guide clinical management in patients with acute ischemic stroke.

A multiparametric stroke MRI protocol should consist of the following:

- MRA to demonstrate vessel occlusion or patency
- T2*-WI (e.g. source images from PWI) to show the presence of or to exclude intracranial hemorrhage

- DWI to show the infarct core and infarct age (ADC maps)
- T2-WI to give a more anatomical image of the brain in stroke patients and to depict microangiopathic changes, edema, old infarcts, other pathology, etc.
- PWI to show the complete area of hypoperfusion and derive the tissue at risk by comparing the results with the findings on DWI

In a simplified approach, it has been hypothesized that DWI more or less reflects the irreversibly damaged infarct core and PWI the complete area of hypoperfusion.[16,30] The volume difference between these two, termed the PWI/DWI mismatch (i.e. PWI minus DWI volume, which is sometimes also given as the ratio PWI/DWI volume), would therefore be a measure of the tissue at risk of infarction or the stroke MRI correlate of the ischemic penumbra. It should be noted that the assessment of mismatch as a percentage may be less reliable than previously thought.[31] On the other hand, if there is no difference in PWI and DWI volumes or even a negative difference (PWI < DWI), this is termed a PWI/DWI match, and according to the model is equivalent to a patient who does not have penumbral tissue because of normalization of prior hypoperfusion or completion of infarction and total loss of the penumbra.[15,28]

Overall, this simple model of PWI/DWI mismatch is acceptably accurate in most acute stroke patients and the findings of stroke MRI are consistent with our pathophysiological understanding.[15,28] It is hoped that by using the mismatch concept, patients can be categorized into two groups: those who may profit from a specific therapy to salvage the penumbra and those in whom ischemic tissue at risk is no longer present. Furthermore, the patient's individual time window due to his or her individual vascular and hemodynamic situation can be taken into account for decision making. The two-zone model does not take into account that the PWI lesion also assesses areas of oligemia that are not in danger. At present, the optimum PWI algorithm to differentiate oligemia from ischemia has not been established. Also, DWI abnormalities are potentially reversible, especially with early reperfusion.[17,32] Partial or complete DWI lesion reversal is independently associated with an excellent outcome.[33] So, currently, we are dealing with a four-zone model, where the true MRI correlate of the ischemic penumbra is the difference between the areas of critical hypoperfusion and irreversibly infarcted DWI lesion.[17] For reasons of practicality, at present, the two-zone model is applied in the clinical setting.

In general, the findings on stroke MRI have been that, the earlier the timepoint of imaging, the less the correlation of DWI and PWI volumes with neurological baseline and outcome scores.[28] The more subacutely stroke MRI is performed, the more likely it becomes that DWI and PWI findings approximate the final infarct size and thus correlate with clinical outcome, which is consistent with older CT and MRI data.[28,34,35] Thus, the baseline DWI and PWI lesion size reflect neither the clinical degree of severity at baseline nor that at outcome, but rather illustrate the potential best- and worse-case scenarios. The clinical and morphological course of hyperacute ischemic infarction is completely open, and thus may be influenced by therapy. Therefore, the mismatch and the evaluation of best or worst outcome should be used to differentiate between those patients who are at a high risk and those who are not. Stroke MRI findings are far more reliable in predicting what fate the patient *may* face if not treated (final stroke size ≈ PWI size) or effectively treated (final stroke size ≤ DWI size). Also, there is a highly significant association of vessel occlusion and presence of a PWI/DWI mismatch (97.5%) and vessel patency and PWI/DWI match in the first hours after stroke. Patients with vessel occlusion and PWI/DWI match in the first hours have probably infarcted their tissue at risk due to poor collaterals or profound drops in blood pressure or oxygenation. In patients with proximal vessel occlusions, a larger area of tissue is at risk, the recanalization rate is lower, and outcome is worse; therefore, vessel patency should be achieved by all means in this patient group. Early recanalization as shown by resolution of a PWI/DWI mismatch, however, leads to smaller infarcts, improved (restituted) perfusion, and a significantly better clinical outcome.[28,30] Here, it seems to be of utmost importance that early reperfusion at 2–4 h after onset of therapy is relevant – not necessarily 'late' reperfusion at 24 h.[36] More research to refine this practical clinical approach and to meet the justified criticism to this simplified model is warranted.[37,38]

Alternative imaging modalities for selection

Doppler/duplex ultrasound

Doppler and Duplex ultrasound (DU) noninvasively and at bedside assesses extracranial and intracranial vessel status.[39] There are several DU-based studies of thrombolytic therapy worth mentioning. Early reports described that rapid recanalization as assessed by DU is associated with a higher rate of clinical improvement and smaller infarcts at outcome.[40] As this series was performed before the approval of thrombolytic therapy, it does not offer data on treated individuals. Christou et al[41] correlated clinical recovery from stroke with the timing of arterial recanalization after therapy with rtPA in 40 patients. Complete recanalization occurred in 12 (30%) patients and partial recanalization in 16 (40%); the timing of recanalization inversely correlated with early improvement in the National Institutes of Health Stroke Scale (NIHSS) Scores, and complete recanalization was common in patients who had follow-up Rankin Scores of 0–1 ($p = 0.006$). No patients had early complete recovery if an occlusion persisted for more than 5 h. Molina et al[42] investigated the timecourse of rtPA-induced recanalization and the relationship between arterial recanalization, infarct volume, and outcome in 72 patients with cardioembolic stroke treated within 3 h from symptom onset (24 treated with rtPA and 48 matched controls). The rate of 6 h recanalization was higher ($p \le 0.001$) in the rtPA group (66%) than in the control group (15%). Infarct volume was 50.2 ± 40.3 ml in rtPA patients and 124.8 ± 81.6 ml in controls ($p \le 0.001$) and was associated strongly ($p \le 0.001$) with duration of MCA occlusion. At 3 months, 14 (58%) rtPA patients and 11 (23%) controls ($p = 0.037$) became functionally independent; this was significantly ($p = 0.002$) related to time to reperfusion. The same authors demonstrated that secondary symptomatic hemorrhage (parenchymal hemorrhage type 2: PH2), as opposed to hemorrhagic conversion or asymptomatic hemorrhage (hemorrhagic infarction types 1 and 2: HI1 and 2; PH1), after thrombolytic therapy, which is associated with a worse clinical outcome, is seen significantly more frequently in patients with late rather than early recanalization.[43] Alexandrov et al[44] monitored consecutive patients receiving intravenous rtPA with transcranial DU,

and documented recanalization in 43 rtPA-treated patients. Recanalization began at a median of 17 min and was completed at 35 min after a rtPA bolus, with a mean duration of recanalization of 23 ± 16 min. Faster recanalization predicted better short-term improvement ($p = 0.03$). Symptomatic hemorrhage occurred in only one patient, who had stepwise recanalization 5.5 h after stroke onset. A pilot multicenter study (DIAS: Duplex-Sonographic Assessment of the Cerebrovascular Status in Acute Stroke) evaluated the potentials and limitations of color-coded duplex sonography (TCCS) for cerebrovascular status assessment in 58 acute stroke patients (rtPA 18; conservative 39; early thrombendarterectomy 1) before and after rtPA therapy.[45] Duplex sonography was performed on admission, 2 h after start of therapy, and 24 h after onset of symptoms. The MCA mainstem was patent in 29 patients (53.7%), occluded in 25 (46.3%), and not assessable in 4. Recanalization of the occluded MCA after 2- and 24 h was diagnosed in 50% and 78% of the patients treated with rtPA and in 0% and 8% in the conservatively treated patients.

In summary, all of these authors demonstrated that rapid arterial recanalization is associated with better short-term and long-term improvement, smaller infarcts, and less chance of secondary hemorrhage (especially PH2). Furthermore, the spontaneous recanalization rate after established vessel occlusion is consistently given as about 15%, whereas the recanalization rate after rtPA is in the range 60–70%. This is in agreement with data from MRI studies[28,46] and illustrates that the greatest effect of thrombolytic therapy is seen when rtPA is given to patients in whom a vessel occlusion has been established. Another phase II trial of ultrasound-enhanced thrombolytic therapy (CLOTBUST) has been presented and has shown this technique to be feasible; a phase III trial is in the planning phase.

Potential disadvantages of DU, however, are its examiner-dependent sensitivity and time consumption, as well as potential problems with uncooperative patients and lack of a transcranial insonation window.

CT/CTA/CTA source images/perfusion-CT

Direct comparison of CT angiography (CTA) and carotid ultrasound suggests that the results from

CTA compare favorably with ultrasound and that CTA can also reliably detect intracranial stenosis, emboli, and aneurysms of moderate or larger size.[47,48] Furthermore, it may easily be performed directly after noncontrast CT. In addition to vessel status, however, CTA source images (CTA-SI) may provide indirect information about the collateral circulation and also improve the contrast of perfused and malperfused brain areas and thereby increase the sensitivity for early ischemic changes not seen on noncontrast scans.[49,50] Analysis of CTA-SI must be clearly differentiated from perfusion-CT, where, in analogy to PWI a contrast bolus tracking method is applied and hemodynamic parameters may be assessed.[51] Wildermuth et al[52] compared CTA and DU in 40 patients with acute stroke in the 3–6 h time window; 20 patients received rtPA. CTA findings were consistent with DU in all patients; the authors concluded that CTA provides important information for the initiation of therapy in patients with acute hemispheric ischemia, such as identification of patients with autolyzed thrombi, or occlusion of the internal carotid artery bifurcation, which may have little potential for benefit from thrombolytic therapy.

Lev et al[53] evaluated the utility of CTA-SI in predicting final infarct volume and clinical outcome in 22 patients with acute MCA stroke who underwent intra-arterial thrombolysis within 6 h of stroke onset. Initial CTA-SI lesion volumes correlated significantly with final infarct volume ($p = 0.0002$) and clinical outcome ($p = 0.01$) – particularly in 10 patients with complete recanalization ($r = 0.97$, $p \leq 0.0001$). Patients with recanalization did not experience infarct growth; those without complete recanalization did. CT/CTA/CTA-SI analysis was a stronger predictor of clinical outcome than was initial NIHSS Score.

Schramm et al[54] investigated the clinical and imaging findings of 23 consecutive patients imaged within 6 h after stroke onset and compared CT/CTA/CTA-SI findings with DWI and MRA. All vessel occlusions detected on CTA were seen on MRA at the same location. Collateral status was determined on the CTA-SI: 7 patients showed good intravascular enhancement of the perilesional vessels; 16 patients showed only poor enhancement around the lesion site. Of the 23 patients, 4 had no initial vessel occlusion but showed small lesions on initial DWI. All but one of these patients had good collaterals. Neither in patients with poor collaterals nor in those with good collaterals

did CTA-SI lesion volumes differ significantly from DWI lesion volumes at baseline. Patients with poor collaterals experienced infarct growth, whereas patients with good collaterals did not, the lesion volume difference being significant ($p = 0.016$). Also, patients with good collaterals uniformly had a significantly better clinical outcome at day 90 as measured by four neurological and outcome scales (NIHSS, Scandinavian Stroke Scale (SSS), Barthel Index, and modified Rankin Score). Therefore, in patients with poor collateral vessel status, CTA-SI may provide similar information to the PWI-DWI mismatch concept.[55] Here, the size of the tissue at risk can be estimated by the difference of the CTA-SI lesion volumes and the brain area supplied by the occluded artery, taking the qualitative assessment of collateral status into account.

Dynamic CT during first pass of an iodine contrast bolus by unidirectional X-ray tube rotation results in images that can be used to construct functional maps of CBV, CBF, or TTP. These functional maps of perfusion-CT provide a high-resolution tool that enables the physician to visualize cerebrovascular parameters and their changes in acute stroke patients. Areas with reduced CBF can be shown immediately after vessel occlusion as high contrast compared with areas with normal perfusion.[51,56,57] A disadvantage is that only part of the brain (currently 2 cm) can be imaged. Furthermore, although perfusion-CT criteria have been established to differentiate irreversible from reversible ischemic damage,[58] the values when compared with MRI yield a substantial standard deviation.[12] While SPECT and especially PET may provide semiquantitative and quantitative hemodynamic data, these modalities are not widely available and thus are primarily of academic interest and probably without any practical implications for the near future.[59,60]

Stroke MRI: current status

Substantial doubts remain regarding the feasibility and practicality as well as the validity of stroke MRI in the clinical setting,[29,61] although it has been shown to the contrary that logistic obstacles can be overcome.[62,63] A dedicated stroke service with multimodal imaging availability around the clock (CT, MRI, and digital subtraction angiography (DSA)) requires a sufficiently large staff, infrastructure such as a stroke service, stroke, or neurocritical care unit, and small distances between emergency room, stroke unit, and imaging facilities to save time. In addition, adequate monitoring has to be available in the MRI scanner. Image quality and information are excellent, and can be optimized by head immobilization and by mild sedation if necessary. Practice and experience with stroke MRI in a dedicated stroke team significantly reduces the time effort for a complete stroke MRI protocol, which need not exceed 15 min, including patient transfer and positioning, and thus facilitates 24 h availability.[62]

Criticisms of stroke MRI are mainly based on a supposed lack of studies assessing sensitivity and specifity of these new imaging methods in a randomized, blinded, and controlled fashion. Also, the use of the term 'imaging gold standard' has added to the controversy, as there is no such thing as an imaging gold standard for acute ischemic stroke due to the lack of correlations of any neuroimaging method with neuropathological findings.[64] Therefore, as a 'quasi gold standard', the diagnosis of ischemic stroke in most studies is established at follow-up with proof of a lesion on either CT or conventional MRI consistent with a clinical syndrome and a comprehensive diagnostic workup.

DWI appears to be far superior to CT in the diagnosis of acute ischemic stroke.[15] While there is still a lack of blinded randomized controlled trials applying DWI in a broad spectrum of patients with suspected stroke,[65] there is good evidence for the superior sensitivity of DWI compared with CT in blinded and randomized evaluations of DWI versus CT in acute ischemic stroke and compared with ICH.[66–68] These trials also avoided a bias against CT common to previous studies, namely that CT was performed 2 h or more before DWI.[69,70] The main advantage of CT is its widespread availability in many hospitals 24 h a day. The sensitivity of CT during the first 6 h of cerebral ischemia was 64% in the ECASS (European Cooperative Acute Stroke Study) reading panel, with an accuracy of 67%. The local investigators of ECASS reached a 40% sensitivity (accuracy 45%) only.[71] Within the first 3 h, the sensitivity of CT decreases to 31% and is not associated with clinical outcome.[72] Fiebach et al[66] compared CT and DWI in 54 patients prospectively randomized for the sequence in which the imaging modalities were performed. The raters yielded on DWI a sensitivity of 91% (95% confidence interval (CI) 88–94%), a specificity of 95%

(75–100%), an accuracy of 91% (89–94%), a positive predictive value of 100% (98–100%), and a negative predictive value of 47% (38–57%). On CT, they reached a sensitivity of 61% (95% CI 52–70%), a specificity of 65% (50–100%), an accuracy of 61% (56–70%), a positive predictive value of 96% (94–100%), and a negative predictive value of 12% (9–17%). Another study, by Saur et al,[67] compared DWI and CT scans in 46 out of 92 acute stroke patients prospectively investigated within 6 h, in whom both imaging modalities had been performed with a time interval of less than 45 min. Ischemic stroke was identified on 33 of 45 CT scans (sensitivity 73%; 95% CI 58–85%) and on 42 of 45 DW images (sensitivity 93%; 95% CI 82–99%). The inter-rater agreement was moderate ($\kappa = 0.57$) for CT and excellent ($\kappa = 0.85$) for DWI. CT studies had a moderate inter-rater agreement for estimation of early infarct signs greater than one-third of the MCA territory ($\kappa = 0.40$), whereas DWI showed good results ($\kappa = 0.68$).

Stroke MRI is also highly accurate in the diagnosis of ICH, which has to be diagnosed or excluded before thrombolytic therapy can be indicated. The appearance of ICH depends on several factors, such as the MRI sequence,[73] the field strength,[74] and the oxygen saturation of hemoglobin and its degradation. Other factors are protein concentration, hydration, form and size of red blood cells, hematocrit, clotting, clot retraction, and clot structure.[73] Hyperacute ICH presents as an unspecific hyperintensity on T2-WI and cannot be seen on T1-WI unless there is a substantial mass effect. However, echo-planar and gradient-echo images or susceptibility-weighted T2*-W images, which are more susceptible to the paramagnetic effects of deoxyhemoglobin may detect hyperacute ICH. Due to the complexity of the appearance of ICH on different sequences at different stages, as opposed to CT, there is a considerable amount of disagreement among clinicians and radiologists as to the role of MRI. Early case series reported the appearance of ICH on T2*-WI.[75–77] In the very first few minutes after symptom onset, the center of the lesion appears heterogeneous on all images (T2-WI, T2*-WI, and T1-WI), which is due to a local predominance of oxyhemoglobin. The periphery of the hematoma is more hypointense on susceptibility-weighted images than on T2-WI, and shows a progressive enlargement over the next few minutes and the first few hours. This is due to a progressive centripetal increase in the concentration of deoxyhemoglobin. There is a surrounding rim, which appears hyperintense on T2-WI and T2*-WI but hypointense on T1-WI and represents perifocal vasogenic edema. A multicenter trial has evaluated the accuracy of stroke MRI for the detection of ICH.[68] Images from 62 ICH patients and 62 nonhemorrhagic stroke patients all imaged within the first 6 h after symptom onset (mean 3 h 18 min) were analyzed in a blinded manner after randomization for the order of presentation. Three experienced readers identified ICH with a 100% sensitivity (95% CI 97.1–100%) and a 100% overall accuracy. Smaller case series also report a good sensitivity of stroke MRI for acute subarachnoid hemorrhage.[78]

Another potential use of stroke MRI is in the identification of patients who carry a high risk of subsequent symptomatic ICH after treatment with rtPA. History of a previous ICH is in general considered to be a contraindication for thrombolytic therapy.[79] However, the detection of older microbleeds on T2*-WI that cannot be detected on CT has not been implemented yet in any treatment guidelines and in only a few institutional protocols (Steven Warach, personal communication). At present, there are conflicting data with regard to the risk of ICH after thrombolytic therapy in patients with microbleeds, so these findings should be applied only in controlled trials to select patients and should not be used as a means to exclude patients from a potentially helpful treatment.[80–82] Other biomarkers, such as early blood–brain barrier disruption (HARM-sign, L Latour personal communication), may allow one to identify patients at risk for reperfusion injury at a timepoint where therapeutic intervention is still possible.[83]

Stroke MRI: from theory to practice

A question that arises is whether patients who would seem to be ideal candidates for thrombolytic therapy really are characterized by the stroke MRI concept: vessel occlusion and PWI/DWI mismatch. A prospective, open-label, nonrandomized multicenter trial (at five university hospitals) examined the MRI baseline characteristics of patients with acute ischemic stroke and studied the influence of intravenous rtPA on MRI parameters and functional outcome in 139 patients (76 rtPA vs 63 controls) within 6 h after symptom onset and on follow-up.[84] The objectives were to define the prevalence and size of mismatch and lesion volumes in acute stroke patients, to assess the effect of rtPA on recanalization rates, and to determine whether the timepoint of thrombolysis and the recanalization rate do have an impact on functional outcome and whether the vascular occlusion pattern is associated with mismatch volume and functional outcome. All patients were studied within a multiparametric stroke MRI protocol within 6 h after symptom onset and for follow-up. Patients were divided into two therapeutic groups: a no-thrombolysis group with conservative treatment and a thrombolysis group with thrombolytic therapy. Baseline characteristics, lesion volumes, mismatch ratio, occlusion types, recanalization, and functional outcome were compared between groups. The two groups did not differ concerning age and sex; however, the initial NIHSS Score was lower ($p = 0.002$) and the time to MRI was longer ($p = 0.002$) in the no-thrombolysis group. Five patients had symptomatic ICH (2 with and 3 without thrombolysis). Ten patients died within the follow-up period of 90 days (4 with and 6 without thrombolysis). The median time to thrombolysis was 180 min (range 45–333 min). Forty-five patients were treated within the 3 h time window and 31 within the 3–6 h window. MRI was performed 180 min (range 75–360 min) after the start of symptoms. A relevant mismatch (mismatch ratio >1.2) was present in 120 of 139 patients (86.3%). MRA demonstrated a vessel occlusion in 90% of patients. The mismatch ratio did not differ ($p < 0.39$), whereas the mismatch volume was smaller in the no-thrombolysis group ($p = 0.032$). The final lesion volume (T2-WI on day 7) was smaller in the thrombolysis group with 35 ml (range 1.6–377 ml) versus 73 ml (range 0–685 ml) ($p = 0.079$). rtPA had a strong effect on recanalization rates ($p < 0.001$). There was no outcome difference between patients treated within 3 h (45 patients) or 3–6 h (31 patients). There was a significantly higher chance of having an independent outcome when treated with rtPA despite the significantly worse baseline NIHSS Score and the greater area of tissue at risk.

Another study, by Kuelkens et al,[85] used a therapy algorithm whereby patients were treated according to the NINDS protocol within the first 3 h (115 patients) and according to stroke MRI findings in the

3–6 h time window (48 patients). The NIHSS Score in the first group was nonsignificantly higher than in the stroke MRI group (12 vs 10.5; $p=0.1$). There was no difference in the rate of symptomatic ICH (5.2% vs 4.2%), but there were significantly more asymptomatic ICH and hemorrhagic conversions in the late-thrombolysis group (1.7% vs 10.4%; $p=0.03$). There was a trend towards a lower mortality in the stroke MRI group (16.5% vs 6.3%; $p=0.08$). Interestingly, the outcome (independent vs dependent or dead, modified Rankin Score 0–2 vs 3–6) of the stroke MRI group was clearly but nonsignificantly better than that of the early group (47% vs 62.5%; odds ratio 0.54, 95% CI 0.27–1.06). The outcome distribution of the early 'NINDS' group parallels that of the original NINDS treatment arm according to the modified Rankin Score percentages. These numbers suggest that with a selection tool such as stroke MRI, the time window for treating stroke with thrombolytic therapy can be substantially widened and can yield even better results when compared with historical studies. There are some differences in between the two groups, such as younger and less severely affected patients in the stroke MRI group, that may have balanced the results in favour of the late group. On the other hand, the natural relationship to time from onset in a patient cohort treated without an ideal selection tool shows that there is no significant treatment effect beyond 290 min.[86] Therefore, the data of Kuelkens et al[85] support the need for a suitable selection tool such as stroke MRI. However, this has first to be firmly established in a randomized trial.

It is a topic of ongoing discussions whether lacunar stroke patients or patients with spontaneous recanalization might benefit from thrombolysis. Some authors argue that, based on the assumption that rtPA exerts its effects through recanalization of larger angiographically visible arteries or that outcome is related to recanalization anyway (none of the large trials assessed recanalization), rtPA should not be withheld in patients with small-vessel disease.[87] Also, the authors of the NINDS study state that is their trial; there was a benefit for lacunar strokes as well as large-vessel or embolic strokes.[88] However, their diagnosis of lacunar stroke was not based on imaging but was merely a clinical assumption at the discretion of the recruiting physician. MRI studies showed that the clinical diagnosis of lacunar stroke is very inaccurate.[89] In a prospective series of 106 patients evaluated with DWI and PWI within 24 h of stroke, Gerraty et al[89] enrolled 19 with a lacunar syndrome (pure motor stroke, ataxic hemiparesis, or sensorimotor stroke). In 13 out of the 19 patients, DWI and PWI altered the final diagnosis of infarct pathogenesis from small-perforating-artery occlusion to large-artery embolism. The authors concluded that lacunes cannot be reliably diagnosed on clinical grounds.[89] Complete reversal of DWI and PWI findings in lacunar stroke after thrombolytic therapy have been described.[90]

One might expand these arguments and ask whether thrombolysis should be limited to patients with DWI/PWI mismatch. Stroke physicians are frequently confronted with stroke patients in whom the exact time of symptom onset is not known – for example those who have a deficit when awakening[91] or who are not in a condition to give the required information due to aphasia or disorientation. At present, patients like these are excluded from thrombolytic therapy even if a CT scan does not demonstrate any or only minor ischemic changes. Accordingly, thrombolysis as an effective therapy may be withheld from patients who might profit from rapid recanalization. Therefore, we suggest that patients presenting with symptoms of acute stroke of unknown onset time should be investigated with stroke MRI and should be given thrombolytic therapy if a vessel occlusion and/or a substantial mismatch are present and T2-WI is negative – maybe even when only a perfusion deficit is present and a very cautiously phrased informed consent can be obtained from the patient or his/her closest relatives.

One has to be aware that these recommendations are not based on prospective randomized data and do not meet the criteria of an officially approved therapy. However, as there is already a substantial and still-growing body of evidence in favor of the recommended procedures, these recommendations may be seen as an expert opinion and provide the rationale for an individual therapeutic approach in an institutional protocol. The fact that an individual therapy based on advanced knowledge is offered that does not meet the criteria of drug approval institutions and therefore may be associated with a higher risk of hazardous if not fatal side-effects must be stressed when informed consent is obtained. Conversely, it should be stated that the drawback of a later onset of therapy may be outweighed by a sophisticated diagnostic imaging procedure telling the physician whether to treat or not to treat. Patients and their relatives should be informed not only about the hazards of thrombolytic therapy within or outside the 3 h time window but also about its potential benefit and thus the risk of *not* being treated.

Future prospects

A further role of stroke MRI in the future is in trial design.[92,93] To demonstrate efficacy in a clinical trial with a treatment time window beyond 3 h, other features of trial design need to be optimized, and proof of pharmacological activity in phase II is needed before lengthy, expensive, labor-intensive, and potentially risky phase III clinical trials are undertaken. The requirement for proof-of-concept phase II studies will prevent the wastefulness of phase III trials that are doomed to futility before they begin. Image-guided phase II studies may answer the question of target biological activity in fewer than 200 patients, the sample size typical of phase II trials. Trends toward benefit using clinical scales at phase II have been notoriously poor predictors of clinical outcomes in phase III trials on much larger samples. It would be unthinkable for clinical trials in cardiology or oncology to enrol patients by bedside clinical impression alone, without objective evidence from diagnostic testing confirming the pathology before inclusion of a patient. Yet this has been the traditional standard by which clinical trials for ischemic stroke have been conducted, because until recently there had been no practical alternative. Stroke MRI parameters such as 'lesion growth' or 'tissue save' have been and are currently being used as surrogate markers for drug efficacy[94,95] in acute stroke studies. The goal of image-based patient selection is to narrow the range of patient characteristics, leading to a more homogeneous sample, reducing within-group variance, and increasing the statistical power (lowering sample size requirement) of the experimental design to demonstrate efficacy. Open clinical trials such as those presented by Röther et al[84] and Külkens et al[85] provide examples of the sample sizes needed when a homogeneous patient group is selected and monitored by stroke MRI (≈ 150 vs 800 patients).

At present, there are only a few trials that use stroke MRI criteria for inclusion and evaluation of surrogate parameters. A stroke MRI-based study on the efficacy of recombinant desmoteplase for treatment of stroke in the 3–9 h time window was positive for the imaging surrogate parameter and will be tested in a phase III study soon.[46] DEFUSE (Diffusion-weighted imaging Evaluation For Understanding Stroke Evolution) (USA) and EPITHET (Echoplanar Imaging Thrombolysis Evaluation Trial) (Australia) are two studies performing MRI-based thrombolysis with rtPA in the 3–6 h time window. Data on DEFUSE are currently not available; for EPITHET, the results of a pilot trial have been published.[96] Combination of rtPA with glycoprotein IIb/IIIa antagonists may be a promising approach and may result in earlier reperfusion and increased vessel patency rates in accordance with cardiological studies.[97] These trials, however, are at present only phase I and II (tirofiban plus rtPA (SATIS: Safety of Tirofiban in Acute Ishemic Stroke), Mario Siebler, personal communication; abciximab plus reteplase (ROSIE: Reopro Retavase Reperfusion of Stroke Safety); eptifibatide plus aspirin, low-molecular weight heparin, and rtPA (ROSIE 2), Steven Warach, personal communication). The ongoing trials section in *Stroke* lists most of these trials.[98]

Conclusions

At present, thrombolytic therapy is still underutilized.[3] Among the major problems are that relatively few candidates meet the clinical and time criteria. Using new imaging technologies such as DWI and PWI in a multiparametric stroke protocol will help to identify and treat patients beyond established time windows with less risk and possibly an increased benefit. Furthermore, these novel techniques can be used for and implemented in the design of pharmaceutical trials, and thereby help to reduce the study size and make the study sample more homogeneous. This may have the effect of reducing the number of negative trials while increasing the number and quality of positive studies, and may therefore be beneficial for developing and establishing new therapies for acute ischemic stroke.

References

1. The National Institute of Neurological Disorders and Stroke rt-PA Stroke Study Group. Tissue plasminogen activator for acute ischemic stroke. N Engl J Med 1995;333:1581–7.
2. Furlan A, Higashida R, Wechsler L, et al. Intra-arterial prourokinase for acute ischemic stroke. The PROACT II study: a randomized controlled trial. Prolyse in Acute Cerebral Thromboembolism. JAMA 1999;282:2003–11.
3. Kaste M. Approval of alteplase in Europe: Will it change stroke management? Lancet Neurol 2003;2:207–8.
4. Lattimore SU, Chalela J, Davis L, et al. Impact of establishing a primary stroke center at a community hospital on the use of thrombolytic therapy: the NINDS Suburban Hospital Stroke Center experience. Stroke 2003;34:E55–7.
5. Grond M, Stenzel C, Schmulling S, et al. Early intravenous thrombolysis for acute ischemic stroke in a community-based approach. Stroke 1998;29:1544–9.
6. Hacke W, Brott T, Caplan L, et al. Thrombolysis in acute ischemic stroke: controlled trials and clinical experience. Neurology 1999;53:S3–14.
7. Brott TG. A combined metaanalysis of NINDS, ECASS I and II, ATLANTIS. In: Proceedings of International Stroke Conference, San Antonio, TX, USA, February 7–9th, 2002.
8. Wardlaw JM, del Zoppo G, Yamaguchi T. Thrombolysis for acute ischaemic stroke. In: The Cochrane Library, Issue 1, 2002. Oxford: Update Software, 2002.
9. Schellinger PD, Kaste M, Hacke W. An update on thrombolytic therapy for acute stroke. Curr Opin Neurol 2004;17:69–77.
10. Astrup J, Siesjö B, Symon L. Thresholds in cerebral ischemia – the ischemic penumbra. Stroke 1981;12:723–5.
11. Ginsberg MD. Adventures in the pathophysiology of brain ischemia: penumbra, gene expression, neuroprotection: the 2002 Thomas Willis Lecture. Stroke 2003;34:214–23.
12. Wintermark M, Reichhart M, Cuisenaire O, et al. Comparison of admission perfusion computed tomography and qualitative diffusion- and perfusion-weighted magnetic resonance imaging in acute stroke patients. Stroke 2002;33:2025–31.
13. Fisher M, Albers GW. Applications of diffusion–perfusion magnetic resonance imaging in acute ischemic stroke. Neurology 1999;52:1750–6.
14. Hacke W, Warach S. Diffusion-weighted MRI as an evolving standard of care in acute stroke. Neurology 2000;54:1548–9.
15. Schellinger PD, Fiebach JB, Hacke W. Imaging-based decision making in thrombolytic therapy for ischemic stroke: present status. Stroke 2003;34:575–83.
16. Warach S, Gaa J, Siewert B, et al. Acute human stroke studied by whole brain echo planar diffusion-weighted magnetic resonance imaging. Ann Neurol 1995;37:231–41.
17. Kidwell CS, Alger JR, Saver JL. Beyond mismatch: evolving paradigms in imaging the ischemic penumbra with multimodal magnetic resonance imaging. Stroke 2003;34:2729–35.
18. Davis S, Fisher M, Warach S. Magnetic Resonance Imaging in Stroke. Cambridge: Cambridge: University Press, 2003.
19. Fiebach JB, Schellinger PD. Stroke MRI. Darmstadt: Steinkopff Verlag, 2003.
20. Mohr JP, Biller J, Hilal SK, et al. Magnetic resonance versus computed tomographic imaging in acute stroke. Stroke 1995;26:807–12.
21. Stejskal EO, Tanner JE. Spin diffusion measurements: spin echoes in the presence of a time-dependent field gradient. J Chem Phys 1965;42:288–92.
22. Le Bihan D, Breton E, Lallemand D, et al. MR imaging of intravoxel incoherent motions: application to diffusion and perfusion in neurologic disorders. Radiology 1986;161:401–7.
23. Röther J, Gass A, Busch E. Diffusion- and perfusion-weighted MRI in cerebral ischaemia – Part 1: Results of animal experiments. Akt Neurol 1999;26:300–8.
24. Latour LL, Warach S. Cerebral spinal fluid contamination of the measurement of the apparent diffusion coefficient of water in acute stroke. Magn Reson Med 2002;48:478–86.
25. Rosen BR, Belliveau JW, Vevea JM, Brady TJ. Perfusion imaging with NMR contrast agents. Magn Reson Med 1990;14:249–65.
26. Fiebach JB, Schellinger PD. Modern magnetic resonance techniques with stroke. Nervenarzt 2002;73:104–17.
27. Baird AE, Lovblad KO, Dashe JF, et al. Clinical correlations of diffusion and perfusion lesion volumes in acute ischemic stroke. Cerebrovasc Dis 2000;10:441–8.
28. Schellinger PD, Fiebach JB, Jansen O, et al. Stroke magnetic resonance imaging within 6 hours after onset of hyperacute cerebral ischemia. Ann Neurol 2001;49:460–9.
29. Powers WJ, Zivin J. Magnetic resonance imaging in acute stroke: not ready for prime time. Neurology 1998;50:842–3.

30. Jansen O, Schellinger PD, Fiebach JB, et al. Early recanalization in acute ischemic stroke saves tissue at risk defined by MRI. Lancet 1999;353:2036–7.

31. Coutts SB, Simon JE, Tomanek AI, et al. Reliability of assessing percentage of diffusion-perfusion mismatch. Stroke 2003;34:1681–3.

32. Kidwell CS, Saver JL, Mattiello J, et al. Thrombolytic reversal of acute human cerebral ischemic injury shown by diffusion/perfusion magnetic resonance imaging. Ann Neurol 2000;47:462–9.

33. Merino JG, Todd JW, Schellinger PD, et al. Reversal of ischemic brain injury in humans. Stroke 2006; submitted for publication.

34. Saver JL, Johnston KC, Homer D, et al. Infarct volume as a surrogate or auxiliary outcome measure in ischemic stroke clinical trials. Stroke 1999;30:293–8.

35. von Kummer R, Allen KL, Holle R, et al. Acute stroke: usefulness of early CT findings before thrombolytic therapy. Radiology 1997;205:327–33.

36. Chalela JA, Kang DW, Luby M, et al. Early magnetic resonance imaging findings in patients receiving tissue plasminogen activator predict outcome: insights into the pathophysiology of acute stroke in the thrombolysis era. Ann Neurol 2004;55:105–12.

37. Fisher M. Reversal of diffusion abnormalities after ischemic stroke: adding difficulty and complexity to the conundrum of acute stroke imaging. Ann Neurol 2002;52:695–6.

38. Fiehler J, Foth M, Kucinski T, et al. Severe ADC decreases do not predict irreversible tissue damage in humans. Stroke 2002;33:79–86.

39. Baumgartner RW, Ringelstein EB. Cerebrovascular ultrasound diagnosis. Ther Umsch 1996;53:528–34.

40. Ringelstein EB, Biniek R, Weiller C, et al. Type and extent of hemispheric brain infarctions and clinical outcome in early and delayed middle cerebral artery recanalization. Neurology 1992;42:289–98.

41. Christou I, Alexandrov AV, Burgin WS, et al. Timing of recanalization after tissue plasminogen activator therapy determined by transcranial Doppler correlates with clinical recovery from ischemic stroke. Stroke 2000;31:1812–16.

42. Molina CA, Montaner J, Abilleira S, et al. Time course of tissue plasminogen activator-induced recanalization in acute cardioembolic stroke: a case–control study. Stroke 2001;32:2821–7.

43. Molina CA, Montaner J, Abilleira S, et al. Timing of spontaneous recanalization and risk of hemorrhagic transformation in acute cardioembolic stroke. Stroke 2001;32:1079–84.

44. Alexandrov AV, Burgin WS, Demchuk AM, et al. Speed of intracranial clot lysis with intravenous tissue plasminogen activator therapy: sonographic classification and short-term improvement. Circulation 2001;103:2897–902.

45. Gerriets T, Postert T, Goertler M, et al. DIAS I: duplex-sonographic assessment of the cerebrovascular status in acute stroke: a useful tool for future stroke trials. Stroke 2000;31:2342–5.

46. Warach S. Early reperfusion related to clinical response in DIAS – phase II, randomized, placebo-controlled dose finding trial of IV desmoteplase 3–9 hours from onset in patients with diffusion–perfusion mismatch. In: Proceedings of ASA – International Stroke Conference, San Diego, CA, 2004.

47. Brant-Zawadzki M, Heiserman JE. The roles of MR angiography, CT angiography, and sonography in vascular imaging of the head and neck. AJNR Am J Neuroradiol 1997;18:1820–5.

48. Lubezky N, Fajer S, Barmeir E, Karmeli R. Duplex scanning and CT angiography in the diagnosis of carotid artery occlusion: a prospective study. Eur J Vasc Endovasc Surg 1998;16:133–6.

49. Lev MH, Nichols SJ. Computed tomographic angiography and computed tomographic perfusion imaging of hyperacute stroke. Top Magn Reson Imaging 2000;11:273–87.

50. Knauth M, Kummer RY, Jansen O, et al. Potential of CT angiography in acute ischemic stroke. AJNR Am J Neuroradiol 1997;18:1001–10.

51. Koenig M, Klotz E, Luka B, et al. Perfusion CT of the brain: diagnostic approach for early detection of ischemic stroke. Radiology 1998;209:85–93.

52. Wildermuth S, Knauth M, Brandt T, et al. Role of CT angiography in patient selection for thrombolytic therapy in acute hemispheric stroke. Stroke 1998;29:935–8.

53. Lev MH, Segal AZ, Farkas J, et al. Utility of perfusion-weighted CT imaging in acute middle cerebral artery stroke treated with intra-arterial thrombolysis: prediction of final infarct volume and clinical outcome. Stroke 2001;32:2021–8.

54. Schramm P, Schellinger PD, Fiebach JB, et al. Comparison of CT and CT angiography source images with diffusion-weighted imaging in patients with acute stroke within 6 hours after onset. Stroke 2002; 33:2426–32.

55. Schramm P, Schellinger PD, Klotz E, et al. Comparison of perfusion computed tomography and computed tomography angiography source images with perfusion-weighted imaging and diffusion-weighted imaging in patients with acute stroke of less than 6 hours' duration. Stroke 2004;35:1652–8.

56. Koenig M, Banach-Planchamp R, Kraus M, et al. CT perfusion imaging in acute ischemic cerebral infarct: comparison of cerebral perfusion maps and

conventional CT findings. Röfo Fortschr Geb Röntgenstr Neuen Bildgeb Verfahr 2000;172:219–26.

57. Koenig M, Kraus M, Theek C, et al. Quantitative assessment of the ischemic brain by means of perfusion-related parameters derived from perfusion CT. Stroke 2001;32:431–7.

58. Wintermark M, Bogousslavsky J. Imaging of acute ischemic brain injury: the return of computed tomography. Curr Opin Neurol 2003;16:59–63.

59. Heiss WD. Best measure of ischemic penumbra: positron emission tomography. Stroke 2003;34: 2534–5.

60. Berrouschot J, Barthel H, Hesse S, et al. Differentiation between transient ischemic attack and ischemic stroke within the first six hours after onset of symptoms by using ^{99m}Tc-ECD–SPECT. J Cereb Blood Flow Metab 1998;18:921–9.

61. Zivin JA, Holloway RG. Weighing the evidence on DWI: caveat emptor. Neurology 2000;54:1552.

62. Schellinger PD, Jansen O, Fiebach JB, et al. Feasibility and practicality of MR imaging of stroke in the management of hyperacute cerebral ischemia. AJNR Am J Neuroradiol 2000;21:1184–9.

63. Buckley BT, Wainwright A, Meagher T, Briley D. Audit of a policy of magnetic resonance imaging with diffusion-weighted imaging as first-line neuroimaging for in-patients with clinically suspected acute stroke. Clin Radiol 2003;58:234–7.

64. von Kummer R. Imaging of stroke pathology without predefined gold standard. Cerebrovasc Dis 2002;14: 270; Author Reply 271.

65. Keir SL, Wardlaw JM. Systematic review of diffusion and perfusion imaging in acute ischemic stroke. Stroke 2000;31:2723–31.

66. Fiebach JB, Schellinger PD, Jansen O, et al. CT and diffusion-weighted MR-imaging in randomized order: DWI results in higher accuracy and lower interrater variability in the diagnosis of hyperacute ischemic stroke. Stroke 2002;33:2206–10.

67. Saur D, Kucinski T, Grzyska U, et al. Sensitivity and interrater agreement of CT and diffusion-weighted MR imaging in hyperacute stroke. AJNR Am J Neuroradiol 2003;24:878–85.

68. Fiebach JB, Schellinger PD, Gass A, et al. Stroke magnetic resonance imaging is accurate in hyperacute intracerebral hemorrhage. A multicenter study on the validity of stroke imaging. Stroke 2004;35:502–7.

69. Gonzales RG, Schaefer PW, Buonanno FS, et al. Diffusion-weighted MR imaging: diagnostic accuracy in patients imaged within 6 hours of stroke symptom onset. Radiology 1999;210:155–62.

70. Fiebach JB, Jansen O, Schellinger PD, et al. Comparison of CT with diffusion-weighted MRI in patients with hyperacute stroke. Neuroradiology 2001;43:628–32.

71. von Kummer R, Bourquain H, Bastianello S, et al. Early prediction of irreversible brain damage after ischemic stroke at CT. Radiology 2001;219:95–100.

72. Patel SC, Levine SR, Tilley BC, et al. Lack of clinical significance of early ischemic changes on computed tomography in acute stroke. JAMA 2001;286:2830–8.

73. Osborn AG. Intracranial hemorrhage. In: Osborn AG (ed). Diagnostic Neuroradiology. St Louis, MO: Mosby-Year Book, 1994:154–198.

74. Zyed A, Hayman LA, Bryan RN. MR imaging of intracerebral blood: diversity in the temporal pattern at 0.5 and 1.0T. AJNR Am J Neuroradiol 1991;12: 469–74.

75. Patel MR, Edelman RR, Warach S. Detection of hyperacute primary intraparenchymal hemorrhage by magnetic resonance imaging. Stroke 1996;27:2321–4.

76. Schellinger PD, Jansen O, Fiebach JB, et al. A standardized MRI stroke protocol: comparison with CT in hyperacute intracerebral hemorrhage. Stroke 1999;30:765–8.

77. Linfante I, Llinas RH, Caplan LR, Warach S. MRI features of intracerebral hemorrhage within 2 hours from symptom onset. Stroke 1999;30:2263–7.

78. Fiebach JB, Schellinger PD, Geletneky K, et al. MRI in acute subarachnoid haemorrhage; findings with a standardised stroke protocol. Neuroradiology 2004; 46:44–8.

79. The European Stroke Initiative. Recommendations for stroke management. Cerebrovasc Dis 2000;10:1–34.

80. Kidwell CS, Saver JL, Villablanca JP, et al. Magnetic resonance imaging detection of microbleeds before thrombolysis: an emerging application. Stroke 2002;33:95–8.

81. Nighoghossian N, Hermier M, Adeleine P, et al. Old microbleeds are a potential risk factor for cerebral bleeding after ischemic stroke: a gradient-echo T2*-weighted brain MRI study. Stroke 2002;33:735–42.

82. Derex L, Nighoghossian N, Hermier M, et al. Thrombolysis for ischemic stroke in patients with old microbleeds on pretreatment MRI. Cerebrovasc Dis 2004;17:238–41.

83. Montaner J, Molina CA, Monasterio J, et al. Matrix metalloproteinase-9 pretreatment level predicts intracranial hemorrhagic complications after thrombolysis in human stroke. Circulation 2003;107:598–603.

84. Röther J, Schellinger PD, Gass A, et al. Effect of intravenous thrombolysis on MRI parameters and functional outcome in acute stroke <6 h. Stroke 2002;33: 2438–45.

85. Külkens S, Schwark C, Schellinger PD, et al. Thrombolysis in ischemic stroke 3 to 6 hours after symptom onset using a MR-based algorithm. In: Proceedings of International Stroke Conference, Phoenix, AZ, USA, February 13–15th, 2003.

86. The ATLANTIS, ECASS and NINDS rt-PA Study Group Investigators. Association of outcome with early stroke treatment: pooled analysis of ATLANTIS, ECASS, and NINDS rt-PA stroke trials. Lancet 2004; 363:768–74.
87. Mohr JP. Thrombolytic therapy for ischemic stroke: from clinical trials to clinical practice. JAMA 2000; 283:1189–91.
88. Hsia AW, Sachdev HS, Tomlinson J, et al. Efficacy of IV tissue plasminogen activator in acute stroke: Does stroke subtype really matter? Neurology 2003;61:71–5.
89. Gerraty RP, Parsons MW, Barber PA, et al. Examining the lacunar hypothesis with diffusion and perfusion magnetic resonance imaging. Stroke 2002;33:2019–24.
90. Chalela JA, Ezzeddine M, Latour LL, Warach S. Reversal of perfusion and diffusion abnormalities after intravenous thrombolysis for a lacunar infarction. J Neuroimaging 2003;13:152–4.
91. Fink JN, Kumar S, Horkan C, et al. The stroke patient who woke up: clinical and radiological features, including diffusion and perfusion MRI. Stroke 2002; 33:988–93.
92. Warach S. Tissue viability thresholds in acute stroke: the 4-factor model. Stroke 2001;32:2460–1.
93. Warach S. Stroke neuroimaging. Stroke 2003;34:345–7.
94. Warach S, Hacke W, Hsu C, et al. Effect of MaxiPost on ischemic lesions in patients with acute stroke: the POST-010 MRI substudy. Stroke 2002;33:383.
95. Warach S, Kaste M, Fisher M. The effect of GV150526 on ischemic lesion volume: the GAIN Americas and GAIN International MRI substudy. Neurology 2000; 54:A87–8.
96. Parsons MW, Barber PA, Chalk J, et al. Diffusion- and perfusion-weighted MRI response to thrombolysis in stroke. Ann Neurol 2002;51:28–37.
97. Seitz RJ, Hamzavi M, Junghans U, et al. Thrombolysis with recombinant tissue plasminogen activator and tirofiban in stroke: preliminary observations. Stroke 2003;34:1932–5.
98. Major ongoing stroke trials. Stroke 2003;34:e61–72.

18

Intra-arterial thrombolysis for acute ischemic stroke

Anthony J Furlan and Herman Zeumer

Intra-arterial thrombolysis

In the 1980s, several reports of intra arterial (IA) thrombolysis therapy in acute ischemic stroke were published.[1–3] The thrombolytic agents used in these early case series were urokinase (UK) and streptokinase (SK). Studies of IA thrombolysis for acute ischemic stroke were initially limited to uncontrolled protocols.[4,5] There was great variability in technique, and efficacy and complication rates varied among the reported series. As a result, in 1996, an American Heart Association (AHA) Special Writing Group published its recommendations for the use of thrombolytics in acute ischemic stroke. Based on the strength of the scientific evidence available at that time, the AHA concluded that IA thrombolysis 'should be considered investigational and only used in the clinical trial setting' and recommended 'further testing of' IA thrombolysis.[6] Advances in microcatheter technology during the 1980s allowed superselective catheterization of even distal branches of occluded intracranial vessels.

Subsequently, the results of the first randomized multicenter controlled trials of IA thrombolysis, PROACT (Prolyse in Acute Cerebral Thromboembolism Trial) I[7] and II,[8] were reported in 1998 and 1999, respectively. PROACT II remains the only randomized controlled multicenter clinical trial to demonstrate the efficacy of IA thrombolysis in patients with acute ischemic stroke of less than 6 h duration due to middle cerebral artery (MCA) occlusion. Trials comparing the IA versus the intravenous (IV) mode of application are not available

and it is not very likely that they will be performed in the future.

General technique of IA thrombolysis

Diagnosis and access

In advance of any procedure, the basic and crucial computed tomography (CT) criterion is to rule out hemorrhage. A complete four-vessel cerebral angiogram, from a transfemoral approach, is necessary to evaluate the site of vessel occlusion, the extent of thrombus, the number of territories involved, and the collateral circulation. Alternatively, a magnetic resonance angiogram (MRA) or a CT angiogram (CTA) can first be done to screen the site of occlusion. A diagnostic catheter is guided into the high cervical segment of the vascular territory to be treated, followed by the introduction of a 2.3-French coaxial microcatheter with a steerable microguidewire. Under direct fluoroscopic visualization, the microcatheter is gently navigated through the intracranial circulation until the tip is embedded within or through the central portion of the thrombus.

Many variations in catheter design and delivery technique have been described.[9] Two types of microcatheter are used most often for local cerebral thrombolysis, depending upon the extent of clot formation. For the majority of intra-arterial cases, a single-endhole microcatheter is used, while for longer segments of clot formation, multiple-sidehole infusion microcatheters are used. Superselective angiography through the microcatheter is performed at regular intervals to assess the degree of clot lysis and to adjust the dosage and volume of the thrombolytic agent. A superselective angiogram is performed, and if there is partial clot dissolution then the catheter is advanced into the remaining thrombus, where additional thrombolysis is performed. Infusion of most of the drug distal to the thrombus into a no-flow vessel has to be avoided. The goal is to achieve rapid recanalization with as little thrombolytic agent as possible to limit the extent of brain infarction and to reduce the risk of hemorrhage. However, common experience indicates that it can take up to 2 h to achieve recanalization after the procedure begins, that thrombolytic agents alone (i.e. without mechanical manipulation) rarely achieve recanalization in less than 30 min, and that recanalization is often incomplete. Among other factors, clot composition plays a key role in the rapidity and degree of recanalization achieved with IA thrombolysis.

Thrombolytic agents

Recombinant prourokinase (rproUK), the thrombolytic agent used in PROACT II (see below), is currently not approved by the US Food and Drug Administration and is not yet commercially available. Although some thrombolytic agents have theoretical advantages over others, there is no proof that one thrombolytic agent is superior to another in terms of safety, recanalization, or clinical efficacy in acute ischemic stroke. Therefore, it is not clear if the results of PROACT II are applicable when agents other than rproUK are used for IA thrombolysis. Commercially available agents include urokinase, recombinant tissue-type plasminogen activator (rtPA), reteplase (rPA) and tenecteplase (tNKase, TNK-rtPA). These thrombolytic agents differ in stability, half-life and fibrin selectivity. Urokinase is not fibrin-selective and therefore can result in systemic hypofibrinogemia. rtPA and rproUK are fibrin-selective and are only active at the site of thrombosis. However, rproUK requires heparin for maximal thrombolytic effect. Newer agents have long half-lives, allowing bolus administration (e.g. rPA), or are more fibrin-selective (e.g. tNKase).

With local fibrinolysis, it is possible to monitor not only the frequency of recanalization but also how fast it occurs. All current single thrombolytic agents often require 30–60 min for recanalization even with direct IA application. Even 325 000 IU urokinase or 40 mg rtPA takes 100 min to recanalize in our experience with 140 patients.[10] A very promising concept involves using Lys-plasminogen with rtPA during local IA infusion.[11] In comparison to rtPA and urokinase alone, adjunctive Lys-plasminogen increased the frequency of recanalizations and reduced the recanalization time. The efficacy of second- and third-generation thrombolytic agents in acute ischemic stroke has not been demonstrated in a randomized controlled trial.

IV heparin

IV heparin is given by most neuro-interventionalists during IA stroke thrombolysis. Systemic anticoagulation with heparin reduces the risk of catheter-related embolism. Also, the thrombolytic effect of some agents such as rproUK is augmented by heparin. Another rationale for antithrombotic therapy is prevention of early reocclusion, which is more common with atherothrombosis than with cerebral embolism. These indications are counterbalanced by the increased risk of brain hemorrhage when heparin is combined with a thrombolytic agent.

The optimal dose of heparin during IA stroke thrombolysis has not been established. PROACT I[7] reported a 27% rate of symptomatic brain hemorrhage when a conventional non-weight-adjusted heparin regimen (100 U/kg bolus, 1000 U/h for 4 h) was employed with IA rproUK. Subsequently a low-dose heparin regimen was used (2000 U bolus, 500 U/h for 4 h), which reduced the symptomatic brain hemorrhage rate with IA rproUK to 7% in PROACT I and 10% in PROACT II. Unfortunately, low-dose heparin also cuts the recanalization rate in half with IA rproUK. Some neuro-interventionalists now employ the PROACT low-dose heparin regimen during IA thrombolysis. However, this dose of heparin does not prolong the activated partial thromboplastin time (aPTT) or activated clotting time (aCT). Other neuro-interventionalists employ weight-adjusted heparin, keeping the aCT between 200 and 300 s.

Other factors influencing outcomes with thrombolysis

Hacke[12] has described an ideal patient for thrombolysis: a young person with good collaterals who has a middle cerebral artery (MCA) occlusion distal to the lenticulostriates due to a fresh fibrin-rich thrombus that passed through a patent foramen ovale. The presence of collateral flow is one of the prime determinants of outcome.[13,14] Good leptomeningeal collaterals may limit the extent of ischemic damage and prolong the therapeutic window. Good collateral flow is also associated with higher rates of reperfusion, presumably by allowing a greater amount of thrombolytic to reach the clot by means of redistribution. Clot composition is a neglected factor in recanalization success rates.[15] Fresh thrombi, which are fibrin- and plasminogen-rich, are easier to lyse than aged atherothrombi, which are more organized and have low fibrin and plasminogen contents and high amounts of platelets and cholesterol. Fresh cardiac emboli may therefore respond better to thrombolysis than atherothrombotic occlusions or calcific emboli.

Risk factors for hemorrhagic transformation

Several series have found no relationship between recanalization and risk of hemorrhage.[16–18] However, these series did not address delayed recanalization or the status of recanalization at the time of brain hemorrhage. The amount of ischemic damage is a key factor in the development of hemorrhage after thrombolysis. Early extensive CT changes and severity of the initial neurological deficit, both of which are indicators of the extent of ischemic damage, are the best predictors of risk of hemorrhagic transformation.[18,19] In ECASS (European Cooperative Acute Stroke Study) I,[20] early CT changes in over one-third of the MCA territory correlated well with the frequency of hemorrhagic infarction. However, the so-called ECASS CT criteria are not present in all cases of hemorrhage and there is considerable inter-reader variability in the interpretation of early CT changes. An analysis of the PROACT II data indicated that patients with early (i.e. <6h) CT infarct volumes greater than 100 ml do

poorly.[21] However, estimated early CT changes (i.e. ECASS criteria) appear less predictive of outcome among homogeneous patients with MCA occlusion compared with patients with mixed sites of arterial occlusion.[21] Given the somewhat conflicting data, it would be prudent either to avoid thrombolysis in patients with clearcut extensive early signs of infarction on CT and a National Institutes of Health Stroke Scale (NIHSS) Score over 20, especially those older than 75, or to emphasize to the family a greatly reduced benefit-to-risk ratio even in <3h patients.

The amount of ischemic damage depends on the duration of occlusion and the degree of collateral blood flow. Both of these factors have been associated with increased hemorrhage risk. Ueda et al[22] found that the amount of residual blood flow, as determined by single photon emission CT (SPECT) scanning, was associated with hemorrhagic transformation, but also used SPECT results to extend the thrombolytic time window beyond 6h in three patients. Improved perfusion after 3h IV rtPA has also been demonstrated with SPECT.[22,23] Apparent diffusion coefficient (ADC) mapping on magnetic resonance imaging (MRI) has also been used to predict hemorrhagic risk.[24]

Several other factors have been associated with hemorrhage after thrombolysis for both stroke and myocardial infarction (MI), including thrombolytic dose, blood pressure, advanced age, prior head injury, and blood glucose.[25–31] A strong relationship between advanced age and hemorrhage was also demonstrated in ECASS and the NINDS (National Institute of Neurological Disorders and Stroke) trial. Although there is no strict age cutoff, physicians need to take into account the increased risk of hemorrhage in patients aged 75 and over when making the decision for thrombolysis for stroke.

Intracerebral hemorrhage (ICH) after thrombolysis for stroke can occur at sites distant from the ischemic region.[32] Cerebral amyloid angiopathy has been implicated as a causative factor for ICH after thrombolysis for MI.[30]

The PROACT trials

Beginning in February 1994, patients were enrolled in the first placebo controlled, double-blinded multicenter trial of IA thrombolysis in acute ischemic stroke, PROACT I.[7] The results were published in 1998. This trial employed rproUK, which is a recombinant single-chain zymogen of an endogenous fibrinolytic, urokinase (uPA).[33] Infusion of rproUK does not result in a systemic dysfibrinogenemia with its associated higher risk of hemorrhagic side-effects. Another clinically relevant characteristic of rproUK is the facilitatory effect of coadministered heparin, which when given with rproUK improves its fibrinolytic efficacy.

In PROACT I, the safety and recanalization efficacy of 6 mg IA rproUK was compared with IA saline placebo in 40 patients with acute ischemic stroke of less than 6 h duration due to MCA occlusion. Only patients with Thrombolysis in Acute Myocardial Infarction (TIMI) grade 0 or grade 1 occlusion of the M1 or M2 MCA on diagnostic cerebral angiography were included. Additional major inclusion criteria included a minimum NIHSS Score of 4 (except for isolated aphasia or hemianopsia) and a maximum NIHSS Score of 30. Major exclusion criteria were uncontrolled hypertension (blood pressure >180/100 mmHg), a history of hemorrhage, recent surgery, or trauma. Early CT changes were not an exclusion criterion. Mechanical disruption of the clot was not permitted, since the goal of the trial was to demonstrate the efficacy and safety of rproUK. In addition to rproUK, patients also received IV heparin. The first 16 patients received 'high-dose' heparin consisting of a 100 IU/kg bolus followed by a 1000 IU/h infusion for 4 h; anticoagulation was prohibited for the following 24 h. Based upon a recommendation from the external safety committee, the heparin regimen was changed after the first 16 patients to a 2000 IU bolus followed by a 500 IU/h infusion for 4 h.

The recanalization rate was 57.7% in the rproUK group and only 14.3% in the placebo group. In the 'high-dose heparin' group, the recanalization rate was 81.8% in the rproUK patients, but the symptomatic ICH rate was 27%. In contrast, in the 'low-dose heparin' group, the recanalization rate was 40% in the rproUK patients, but the ICH rate decreased to 6%. Overall, symptomatic ICH occurred in 15.4% of treatment patients and in 14.3% of patients who received placebo. Although not a clinical efficacy trial, there appeared to be a 10–12% increase in excellent outcomes in the IA rproUK group as compared with the control group.

The follow-up clinical efficacy trial, PROACT II, was launched in February 1996 and the results were published in December 1999.[8] PROACT II was a randomized, controlled, multicenter trial, but differed from PROACT I in that an open-label design with blinded follow-up was used. Patient selection was essentially the same as in PROACT I, with the major exception that patients with early signs of infarction in greater than one-third of the MCA territory (the so-called ECASS criteria[17]) on the initial CT scan were excluded. Additionally, a dose of 9 mg of rproUK was used instead of 6 mg, and 'low-dose heparin' was used in the treatment and control groups. A total of 180 patients were randomized to receive either 9 mg of IA rproUK plus low-dose IV heparin or low-dose IV heparin alone. The patients in PROACT II had a very high baseline stroke severity, with a median NIHSS Score of 17. The median time from onset of symptoms to initiation of IA thrombolysis was 5.3 h.

The primary outcome measure was the proportion of patients who achieved a modified Rankin Score of 2 or less at 90 days, which signifies slight or no neurological disability. For the rproUK-treated group, there was a 15% absolute benefit ($p = 0.043$). The benefit was most noticeable in patients with a baseline NIHSS Score between 11 and 20. On average, seven patients with MCA occlusion would require IA thrombolysis for one to benefit. Recanalization rates were 66% at 2 h for the treatment group and 18% for the placebo group ($p < 0.001$). Symptomatic ICH occurred in 10% of the r-proUK group and 2% of the control group. Considering the later time to treatment and greater baseline stroke severity in PROACT II, the symptomatic ICH rate compared favorably with the IV rtPA trials (6% in the NINDS trial, 9% in ECASS II, and 7% in ATLANTIS (Atleplase Thrombolysis for Acute Noninterventional Therapy in Ischemic Stroke)). As in the NINDS trial, in PROACT II, despite the higher ICH rate, patients benefited overall from therapy, and there was no excess mortality (rproUK 24%, control 27%).

Carotid territory IA thrombolysis: special features

The majority of hemispheric vessel occlusions are due to embolism. In thrombolysis trials, the 30-day mortality rate in hemispheric stroke is between 15% and 20% and is not significantly different between treatment and placebo. Thrombolytic treatment has had no impact on survival, but rather improves the clinical outcome in patients with less than massive strokes. Most successful recanalizations of the carotid circulation involve the MCA. Recanalization of the internal carotid artery (ICA) origin is seldom achieved, even with direct IA approaches. Some interventionalists advocate passing the catheter through the obstructing thrombus to access the MCA. Occlusion of the carotid 'T' eliminates the posterior communicating artery and ophthalmic artery collaterals, so that leptomeningeal collaterals and the anterior communicating artery often are not sufficient to save major parts of the hemisphere even for a short period of time.[34,35] Recanalization of the carotid 'T' is difficult and rarely leads to good clinical results; such patients are commonly excluded from clinical trials.

Vertebrobasilar IA thrombolysis: special features

In the posterior circulation, two special conditions have to be kept in mind. First, the natural history of acute basilar occlusion is extremely poor, with mortality rates in the range 83–91%.[36,37] Second, atherothrombotic occlusions of the basilar artery are relatively more common than embolic occlusions.[35] Hence, there is often a need for angioplasty of an underlying basilar artery atherostenosis. Accordingly, IA thrombolysis is preferred in patients with acute basilar artery occlusion. In a compilation of reported cases of vertebrobasilar (VB) thrombolysis, the mortality rate in patients failing recanalization was 90%, compared with 31% in patients achieving at least partial reperfusion.[36] Approximately 278 cases have been reported, with an overall basilar recanalization rate of 60%. Good outcomes are strongly associated with recanalization after thrombolytic therapy. The majority of patients with successful VB recanalization have mild or moderate disability, compared with less than 14% of patients whose vessels remained occluded.[38]

Distal basilar artery occlusions have a higher recanalization rate because they often consist of soft emboli, which are easier to lyse than atherosclerosis-related thrombi.[39] In addition, the high rate of reocclusion worsens the prognosis of mid or lower basilar atherothrombosis. Excellent results support the use of angioplasty for stabilizing atherothrombotic

recanalization.[40–42] Short-segment occlusions are easier to lyse than longer-segment occlusions. Patients who are younger have higher recanalization rates, probably due to the increased incidence of embolic occlusions seen in this age group.

The time window for thrombolysis was thought to be longer in the posterior circulation. Many series have included patients up to 72 h after symptom onset.[42] However, thrombolysis with such prolonged time windows makes sense only in patients with prolonged stuttering courses, such as VB patients with chronic atherothrombotic disease in whom collaterals have developed over time. Except in such cases with favorable hemodynamic conditions, treatment exceeding the 6 h window has a very poor prognosis, especially in the presence of coma or tetraparesis for several hours.[35]

The importance of signs of infarction on CT in the brainstem and other posterior circulation locations is controversial.[43] The decision must be made individually regarding the lethal thread and the clinical status related to the CT findings. A clearly hypodense, destroyed brainstem in a comatose, reflexless individual is certainly not an indication.

Investigational endovascular acute stroke therapies

Combination and mechanical reperfusion therapy in acute stroke

Initial studies of thrombolytic therapy in acute ischemic stroke involved a single pharmacological agent given either IV or IA. The NINDS trial[44] led to FDA approval of IV rtPA, but only for patients with stroke of less than 3 h duration, which has limited its widespread use. PROACT II[45] demonstrated clinical efficacy with IA rproUK in patients with MCA occlusion of less than 6 h duration, but rproUK did not receive FDA approval based on this single randomized trial. Nonetheless, the principle of IA thrombolysis has been widely endorsed as a reasonable option in selected patients with acute ischemic stroke of up to 6 h duration.[46–48]

Unfortunately, neither IV nor IA thrombolysis using only a single pharmacological agent is an efficient way to rapidly recanalize occluded major brain arteries. Even when it works, IV or IA rtPA takes at least 15–30 min to reopen an occluded major vessel such as the MCA, and there is no evidence that other available thrombolytic agents are faster. Occlusion in large vessels such as the ICA and basilar artery are resistant to IV or IA thrombolysis with one agent. Recent transcranial Doppler (TCD) studies after IV rtPA suggest only a 30% complete recanalization rate for MCA occlusion, a 48% partial recanalization rate, and a 27% reocclusion rate.[49] The MCA complete recanalization rate with IA rproUK was only 20% after 2 h, with a 63% partial recanalization rate and a 10% reocclusion rate within the first hour of treatment.[45] The low rate of complete recanalization and the high rate of reocclusion with stroke thrombolysis is not surprising considering that not even aspirin is allowed for 24 h after IV rtPA.

Faster and more complete recanalization should translate into better patient outcomes. To achieve this, the trend in acute coronary syndromes (ACS) has been to employ multiple pharmacological agents and, increasingly, percutaneous coronary intervention (PCI). The impetus, as in stroke, is the more rapid and complete recanalization of occluded or stenosed coronary arteries. The standard treatment in many ACS patients includes antiplatelet therapy with aspirin and clopidogrel, antithrombotic therapy with heparin or low-molecular-weighted heparin (LMWH), and direct PCI.[50] In ACS, the TIMI 14 trial[14] reported the highest TIMI grade 3 complete recanalization rates with reduced-dose IV rtPA combined with the glycoprotein (GP) IIb/IIIa antagonist abciximab. However, the rate of brain hemorrhage was increased in patients aged over 75 receiving reduced-dose reteplase and abciximab in the GUSTO (Global use of Strategies to Open Occluded Coronary Artery) V trial.[52]

If we are to improve the efficiency of acute stroke thrombolysis, we shall also need to develop multimodal combination therapies while simultaneously reducing the risk of brain hemorrhage. The PROACT I study demonstrated that the recanalization efficacy and safety of rproUK were affected by the concomitant use of heparin.[53] A major stimulus to the development of stroke thrombectomy devices has been to improve the speed and completeness of recanalization compared with an IA drug alone. In the MERCI (Mechanical Embolus Removal in Cerebral Ischemia) trial, vessels were opened faster with the MERCI retriever system, but the recanalization efficacy

(TIMI grade 2/3) and safety results achieved with the MERCI retriever system alone were very similar to the results achieved with IA rproUK in PROACT II.[54–56] Indeed, the MCA recanalization rate in the MERCI trial was 45%, compared with 66% in PROACT II. In the MERCI trial, 17 patients also received thrombolytics when the device failed to recanalize the vessel, but the outcomes in these patients were not reported.

There are numerous anecdotal reports of combination reperfusion therapies in acute stroke employing various IV and IA drugs and devices.[57–61] The only published clinical trials designed to specifically investigate combination reperfusion therapy in acute stroke are the EMS (Emergency Management of Stroke) study[62] and the follow-up IMS (Interventional Management of Stroke) I study.[63] The EMS study investigated the feasibility, safety, and efficacy of reduced-dose (0.6 mg/kg) IV rtPA combined with up to 20 mg IA rtPA in patients with stroke of less than 3 h duration. Thirty-five patients were randomly assigned to either the IV/IA group or the placebo/IA group. Recanalization was achieved in 54% of the IV/IA group and 10% of the IA group. There was no significant difference in the rate of symptomatic brain hemorrhage between the two groups at 72 h (11.8% IV/IA vs 5.5% placebo/IA). The investigators concluded that IV/IA rtPA was feasible and safe, and appeared to result in better recanalization than IA alone. However, there was no difference in the 90-day clinical outcomes between the two treatment groups.

The follow-up IMS I study treated 80 patients with less than 3 h stroke with 0.6 mg/kg IV rtPA combined with up to 22 mg IA rtPA and compared clinical outcome at 90 days with placebo subsets derived from the NINDS rtPA stroke trial. The rate of symptomatic brain hemorrhage in IMS I was 6.3%, which was similar to the 6.6% rate in the NINDS trial. IMS I patients had a significantly better clinical outcome at 90 days compared with NINDS placebo patients.

The ongoing IMS II study again employs reduced-dose IV rtPA combined with IA rtPA, but now delivered through an ultrasonic EKOS catheter in an attempt to accelerate thrombolysis. External ultrasound has also been shown to enhance IV rtPA in the CLOTBUST (Combined Lysis of Thrombus in Brain Ischemia Using Transcranial Ultrasound and Systemic tPA Trial) study.[64] In CLOTBUST, complete MCA recanalization with dramatic clinical recovery occurred in

49% of patients receiving IV rtPA combined with transcranial ultrasound, versus 30% in patients receiving IV rtPA only. Other clinical trials of combination rtPA and GPIIb/IIIa inhibitors, some based on perfusion brain imaging, are underway (ROSIE (ReoPRO Retavase Reperfusion of Stroke Safety Study) and CLEAR (Combination Approach to Lysis Utilizing Eptifibatide and rt-PA in Acute Ischemic Stroke)). There have also been very limited studies of combination cytoprotective and reperfusion therapy in acute stroke (lubeluzole[65] and CoolAID[66]). Until randomized clinical efficacy trials can be completed, combination reperfusion therapies for acute stroke will remain experimental for the foreseeable future.

Current status and future of IA thrombolysis: personal perspectives

Since a clinical trial comparing IV with IA or combination thrombolysis will be difficult to perform and IV rtPA under 3 h remains the only FDA-approved acute stroke therapy, deciding on the best approach to reperfusion in an individual patient must take into account numerous factors discussed above.[67,68] The advantages of local fibrinolysis include precise angiographic information, control of the progress of recanalization (including the option to use mechanical devices), lower systemic thrombolytic activity, and higher recanalization rates for large-vessel occlusions. The risk of serious procedural complications was not as high in PROACT I and II, and cerebral angiography in experienced centers is associated with rates of permanent complications and death of only 0.1% and 0.02%, respectively. On the other hand, IA thrombolysis requires access to a team of physicians (an interventionalist and tertiary stroke team) capable of performing IA thrombolysis. Such expertise is not readily available in many developing countries or communities across Europe and the USA, and is usually limited to large academic centers. Treatment delays are also inherent to IA thrombolysis. In PROACT II, the median time to drug infusion from stroke onset was 5.3 h and the average time from arrival to the hospital to the initiation of IA rproUK was 3 h. IA thrombolysis also involves costs and procedural risks not inherent to IV thrombolysis. As the

total number of IA-treated patients is small, not much is known about drug and dose efficacy relations. An IA web registry has recently been established to gather more information.[69]

IV thrombolysis has the important advantages of time, ease of administration, and widespread availability. However, currently less than 5% of acute stroke patients receive IV rtPA, mainly because of the 3 h treatment window. The difficulty in demonstrating a benefit from IV thrombolysis beyond 3 h from stroke onset arises from a number of factors. The proportion of patients with major stroke who have salvageable brain decreases with time, while the brain hemorrhage rate with thrombolysis increases. A worse than expected outcome due to the inclusion of patients with early signs of infarction on CT contributed to the negative results of ECASS I. Conversely, a better than expected outcome made it difficult to demonstrate a benefit in ECASS II when such patients were excluded. In the IV thrombolysis trials, vascular imaging studies were not performed, so that neither the sites of arterial occlusion nor the recanalization rates are known. Patients with ischemic stroke of less than 6 h duration have a wide variety of occlusion sites, and 20% have no visible occlusion, despite similar neurological presentations.

The key issue is to achieve complete recanalization as quickly as possible. A good clinical outcome is significantly related to recanalization regardless of how it is achieved. The factors that determine individual susceptibility to ischemia are not completely understood, and clearly there is a great deal of variability in time to irreversible damage among individuals, i.e. there are many therapeutic windows. Greater recanalization efficacy is taken as an explanation of why the time window for successful IA thrombolysis may be longer than for IV administration. Based on PROACT II, a 6 h window appears to be a realistic goal for IA therapy in anterior circulation ischemia. However, in PROACT II, only patients with MCA occlusions were treated – an occlusion type in which the probability of good collateralization is high, recanalization occurs frequently and the possibility of recanalization 'in time' is greatest. Patient selection contributed greatly to the degree of efficacy in PROACT, and this is now a central challenge in acute reperfusion therapy.

It is increasingly obvious that selecting reperfusion therapy based only on time from stroke onset, a neurological examination score, and a routine CT scan is inadequate. Since the evolution of new-generation MRI scanners, and with the development of multislice spiral CT, a great variety of information can now be made available within minutes describing the anatomical and pathophysiological situation of an acute stroke patient in great detail. This offers the opportunity to make highly selective treatment decisions.[70–72] The DIAS (Desmoteplase in Acute Stroke) trial was the first randomized trial to select patients for IV thrombolysis based on a 20% MRI perfusion–diffusion mismatch up to 9 h from stroke onset.[73] The preliminary results suggest that physiological perfusion imaging will improve patient selection for therapy beyond the current 3 h IV rtPA window.

References

1. Nenci GG, Gresele P, Taramelli M, et al. Thrombolytic therapy for thromboembolism of vertebrobasilar artery. Angiology 1983;34:561–71.
2. del Zoppo GJ, Ferbert A, Otis S, et al. Local intra-arterial fibrinolytic therapy in acute carotid territory stroke: a pilot study. Stroke 1988;19:307–13.
3. Hacke W, Zeumer H, Ferbert A, et al. Intra-arterial thrombolytic therapy improves outcome in patients with acute vertebrobasilar occlusive disease. Stroke 1988;19:1216–22.
4. Zeumer H, Freitag HJ, Zanella F, et al. Local intra-arterial fibrinolytic therapy in patients with stroke: urokinase versus recombinant tissue plasminogen activator (rt-PA). Neuroradiology 1993;35:159–62.
5. Nesbit GM, Clark WM, O'Neil OR, Barnwell SL. Intracranial intra-arterial thrombolysis facilitated by microcatheter navigation through an occluded cervical internal carotid artery. J Neurosurg 1996;84: 387–92.
6. Adams HP, Brott TC, Furlan AJ, et al. Guidelines for Thrombolytic Therapy for Acute Stroke: A Supplement to the Guidelines for the Management of Patients with Acute Ischemic Stroke, A Statement for Healthcare Professionals From a Special Writing Group of the Stroke Council, American Heart Association. Circulation 1996;94:1167–74.
7. del Zoppo GJ, Higashida RT, Furlan AJ, et al. PROACT: a phase II randomized trial of recombinant pro-urokinase by direct arterial delivery in acute middle cerebral artery stroke. Stroke 1998;29:4–11.
8. Furlan A, Higashida R, Wechsler L, et al. Intra-arterial prourokinase for acute ischemic stroke – the PROACT II study: a randomized controlled trial. JAMA 1999; 282:2003–11.
9. Higashida RT, Halbach VV, Tsai FY, et al. Interventional neurovascular techniques in acute thrombolytic therapy for stroke. In: Yamagushi T, Mori E, Minematsu K, del Zoppo GJ (eds). Thrombolytic Therapy in Acute Ischemic Stroke III. Tokyo: Springer-Verlag, 1995: 294–300.
10. Eckert B, Koch C, Thomalla G, et al. Acute basilar artery occlusion treated with combined IV abciximab and IA t-PA: report of 3 cases. Stroke 2002;33:1424–7.
11. Freitag HJ, Becker VU, Thie A, et al. Lys-plasminogen as an adjunct to local intra-arterial fibrinolysis for carotid territory stroke: laboratory and clinical findings. Neuroradiology 1996;38:181–5.
12. Hacke W. Thrombolysis: stroke subtype and embolus type. In: del Zoppo GJ, Mori E, Hacke W (eds). Thrombolytic Therapy in Acute Ischemic Stroke II. Berlin: Springer-Verlag, 1993:153–9.
13. von Kummer R, Holle R, Rosin L, et al. Does arterial recanalization improve outcome in carotid territory stroke? Stroke 1995;26:581–7.
14. Ringelstein EB, Biniek R, Weiler C, et al. Type and extent of hemispheric brain infarctions and clinical outcome in early and delayed middle cerebral artery recanalization. Neurology 1991;42:289–98.
15. Chimowitz M, Pessin M, Furlan A, et al. The effect of source of cerebral embolus on susceptibility to thrombolysis. Neurology 1994;44(Suppl 2):A356 2(abst).
16. von Kummer R, Hacke W. Safety and efficacy of intravenous tissue plasminogen activator and heparin in acute middle cerebral artery stroke. Stroke 1992;23: 646–52.
17. Mori E, Yoneda Y, Tabuchi M, et al. Intravenous recombinant tissue plasminogen activator in acute carotid artery territory stroke. Neurology 1992;42:976–82.
18. Levy DE, Brott TG, Haley EC, et al. Factors related to intracranial hematoma formation in patients receiving tissue-type plasminogen activator for acute ischemic stroke. Stroke 1994;25:291–7.
19. Bozzao L, Angeloni U, Bastianello S, et al. Early angiographic and CT findings in patients wtih hemorrhagic infarction in the distribution of the middle cerebral artery. AJNR Am J Neuroradiol 1991;12:1115–21.

20. Hacke W, Kaste M, Fieschi C, et al. Intravenous thrombolysis with recombinant tissue plasminogen activator for acute hemispheric stroke. The European Cooperative Acute Stroke Study (ECASS). JAMA 1995;274:1017–25.

21. Roberts HC, Dillon WP, Furlan AJ, et al. Computed tomographic findings in patients undergoing intra-arterial thrombolysis for acute ischemic stroke due to middle cerebral artery occlusion: results from the PROACT II trial. Stroke 2002;33:1557–65.

22. Ueda T, Hatakeyama T, Kumon Y, et al. Evaluation of risk of hemorrhagic transformation in local intra-arterial thrombolysis in acute ischemic stroke by initial SPECT. Stroke 1994;25:298–303.

23. Alexandrov AV, Bratina P, Grotta JC. TPA associated reperfusion after acute stroke demonstrated by HMPAO-SPECT. Stroke 1998;29:288 (abst).

24. Kidwell CS, Saver JL, Duckwiler G, Starkman S, et al. Predictors of hemorrhagic transformation following intra-arterial thrombolysis. Stroke 2001;32:319 (abst).

25. Gore JM, Sloan M, Price TR, et al. Intracerebral hemorrhage, cerebral infarction, and subdural hematoma after acute myocardial infarction and thrombolytic therapy in the Thrombolysis in Myocardial Infarction study. Thrombolysis in myocardial infarction, phase II, pilot and clinical trial. Circulation 1991;83:448–59.

26. Selker HP, Beshansky JR, Schmid CH, et al. Presenting pulse pressure predicts thrombolytic therapy-related intracranial hemorrhage, Thrombolytic Predictive Instrument (TPI) project results. Circulation 1994;90:1657–61.

27. Simoons ML, Maggioni AP, Knatterud G, et al. Individual risk assessment for intracranial haemorrhage during thrombolytic therapy. Lancet 1993;342:1523–8.

28. Gebel JM, Sila CA, Sloan MA, et al. Thrombolysis-related intracranial hemorrhage: a radiographic analysis of 244 cases from the GUSTO-1 trial with clinical correlation. Stroke 1998;29:563–9.

29. Larrue V, von Kummer R, del Zoppo G, et al. Hemorrhagic transformation in acute ischemic stroke, potential contributing factors in the European Cooperative Acute Stroke Study. Stroke 1997;28:957–60.

30. Sloan MA, Price TR, Petito CK, et al. Clinical features and pathogenesis of intracerebral hemorrhage after rt-PA and heparin therapy for acute myocardial infarction: the Thrombolysis in Myocardial Infarction (TIMI) II pilot and randomized clinical trial combined experience. Neurology 1995;45:649–58.

31. Kase CS, Furlan AJ, Wechsler LR, et al. Cerebral hemorrhage after intra-arterial thrombolysis for ischemic stroke. The PROACT II trial. Neurology 2001;57:1603–10.

32. The NINDS t-PA Stroke Study Group. Intracerebral hemorrhage after intravenous t-PA therapy for ischemic stroke. Stroke 1997;28:2109–18.

33. Credo RB, Burke SE, Barker WM, et al. Recombinant glycosylated pro-urokinase: biochemistry, pharmacology, and early clinical experience. In: Sasahara AA, Loscalzo J (eds). New Therapeutic Agents in Thrombosis and Thrombolysis. New York: Marcel Dekker, 1997:561–89.

34. Kucinski T, Grzyska U, Groden C, et al. Intracranial arterial occlusion site predicts outcome in carotid artery stroke. Radiology 1999;213(P):394.

35. Eckert B, Kucinski T, Fiehler J, et al. Local intra-arterial fibrinolysis in acute hemispheric stroke: effect of occlusion type and fibrinolytic agent on recanalization success and neurological outcome. Cerebrovasc Dis 2003;15:258–63.

36. Hacke W, Zeumer H, Ferbert A, et al. Intra-arterial thrombolytic therapy improves outcome in patients with acute vertebrobasilar occlusive disease. Stroke 1988;19:1216–22.

37. Hoffman AI, Lambiase RE, Haas RA, et al. Acute vertebrobasilar occlusion: treatment with high-dose intraarterial urokinase. AJR Am J Roentgenol 1999;172:709–12.

38. Katzan IL, Furlan AJ. Thrombolytic therapy. In: Fisher M, Bogousslavsky J (eds). Current Review of Cerebrovascular Disease, 3rd edn. Boston: Butterworth–Heinemann, 1999:185–93.

39. Cross DT, Moran CJ, Akins P, et al. Relationship between clot location and outcome after basilar artery thrombolysis. AJNR Am J Neuroradiol 1997;18:1221–8.

40. Matsumoto K, Satoh K. Intraarterial therapy in acute ischemic stroke. In: Yamaguchi T, Mori E, Minematsu K, et al (eds). Thrombolytic Therapy in Acute Ischemic Stroke III. Tokyo: Springer-Verlag, 1995:279–87.

41. Clark W, Barnwell S, Nesbit G, et al. Efficacy of intra-arterial thrombolysis of basilar artery stroke. J Stroke Cerebrovasc Dis 1997;6:457(abst).

42. Wijdicks EF, Nichols DA, Thielen KR, et al. Intra-arterial thrombolysis in acute basilar artery thromboembolisms: the Initial Mayo Clinic experience. Mayo Clin Proc 1997;72:1005–13.

43. Becker KJ, Purcell LL, Hacke W, et al. Vertebrobasilar thrombosis: diagnosis, management, and the use of intra-arterial thrombolytics. Crit Care Med 1996;24:1729–42.

44. The National Institute of Neurological Disorders and Stroke rt-PA Stroke Study Group. Tissue plasminogen activator for acute ischemic stroke. N Engl J Med 1995;333:1581–7.

45. Furlan A, Higashida R, Wechsler L, et al. Intra-arterial prourokinase for acute ischemic stroke – the PROACT II

study: A randomized controlled trial. JAMA 1999; 282:2003–11.

46. ECC Guidelines. Part 7: The Era of Reperfusion. Section 2: Acute Stroke. Circulation 2000;102:1–204.

47. Emergency interventional stroke therapy: a Statement from the American Society of Interventional and Therapeutic Neuroradiology and Society of Cardiovascular and Interventional Radiology. AJNR Am J Neuroradiol 2001;22:54.

48. Adams HP Jr, Adams RJ, Brott T, et al. Stroke Council of the American Stroke Association. Guidelines for the early management of patients with ischemic stroke: a scientific statement from the Stroke Council of the American Stroke Association. Stroke 2003;34:1056–83.

49. Alexandrov AV, Grotta JC. Arterial reocclusion in stroke patients treated with intravenous tissue plasminogen activator. Neurology 2002;59:862–7.

50. ACC/AHA Guidelines on Management of Patients with STEMI: Hospital and Long-Term Management. http://www.acc.org/clinical/guidelines/stemi/index.htm.

51. Antman EM, Giugliano RP, Gibson CM, et al, for the Thrombolysis in Myocardial Infarction (TIMI) 14 Investigators. Abciximab facilitates the rate and extent of thrombolysis: results of Thrombolysis in Myocardial Infarction (TIMI) 14 trial. Circulation 1999;99:2720–32.

52. Lincoff AM, Califf RM, Van de Werf F, et al. Mortality at 1 year with combination platelet glycoprotein IIb/IIIa inhibition and reduced-dose fibrinolytic therapy vs conventional fibrinolytic therapy for acute myocardial infarction: GUSTO V randomized trial. JAMA 2002;288:2130–5.

53. Smith WS, Sung G, Starkman S, et al, for the MERCI Trial Investigators Safety and Efficacy of Mechanical Embolectomy in Acute Ischemic Stroke: Results of the MERCI Trial. Stroke, Jul 2005;36:1432–1438.

54. del Zoppo GJ, Higashida RT, Furlan AJ, et al, the PROACT Investigators. PROACT: a phase II randomized trial of recombinant pro-urokinase by direct arterial delivery in acute middle cerebral artery stroke. Stroke 1998;29:4–11.

55. Smith WS, Sung G, Starkman S, et al. Safety and efficacy of mechanical embolectomy in acute ischemic stroke: results of the MERCI trial. stroke 2005;36:1432–8.

56. Becker KJ, Brott TG, Approval of the MERCI clot retriever: a critical view. Stroke 2005;36:400–3.

57. Tomsick TA. Mechanical embolus removal. A new day dawning. Stroke 2005;36:1439–40.

58. Noser EA, Shaltoni HM, Hall CE, et al. Aggressive mechanical clot disruption: a safe adjunct to thrombolytic therapy in acute stroke? Stroke 2005;36:292–6.

59. Lee KY, Kim DI, Kim SH, et al. Sequential combination of intravenous recombinant tissue plasminogen activator and intra-arterial urokinase in acute ischemic stroke. AJNR Am J Neuroradiol 2004;25:1470–5.

60. Pelz D, Andersson T, Lylyk P, et al. Stroke Review: Advances in Interventional Neuroradiology 2004. Stroke 2005;36:211–14.

61. Lee DH, Jo KD, Kim HG, et al. Local intraarterial urokinase thrombolysis of acute ischemic stroke with or without intravenous abciximab: a pilot study. J Vasc Interv Radiol 2002;13:769–74.

62. Lewandowski CA, Frankel M, Tomsick TA, et al. Combined intravenous and intra-arterial r-TPA versus intra-arterial therapy of acute ischemic stroke: Emergency Management of Stroke (EMS) bridging trial. Stroke 1999;30:2598–2605.

63. The IMS Study Investigators. Combined intravenous and intra-arterial recanalization for acute ischemic stroke: the Interventional Management of Stroke Study. Stroke 2004;35:904.

64. Alexandrov AV, Molina CA, Grotta JC, et al. CLOTBUST Investigators. Ultrasound-enhanced systemic thrombolysis for acute ischemic stroke. N Engl J Med 2004;351:2170–8.

65. Grotta J. Combination therapy with lubeluzole and t-PA in the treatment of acute ischemic stroke. Presented at the AHA 23rd International Joint Conference on Stroke, February 1998.

66. De Georgia MA, Krieger DW, Abou-Chebl A, et al. Cooling for acute ischemic brain damage (CoolAID): a feasibility trial of endovascular cooling. Neurology 2004;63:312–17.

67. ECC Guidelines. Part 7: The Era of Reperfusion. Section 2: Acute Stroke. Circulation 2000;102:1–204.

68. Emergency Interventional Stroke Therapy: a Statement from the American Society of Interventional and Therapeutic Neuroradiology and Society of Cardiovascular and Interventional Radiology. AJNR Am J Neuroradiol 2001;22:54.

69. INSTOR: Interventional Stroke Therapy Outcomes. Registry. www.strokeregistry.org.

70. Keir SL, Wardlaw JM. Systematic review of diffusion and perfusion imaging in acute ischemic stroke. Stroke 2000;31:2723–31.

71. Fisher M, Albers GW. Applications of diffusion–perfusion magnetic resonance imaging in acute ischemic stroke. Neurology 1999;52:1750–6.

72. Hacke W, Warach S. Diffusion-weighted MRI as an evolving standard of care in acute stroke. Neurology 2000;54:1548–9.

73. Hacke W, Albers G, Al-Rawi Y, et al, for the DIAS Study Group. The Desmoteplase in Acute Ischemic Stroke Trial (DIAS): a phase II MRI-based 9-hour window acute stroke thrombolysis trial with intravenous desmoteplase. Stroke 2005;36:66–73.

19

Various combined approaches: present and future

Danilo Toni, Svetlana Lorenzano, Romesh Markus, and Geoffrey Donnan

Introduction

A meta-analysis of large randomized controlled trials of thrombolysis[1] has demonstrated the substantial efficacy of this approach, particularly with intravenous (IV) recombinant tissue-type plasminogen activator (rtPA), but has also highlighted some worrisome side-effects and limits that definitely hamper its wider use in clinical practice. Symptomatic and even fatal hemorrhagic transformation and reperfusion damage still appear to be the most feared possible consequences of treatment – although this may be more the case for non-experts than for clinicians familiar with thrombolysis.[2] As with the experience of cardiologists, the rate and degree of arterial recanalization and the potential occurrence of arterial re-occlusion are generally seen as critical aspects limiting the efficacy of thrombolysis.

However, the main limitation on the routine use of thrombolysis is the very narrow therapeutic window that is available: 120–140 min after stroke onset in the NINDS (National Institute of Neurological Disorders and Stroke) Study,[3] or up to a maximum of 240–270 min as suggested by a pooled analysis of individual data from the NINDS study and ECASS I and II (European Cooperative Acute Stroke Study). In this chapter, we shall review the possibility of overcoming these obstacles by combining thrombolysis with other drugs, starting from the standpoint of the proposed combination and then discussing its rationale.

Combined intravenous and intra-arterial thrombolysis

The door-to-needle interval time for IV thrombolysis is theoretically shorter than that for intra-arterial (IA) thrombolysis. However, it is associated with low recanalization rates – particularly of larger more proximal vessels, such as the basilar artery, the internal carotid artery (ICA) and the proximal middle cerebral artery (MCA). In fact, the recanalization rate of proximal arterial occlusion by IV rtPA ranges from 10% for ICA occlusion to 30% for proximal MCA occlusion.[4]

On the other hand, IA treatment allows greater diagnostic precision (angiography performed before local IA thrombolysis can document arterial occlusion and provides information on collateral flow) and effective lysis of blood clots with higher rates of recanalization. Moreover, local thrombolysis leads to a higher concentration of the drug in the affected vascular territory, with a lower total drug dose than that used for IV therapy, and a potential lower risk of intracerebral hemorrhage.[5] However, therapy has the disadvantage of requiring technical expertise that is not widely available, and a longer delay to initiation of treatment.

Given these premises, an IV/IA approach might have the potential of combining the advantages of IV thrombolysis (fast and easy to use) with the advantages of IA treatment (higher rate of recanalization), in order to maximize the speed and frequency of recanalization and to minimize potential side-effects by giving lower doses of drug. Early treatment with this combination has been tested in several studies involving acute ischemic stroke patients (Table 19.1).

One of the first attempts was made by Freitag et al,[6] who tested a combination of 10 mg of IV rtPA with 2500 IU of IA lys-plasminogen (i.e. plasmin) in 20 patients with acute stroke in the carotid distribution. The recanalization time and recanalization rate were superior to those of patients treated with urokinase or rtPA alone. Moreover, a higher percentage of the patients receiving the combined treatment had a final Barthel Index score between 90 and 100 as compared with those given urokinase or rtPA alone, with hemorrhagic transformation without clinical deterioration in 25% of the former and 12% of the latter and only one case of hematoma with clinical deterioration in the single-drug group.

Subsequent studies tested the combination of IV rtPA with IA rtPA or IA urokinase. The EMS (Emergency Management of Stroke) Bridging Trial[7] was the first pilot study to compare the safety and efficacy of combined IV/IA rtPA verses IA rtPA alone within 3 h of stroke onset. This was a double-blinded, randomized, placebo-controlled, multicenter study, which, according to the inclusion and exclusion criteria used in the NINDS trial,[8] enrolled 17 patients into the IV/IA group and 18 into the placebo/IA group. In the combined treatment arm, patients received 0.6 mg/kg of IV rtPA (60 mg maximum; 10% of the dose as a bolus over 1 min and the remainder over 30 min) plus IA rtPA by infusion at a rate of 10 mg/h (20 mg maximum). In the other treatment arm, patients received IV placebo in an identical manner to the former group, followed by an IA infusion of rtPA at a rate of 10 mg/h (20 mg maximum over 2 h). No IV heparin infusion or oral anticoagulants were administered during the first 24 h, while 4000 IU of heparin were given as an IV bolus at the beginning of the IA procedure. The mean time to IV treatment was 2.6 h, and that to IA therapy was 3.3 h. The median baseline National Institutes of Health (NIHSS) Score of patients allocated to the combined group was 16, as compared with 11 for patients receiving IA rtPA alone, indicating a more severe neurological deficit of the former even when compared with patients enrolled in the NINDS trial[8] and ECASS I and II.[9,10]

At baseline angiography performed after IA infusion of rtPA or placebo, no difference was found between the two groups with regard to the frequency of IA thrombus, mainly located in MCA M1 or M2 tracts. Partial or complete recanalization was more frequent in patients in the combined arm (53% vs 28% in the IA thrombolysis-alone group), suggesting that this approach might be particularly applicable for patients with persistent thrombus after IV rtPA. Unfortunately, the higher rate of recanalization was not associated with a significantly improved clinical outcome, since at 3-month follow-up, 53% of patients in the combined group and 44% in the IA rtPA group were dead/dependent (modified Rankin Score (mRS) ≥ 3). The safety of the combined approach was acceptable, symptomatic intracerebral hemorrhage (ICH) occurring in 12% of cases, as compared with 6% in the IA rtPA-alone arm. However, no inference regarding efficacy and safety is possible, because of the small number of enrolled patients, the excess of adverse events (8, mainly cardiac) unrelated to treatment assignment in the combined treatment arm, and the above-mentioned imbalance of randomization, with enrolment of more severe patients in the combined treatment arm.

In a retrospective analysis of 20 consecutive patients with carotid artery distribution strokes treated with a combined IV/IA rtPA approach, Ernst et al[11] reported very positive results. Patient selection criteria were those of the NINDS study,[8] and the median NIHSS Score at admission was 21. Initially, rtPA was given IV 0.6 mg/kg (maximum dose 60 mg), with 15% of the dose given as a bolus, followed by a continuous IV infusion over 30 min. All 20 patients underwent angiography, and 16 of them also received local IA rtPA (0.3 mg/kg, maximum dose 24 mg) over a maximum of 2 h. A heparin bolus ranging from 2000 to 4000 IU was administered to 11 of the 16 patients receiving local IA rtPA, while an IV heparin infusion was given globally to 10 of the 20 patients (see below). The mean time to IV treatment was 2.02 h and that to IA therapy was 3.3 h. Sixty-nine percent of patients had partial or complete recanalization, and, despite the high baseline NIHSS Score at 3-month follow-up, 63% of patients had an mRS of 0–2 while 10% were dead. Even a subgroup of 5 patients (25%) with carotid terminus occlusions, including 2 patients with cervical ICA occlusions, did well, reaching an mRS of 0 in 4 cases and of 2 in the remaining one. The rate of symptomatic hemorrhage was 5%, being similar to the overall hemorrhagic rate reported in the

Table 19.1   Clinical studies combining intravenous (IV) with intrarterial (IA) thrombolysis

Authors	No. of patients	NIHSS Score on admission	Treatment dose	Mean time to treatment	Partial/complete recanalization	Symptomatic ICH	Deaths	Outcome measures
Lewandowski et al[7] (randomized double-blinded placebo-controlled multicenter phase I study)	35:			2.6 h to IV 3.3 h to A				RS 0–2 at 3 months:
	17 IV/IA rtPA	16 (median)	0.6 mg/kg of IV rtPA + 20 mg max. of IA rtPA		9 (53%)	2 (12%)	5 (29%)	8 (47%) (IV/IA)
	18 placebo/IA rtPA	11 (median)	placebo + 20 mg max. of IA rtPA		5 (28%)	1 (6%)	1 (6%)	10 (56%) (placebo/IA)
Ernst et al[11] (retrospective analysis)	20:	21 (median)		2.02 h to IV 3.3 h to IA		1 (5%)	2 (10%)	RS 0–2 at 3 months:
	16 IV/IA rtPA		0.6 mg/kg of IV rtPA + 24 mg max. of IA rtPA		11 (69%)			10 (63%) (IV/IA rtPA)
	4 IV rtPA		60 mg max. of IV rtPA					
Suarez et al[15] (open-label study)	45:			2.10 h to IV 3.2 h to IA		2 IV rtPA alone (4.4% of whole series)	7 (15% of whole series)	BI ≥ 95 at 3 months:
	13 IV rtPA/IA UK	13 (mean)	0.6 mg/kg of IV rtPA + 750 000 IA UK		18 (75%) IV/IA thrombly		1 (8%)	12 (92%) (IV rtPA/IA UK)
	11 IV rtPA/IA rtPA	12 (mean)	0.6 mg/kg of IV rtPA + 30 mg IA rtPA				3 (27%)	7 (64%) (IV/IA rtPA)
	21 rtPA alone	8 (mean)	0.6 mg/kg of IV rtPA				3 (14%)	14 (66%) (IV rtPA alone)
Hill et al[16] (prospective, open-label study)	7:	18 (median)		1.40 h to IV 5.10 h to IA	6 (86%)	0	0	NIHSS Score ≤ 3 at 3 months: 4 (67%)
	6 IV/IA rtPA		0.9 mg/kg IV rtPA + 20 mg max. IA rtPA					
	1 IV rtPA alone		0.9 mg/kg IV rtPA					
Keris et al[17] (open-label study)	45:							RS 0–3 at 1 year:
	12 IA/IV rtPA	25 (mean)	25 mg max. of IA rtPA + 25 mg max. of IV rtPA	3.49 h to IA	6 (50%)	0	2 (17%)	10 (83%) (IA/IV rtPA)
	33 conventional therapy	24 (mean)					21 (64%)	11 (33%) (control group)
Zaidat et al[13] (retrospective analysis)	18 with carotid terminus occlusion:							RS 0–2 at 3 months:
	5 IA/IV rtPA	15 (median)	0.6 mg/kg of IV rtPA + 30 mg max. of IA rtPA	2.23 h to IV rtPA 2.55 h to IA rtPA	4 (80%)	1 (20%)	1 (20%)	1 (20%), NS
	13 IA UK	15 (median)	1.5 MU UK	4 h to IA UK	8 (62%)	2 (15%)	8 (62%)	1 (8%), NS

NIHSS, National Institutes of Health Stroke Scale; ICH, intracerebral hemorrhage; rtPA, recombinant tissue-type plasminogen activator; UK, urokinase; RS, Rankin Score; BI, Barthal Index; NS, not significant.

NINDS[8] and PROACT II (Prolyse in Acute Cerebral Thomboembolism)[12] studies, but better than the 17% hemorrhagic rate in patients with NIHSS Score >20 reported in the NINDS study.

Ernst et al[11] concluded that the advantages of giving combined thrombolysis starting with IV rtPA include a shorter time to initiate therapy, as well as the possibility that IV rtPA alone is sufficient for cure, as they observed in 3 (15%) patients who significantly improved during angiography, with evidence of partial recanalization, and did not receive IA rtPA. Moreover, it is evident that IV rtPA may potentiate the efficacy of IA thrombolysis, as suggested by the high recanalization rate achieved.

A good clinical outcome was also seen in 5 patients with carotid terminus occlusion who received IV/IA thrombolysis in the retrospective study published by Zaidat et al.[13] They found complete recanalization in 80% of cases, as compared with 62% of 13 patients with similar arterial occlusion treated by the same group with IA thrombolysis alone, while symptomatic hemorrhage was evident in 20% of the former and 15% of the latter, and the mortality rates were respectively 20% and 62%. However, because of the small number of treated patients and the retrospective and uncontrolled nature of the study,[14] caution should be exercised in its interpretation. It does, however, stress the need for larger randomized, controlled trials.

An interesting development in this field is the better selection of patients to be submitted to combined IV/IA thrombolysis with the use of modern magnetic resonance imaging (MRI) techniques.

In an open-label study over a period of 6 years, Suarez et al[15] evaluated 45 patients within 3h of stroke onset, clinically selected according to the NINDS study criteria. The mean NIHSS Score at admission was 12. All patients were treated with IV rtPA 0.6 mg/kg (maximum dose 60 mg), with 10% of the dose as a bolus over 1 min and the remainder over 30 minutes, and then underwent emergency MRI with diffusion-weighted (DWI) and perfusion-weighted (PWI) sequences. Twenty-four patients presented PWI/DWI mismatches and underwent cerebral angiography and IA thrombolysis (13 with urokinase and 11 with rtPA). Twenty-one patients received only the initial IV rtPA because of normal MRI findings, normal angiographic findings after abnormal MRI results, evidence of subcortical matched PWI/DWI defects, complete ICA occlusion, or complete improvement before angiography. The mean time to IV treatment was 2.10 h, and that to IA therapy was 3.2 h. Recanalization was observed in 75% of patients treated with combined IV/IA thrombolysis, and was complete in half of the cases. Eighty-eight percent of the observed occlusions were in the MCA territory. Symptomatic ICH was detected in only 2 (4.4% of the whole series) patients receiving IV rtPA alone. Fifteen percent of the patients died while in the hospital, while 77% of the survivors had good outcomes (Barthel Index ≥95) 3 months after treatment. Although this study lacks a true control population (the IV rtPA-only group simply represented patients excluded from IA rtPA treatment) and adequate sample size, the results are encouraging as compared with those of treated patients in clinical trials of IV, IA, or combined thrombolysis. The most intriguing implication of this study, however, is the observation that DWI and PWI can help identify patients with acute ischemic strokes and small diffusion changes who had previously received IV rtPA but remained with brain tissue at risk because of persisting vascular occlusions, which may require more aggressive treatment with IA therapy.

A similar approach was adopted by Hill et al[16] in a small prospective open-label study. Seven patients, initially treated with full-dose IV rtPA (0.9 mg/kg, maximum dose 90 mg, with 10% as a bolus followed by an infusion over 60 min) were found to have persistent occlusion of the symptomatic artery on magnetic resonance angiography (MRA) or transcranial Doppler ultrasound (TCD) and PWI/DWI mismatch. Of these, 6 received IA rtPA (maximum dose 20 mg) and one underwent angioplasty. Angiographic recanalization was achieved in 6 patients (86%), of whom 4 (67%) achieved good neurological outcomes (NIHSS Score ≤3) at 90 days. The mean time to IV thrombolysis was 1.40 h and that to IA treatment was 5.10 h. There was no incidence of symptomatic ICH or significant extracerebral hemorrhage.

Finally, it is worth mentioning the study by Keris et al,[17] who tested a combined but reversed approach, by giving first IA and then IV rtPA. The rationale was to obtain the highest possible arterial recanalization with local IA therapy, while continuous infusion of IV rtPA should serve to increase the efficacy of treatment. They treated 12 patients with the IA/IV approach and compared them with 33 control patients who received conventional treatment. The selection criteria were those of the NINDS study and the mean baseline NIHSS Scores were 25 in the combined group and 24 in the control group. In the treatment arm, patients received a maximum of 25 mg IA rtPA, within a mean of 3.49 h of stroke onset, followed by 25 mg IV rtPA within 6 h of stroke onset.

Despite the relatively low dose of rtPA, hemorrhagic conversion was almost three times more common in the thombolysis group than in the control group (17% vs 6%), but in no case was it symptomatic. During the first 30 days, 48% of patients in the control group and 17% in the thrombolysis group died, and this difference was even more marked at 12 months (64% vs 17%). Good outcome (mRS ≤ 3) at 1 month was observed in 67% of treated patients and 21% of controls, and at 12 months in 83% and 33% of patients, respectively. Again, these data must be regarded with caution, due to the small sample of patients studied and to some imbalance in baseline characteristics (greater age and a higher frequency of atrial fibrillation and hypertension in the control group).

In conclusion, all of the studies reviewed show that patients treated with combined IV and IA thrombolysis are more likely to have partial or complete reperfusion of an occluded intracerebral artery associated, in most cases, with an improved clinical outcome. Furthermore, the incidence of ICH is not significantly increased, which suggests that this approach is technically feasible and may be safe. However, additional larger studies are needed to determine the safety and effectiveness of this approach to acute ischemic stroke therapy. Such studies should also address the cost/benefit ratio and quality of life, given the major investment in time, personnel, and equipment required by combined IV/IA techniques.[7]

Combined thrombolysis and antithrombotic therapy

While the rate of arterial recanalization and its relationship to clinical outcome are obviously taken into account in all studies of IA thrombolysis,[18] they have been investigated in only a few clinical studies of IV thrombolysis,[19,20] and no study has related clinical outcome to arterial reocclusion. These events appear to play a major role in coronary revascularization, so that antithrombotic treatments are always given after thrombolysis. One could argue that the pathophysiology of coronary occlusion is different from that of intracerebral arteries, in situ thrombosis being the main cause in the former, while more frequently embolism from a cardiac or an arterial source leads to stroke.[21,22] Hence, in stroke, reocclusion of an intracerebral artery should not be a major problem, unless a very early new embolism from the same source occurs.

Nevertheless, based on the cardiac experience, arterial recanalization and reocclusion are seen by many researchers as a key issue in thrombolysis for stroke and the concomitant use of antithrombotic agents.

Thrombolysis plus antiplatelet agents

The preceding argument formed the rationale for combining thrombolysis and aspirin in MAST-I (Multicenter Acute Stroke Trial – Italy).[23] In this trial, 622 patients were randomized within 6 h of stroke to streptokinase (SK) plus 300 mg of aspirin, 300 mg of aspirin alone, or standard therapy. The results are well known: patients treated with the combination of SK and aspirin had significant increases in both the 10-day fatality rate and intracerebral hematoma, as compared with controls. A post hoc analysis of that study[24] confirmed the negative interaction of the combined therapy, demonstrating that the increase in early case fatality was due to treatment and not to other variables. The main reason for trial failure was likely the higher risk of death associated with cerebral hemorrhage in patients receiving aspirin, consequent to platelet dysfunction and bleeding time prolongation induced by aspirin.[25,26] Although a high proportion of patients died early without a second computed tomography (CT) scan in the combined group, there were comparable rates of hemorrhagic transformation in the two groups (SK plus aspirin and SK alone) at repeat CT scan analysis. Moreover, since CT scan data were incomplete, the contribution of other factors, such as the development of cerebral edema, cannot be excluded. In fact, in a post hoc study on the same population of patients,[27] it was demonstrated that edema contributed to the prediction of an unfavorable outcome in patients with hemorrhagic transformation in MAST-I. The risk of death increased 3 days after randomization, when cerebral edema is usually worst, particularly in patients with very severe neurological deficit. It is therefore possible that both hemorrhage and edema contributed to the higher case fatality in patients treated with combined therapy, suggesting that too severely impaired patients were entered into the study.

The Thrombolysis in Acute Stroke Pooling Project Group[28] pooled individual patient data from MAST-I,[23] ASK,[29] MAST-Europe,[30] and the Glasgow Trial.[31] Concomitant use of aspirin with SK had a significantly detrimental effect on the risk of 3-month death, but not on the risk of death or severe disability. The authors commented that the negative effect of the combination of aspirin and SK on mortality rates was compensated by a positive effect on functional outcome in surviving patients. The same results were observed when the analysis was extended to any antiplatelet drug taken during or up to 48 h after thrombolysis.

These clinical data are not explained by experimental studies. Here, the picture is further complicated by the observation of antagonism of rtPA-mediated thrombolysis by aspirin. In a study on the effect of aspirin on the kinetics of cerebral clot lysis in a rabbit model of stroke, Thomas et al[32] found that IV aspirin causes a paradoxical attenuation of cerebrovascular thrombolysis. Given that aspirin can have significant effects on vascular cyclooxygenase levels that can last for 24 h or more, the authors suggested a decreased capacity for PGI_2(prostacyclin) production as a possible explanation. PGI_2 is the most abundant vasodilator prostaglandin in cerebral vessels[33] and contributes to the maintainance of cerebral blood flow.[34] Consequently, the cerebral vasculature, when stressed by an embolic stroke, might be unable to efficiently redirect blood flow around the clot through hemodynamic changes such as opening collaterals or increasing the luminal diameter of the embolized vessel. This loss of cerebrovascular regulation would greatly restrict the access of rtPA to the embolus, thus reducing the rate at which lysis takes place. In agreement with this hypothesis, Bednar and Gross[35] demonstrated that high-dose aspirin causes a reduction in cerebral blood flow (CBF) by approximately 20% in a rabbit model, and that the reversal of the aspirin antagonism of rtPA thrombolysis is feasible with nitric oxide (NO) donors (nitroglycerin or nitroprusside) or with the β_1 antagonists atenolol (NO-dependent) and hydralazine (NO-independent). These antihypertensive agents

are able to increase regional CBF and rtPA-mediated clot lysis despite aspirin pretreatment, suggesting a common mechanism for these agents in reversing aspirin antagonism of thrombolysis.[36,37]

A possible alternative hypothesis is that PGI_2 may stimulate fibrinolysis through the release of endogenous tPA from the vessel wall.[38] In confirmation of the PGI_2 inhibition hypothesis, Thomas et al[32] reversed the effects of aspirin on clot lysis by giving iloprost, a PGI_2 analog that may act as a substitute for endogenous PGI_2 production. An editorial comment by Ellis[39] on the article by Thomas et al,[32] however, stressed that caution should be used in interpreting the mechanism of action of aspirin in the inhibition of clot lysis.

It is of interest that in the same rabbit stroke model, pretreatment with ticlopidine followed by rtPA significantly reduced brain infarct size, and the administration of ticlopidine did not affect clot lysis or CBF as compared with rtPA alone.[40,41]

Incidentally, considering the large population base currently using antiplatelet agents, these data, rather than giving indications on the risk/benefit ratio of emergent cotreatment with antiplatelet agents and thrombolysis, stress that antiplatelet agents used for stroke prevention may influence the success rate of thrombolysis.

The platelet glycoprotein (GP)IIb/IIIa receptor inhibitors are a new class of very powerful platelet function antagonists (discussed in detail in Chapter 10). For the purposes of the present discussion, it is useful to recall that their mechanism of action categorizes them as a type of thrombolytic agent. In fact, after activation, platelets can facilitate thrombin generation by several mechanisms. Activated platelets undergo a conformational change that provides a catalytic surface upon which thrombin is formed from prothrombin.[42] Activated platelets also release an activated form of factor V from α-granules[43] and activate many coagulation factors, such as factors VIII, XI, and XII. Finally, activated platelets activate fibrin mesh formation by activating factor XIII (fibrin stabilization factor)[44] and releasing plasminogen activator inhibitor 1(PAI-1), together with other vasoconstricting substances.[45] In addition, thrombin itself is the most potent stimulant for platelet activation,[45] thus facilitating further platelet activation. These processes induce a cascade reaction that causes explosive thrombin generation. Activated GPIIb/IIIa receptors have a high binding affinity for fibrinogen and other adhesive proteins that make platelets crosslink one to another (aggregation).[45] Hence, GPIIb/IIIa inhibitors, by antagonizing the mentioned mechanisms, may not only prevent the development of a thrombus but also dissolve the thrombus immediately. A newly formed thrombus during coronary angiography can be dissolved by IV abciximab.[46] This agent dissolves the thrombus by displacing fibrinogen from the GPIIb/IIIa receptor in a dose-dependent manner, because abciximab has a greater affinity for the receptor than fibrinogen dose. Inhibition of PAI-1 synthesis and increased elaboration of urokinase-type plasminogen activator (uPA) are other possible mechanisms.[46] Additional data suggest that GPIIb/IIIa antagonists may improve flow in both the coronary and cerebral microcirculations.[47,48]

Whatever the mechanism of action, it is of interest that angiographic studies in acute myocardial infarction showed that the combination of abciximab, aspirin, and adjusted-dose heparin reopens 40–50% of occluded coronary vessels.[49,50] Again in the setting of myocardial infarction, the combination of abciximab, aspirin, and adjusted-dose heparin, supplemented by a reduced dose of rtPA or reteplase, yielded coronary patency rates better than 80% (i.e. Thrombolysis in Myocardial Infarction (TIMI) flow grade 2 or 3).[49,51]

Theoretically, reducing the dose of a thrombolytic agent by exploiting the adjuvant effects of antiplatelet agents such as abciximab should also be important in stroke in order to achieve a higher rate of arterial recanalization and to minimize the risk of arterial reocclusion without increasing that of hemorrhagic transformation. Unfortunately, experience with this combined treatment in stroke patients is limited, and only case reports are available.

In patients with acute basilar artery occlusion, IV abciximab associated with IA thrombolysis was safe and effective in achieving complete arterial recanalization.[52,53]

IA administration of abciximab combined with IA thrombolysis has also been reported to be effective in the recanalization of an occluded MCA or anterior cerebral arteries or even of an intracerebral ICA, without causing hemorrhagic transformation.[54] The potential advantage of this approach is the much smaller amount of abciximab that need be used compared with IV administration, and hence the lower risk of hemorrhagic events. Locally delivered abciximab facilitates thrombolysis by saturation of GPIIb/IIIa receptors on the platelets of target thrombi, without saturation of whole-body platelet receptors. Theoretically, once GPIIb/IIIa receptors of locally adhered platelets are saturated, newly replenishing platelets from the systemic circulation cannot initiate the cascade reaction of explosive thrombin generation, because platelets must aggregate at the target lesion before their activation, but receptors for the aggregation at the lesion are already blocked.

In conclusion, although the number of reported patients is very limited, abciximab in combination with thrombolysis might be a promising therapeutic approach, which is worth being tested in a randomized controlled trial.

Thrombolysis plus anticoagulants

In thrombolytic treatment of myocardial infarction, adjunctive anticoagulation with heparin appears to improve arterial patency.[55] This therapeutic concept has been transferred to ischemic stroke in some studies of IA[11,12,17,22] and IV[28,56–60] thrombolysis (Table 19.2).

In the PROACT study,[17] all of the 40 enrolled patients received IV heparin immediately after recombinant prourokinase (rproUK) or placebo. The first 16 patients received a 100 IU/kg bolus followed by a 1000 IU/h constant infusion ('high heparin') for 4 h. Thereafter, on the recommendation of the External Safety Committee, the heparin regimen was modified to a 2000 IU bolus and 500 IU/h infusion ('low heparin') for the remaining patients. This study design does not allow a direct evaluation of the possible additional effects of heparin, since this would require a comparison between rproUK plus heparin and rproUK alone. However, a contribution of adjunctive IV heparin can be hypothesized, considering that the recanalization rate following IA rproUK plus high-dose heparin was 82%, as compared with 40% following IA rproUK plus low-dose heparin. Unfortunately, side-effects were also significantly different, symptomatic hemorrhagic transformation amounting to 27% in the high-dose heparin group and to 6.7% in the low-dose heparin group.

In the PROACT II study,[12] in an attempt to increase the recanalization rate while limiting symptomatic

Table 19.2 Clinical studies combining thrombolysis with anticoagulants

Authors	No. of patients	NIHSS Score on admission	Treatment dose	Time to treatment	Partial/complete recanalization	Symptomatic ICH	Deaths	Outcome measures
von Kummer and Hacke[56] (open prospective single-site study)	32	≥18	100 mg IV rtPA + bolus of 5000 U heparin followed by infusion of 1000–1500 U/h within 6 h	3.8 h (mean)	11 (34%) within 90 min; 53% within 12–24 h	3 (9%) (fatal)	9 (28%)	Good: 14 (44%) Poor: 9 (28%)
PROACT (del Zoppo et al[22]) (randomized double-blinded, placebo-controlled multicenter trial)	40:							RS 0–1 at 3 months:
11 IA rproUK + high-dose heparin		17 (median) (IA rproUK/heparin)	6 mg rproUK + heparin 100 IU/kg bolus +1000 IU/h for 4 h	5.4 h (median)	9 (82%)	3 (27%)	7 (27%) (rproUK/heparin)	8 (31%) (rproUK/heparin)
15 IA rproUK + low-dose heparin			6 mg rproUK + heparin 2000 IU bolus +500 IU/h for 4 h		6 (40%)	1 (6.7%)		
5 placebo + high-dose heparin		19 (median) (placebo/heparin)	Placebo+heparin 100 IU/kg bolus +1000 IU/h for 4 h	5.7 h (median)	0 (0%)	1 (20%)	6 (43%) (placebo/heparin)	3 (21%) (placebo/heparin)
9 placebo + low-dose heparin			Placebo+heparin 2000 IU bolus + 500 IU/h for 4 h		2 (22%)	0 (0%)		
PROACT II (Furlan et al[12]) (randomized controlled multicenter open-label clinical trial with blinded follow-up)	180:							RS 0–2 at 3 months:
121 IA rproUK + low-dose heparin		17 (median)	110 pts: 9 mg rproUK + 2000 IU bolus and 500 IU/h infusion of IV heparin for 4 h	5.3 h (median) to rproUK	66%	10.2%	18%	48 (44%)
59 low-dose heparin alone		17 (median)	2000 IU bolus and 500 IU/h infusion of IV heparin for 4 h		18%	2%	12%	15 (25%)

Table 19.2 (*Continued*)

Authors	No. of patients	NIHSS Score on admission	Treatment dose	Time to treatment	Partial/complete recanalization	Symptomatic ICH	Deaths	Outcome measures
Grond et al[59] (prospective, open-label single-center study)	100	12 (median)	0.9 mg/kg iv rtPA +1000 IU/h heparin infusion	2.4 h (mean)		6 (6%)	12 (12%)	BI≥95 at 3 months: 53 (53%)
Rudolf et al[60] (prospective, open-label single-center study)	300 (275 treated) 122 IV rtPA +low-dose heparin 153 IV rtPA +high-dose heparin	11 (median)	0.9 mg/kg IV rtPA +immediate anticoagulation: 122 pts received <10000 IE/day 153 pts received >10000 IE/day			4/122 (3%) 9/153 (6%)	38/275 (14%)	RS 0–2 at 3 months: 151/275 (55%)
Trouillas et al[58] (open nonrandomized study)	100	18 (mean)	0.8 mg/kg IV rtPA; IV heparin administered according to three protocols: 31 pts: immediate IV unfractioned heparin at initial dose of 300 IU/kg 41 pts: delayed heparinization at 24+6 h after day-1 CT 9 pts: nadroparin immediately at a dose of 3075 anti-Xa IU	3.56 h (mean)		2 (2%) (fatal) 2 (2%)	6 (6%)	RS 0–1 at 3 months: 45 (45%)

NIHSS, National Institutes of Health Stroke Scale; ICH, intracerebral hemorrhage; IA, intra-arterial; IV, intravenous; proUK, recombinant prourokinase; rtPA, recombinant tissue-type plasminogen activator; RS, Rankin Score; BI, Barthel Index.

ICH, the total dose of rproUK was increased from 6 mg to 9 mg given over 2 h while using the same low-dose heparin as in PROACT I. Compared with patients receiving only low-dose IV heparin, patients with ischemic stroke caused by MCA occlusion treated with IA rproUK plus heparin were 58% more likely to have slight or no neurological disability at 90 days. Compared with the rproUK plus low-dose heparin in PROACT I, the higher rproUK dose in PROACT II improved recanalization efficacy (with partial and complete recanalization at 2 h angiogram in 66% vs 40% of cases), but also increased the rate of symptomatic ICH (10.2% vs 6.7%). Also, in this study, it is not clear whether heparin contributed to the ICH, but this appears to be unlikely because the level of anticoagulation reached was subtherapeutic, without prolongation of the activated partial thromboplastin time (aPTT) beyond the normal range, and the same low-dose heparin was given to both rproUK-treated patients and controls.[61]

Low-dose subcutaneous (SC) heparin (5000 IU of heparin after the first CT, followed by 5000 IU SC tid) was also administered to patients treated with IV/IA rtPA in the study by Keris et al,[17] while high-dose IV heparin was given to 3 of the 4 patients receiving IV rtPA alone, and to 7 of the 16 patients receiving combined IV/IA rtPA in the series of Ernst et al.[11] Although Keris et al[17] commented that the combined approach produced a response to a modest coadministration of heparin for maintenance of intra-arterial catheters and as another prophylaxis of thrombosis, in neither of these studies was an analysis of the possible risk/benefit ratio of the additional heparin infusion made. Hence, at present, the most that we can say is that the evidence of recanalization efficacy demonstrated in the two PROACT trials, and the safety of the low dose of IV heparin, support further investigation of the clinical efficacy and safety of IA thrombolysis combined with anticoagulant therapy.

With regard to the safety and efficacy of IV thrombolysis in combination with heparin, one of the first studies was that published by von Kummer and Hacke.[56] This was an open prospective single-site study in which 32 patients with severe hemispheric stroke syndrome (NIHSS Score ≥ 18), caused by angiographically proven MCA and/or intracranial ICA occlusion, were treated with 100 mg alteplase by IV infusion over 90 min within a mean of 3.8 h after symptom onset. Simultaneously with alteplase,

a bolus of 5000 IU of heparin was given, followed by a continuous infusion in order to double the aPTT. Reperfusion was assessed by digital subtraction angiography (DSA) in all patients immediately after treatment and by transcranial Doppler monitoring (in 30 patients) and/or a third angiogram (in 5 patients) performed 12–24 h later. Complete or partial reperfusion was observed in 34% of patients 90 min after the initiation of alteplase infusion, and in 53% within 12–24 h. Reocclusion was documented in one patient by postmortem study. Fatal parenchymal hemorrhage was observed in 3 (9%) patients who had a large MCA infarct and in 2 cases who had not recanalized. Lacking a control rtPA-alone group, this study did not provide data on the potential efficacy of additional heparin in terms of recanalization rate and prevention of reocclusion, while the relatively low incidence of parenchymal hemorrhage led the authors to suggest that this combined approach was substantially safe.

The largest single-center series of patients receiving combined IV rtPA and heparin is that reported by the University of Köln group. In their first report,[59] they described 100 patients treated within 3 h of stroke onset with IV rtPA (0.9 mg/kg, 10% bolus, 90% over 60 min), followed by IV heparin aimed at increasing the aPTT to 1.5–2 times standard normal values. The heparin infusion was maintained for approximately 10 days. The key results of this study are a rate of symptomatic hemorrhagic transformation of 6% (1% fatal) and a Barthel Index of 95–100 reached by 53% of patients at 3-month follow-up, as compared with 50% of rtPA-treated patients in the NINDS study.[8] Besides other factors, such as early CT signs of the infarct and a past medical history of myocardial infarction, a significant relationship between aspirin pretreatment and intracerebral hemorrhage was also found in this study. This might suggest that the combination of aspirin, rtPA, and high-dose heparin should be avoided.

However, in the subsequent extension of their open study to 300 consecutive patients,[60] a logistic regression analysis showed no correlation between hemorrhagic complications and aspirin pretreatment, or post-thrombolytic heparin. At 3-month follow-up, 53% of patients were independent (mRS 0–2). The study did not include a parallel control group, and hence cannot provide evidence for the efficacy of combined treatment, but it supports the feasibility and safety of IV thrombolysis associated with immediate heparin therapy.

An interestingly different approach was adopted by Trouillas et al,[57,58] who treated 100 patients with 0.8 mg/kg of rtPA (10% bolus, and the remainder over 90 min) within 7 h of stroke onset. Of these, 81 were subsequently anticoagulated according to three protocols: (1) 31 patients received immediate IV heparin at a dose aimed at raising the aPTT to 1.5 times baseline values; (2) 41 patients received delayed IV heparin, at the same dose as group 1, starting 24 + 6 h after rtPA and immediately after day 1 CT; (3) 9 patients were given SC nadroparin immediately after thrombolysis, at a dose of 3075 anti-factor Xa IU.

At 3-month follow-up, 45% of patients had a good outcome (mRS 0–1). Seven percent of the patients (half of whom had received immediate heparin) had secondary parenchymal hematoma; in 2 cases this was immediate, while in the remaining 5 it was delayed but always occurred within 24 h. Three of these 5 patients with delayed parenchymal hemorrhage had received immediate heparin, while the remaining 2 had been treated with SC nadroparin. No parenchymal hemorrhage occurred in patients receiving delayed IV heparin. The authors concluded that their study confirmed the potential danger of heparin use during the first 24 h after thrombolysis. It must be noted, however, that the nadroparin dose was subtherapeutic, and hence this statement may be debatable for parenchymal haemorrhages observed in the rtPA-plus-nadroparin group.

A final comment here relates to the previously mentioned Thrombolysis in Acute Stroke Pooling Project,[28] which, besides the effects of the combination of IV SK and aspirin, also analyzed the effect of concomitant anticoagulant therapy within 48 h of stroke onset. Heparin was given to 26% of patients in the SK group and 37% of those in the control group – this marked imbalance may be explained by the fact that anticoagulant treatment was not randomized but was added according to the choice of the treating physician, perhaps in the less severely affected patients. However, the risk of 3-month mortality in the SK group not receiving additional heparin was increased by 56%, as compared with a 4% increase in SK patients receiving additional heparin. The same trend was observed for early deaths and death/disability at trial completion.

Hence, although the results of these disparate studies are quite controversial, at least the safety of the combined approach appears to be substantially confirmed. This should, therefore, encourage investigators to conduct controlled trials to assess the potential benefit of combined therapy of thrombolysis and heparin compared with thrombolysis alone.

Paradoxically, it is worth stressing that the rationale for the additional use of heparin is weak. Insight into this controversial point is suggested by a study on the kinetics of hemostatic abnormalities induced by acute ischemic stroke.[62] Twenty-three patients treated with rtPA, followed by IV high-dose heparin within 1–2 h (18 patients) or 24 h (5 patients), were compared with 21 stroke patients given low-dose heparin (3×5000 IU/day SC, 10 patients) or high-dose heparin (5000 IU IV bolus, followed by a 1000 IU/h infusion, PTT 65–90 s, 11 patients). In addition, 50 age- and risk factor-matched subjects and 75 patients without vascular risk factors were included as additional control groups. The markers of coagulation activation taken into account were D-dimer antigen (which is an indicator of the formation of factor XIIIa crosslinked fibrin), fibrin monomer (which is the product of the thrombin-mediated cleavage of fibrinopeptide A from fibrinogen), prothrombin fragment fibrinopeptide 1.2 (which is co-released with each thrombin molecule from prothrombin by factor Xa), and thrombin–antithrombin III (ATIII) complex (which is the product of a complex formation between active thrombin and ATIII).

In short, the study showed massive coagulation activation within the first hours after rtPA treatment that lasted for up to 72 h. In contrast, acute ischemic stroke itself had only minor effects on hemostasis. This systemic procoagulant activation following rtPA may be explained by exposure of clot-bound thrombin and factor Xa as the clot undergoes lysis. The platelet activation by rtPA shown in vitro[63] may be an alternative explanation. These results are consistent with observations of procoagulant tendencies induced by thrombolysis in myocardial infarction.[64–66] Importantly, concentrations of hemostatic markers did not differ significantly between patients treated with high- or low-dose heparin, nor was their massive increase after rtPA prevented by heparin. Since the authors did not study the effects of rtPA treatment in the absence of any heparin anticoagulation, it cannot be excluded that this condition would have been associated with an even more pronounced activation of coagulation. However, such failure of intravenous heparin to suppress thrombin activity has also been observed after coronary thrombolysis.[67] A possible explanation is the observation that heparin–ATIII binding sites on thrombin are masked when this enzyme is bound to fibrin on the blood clot.[68] Hence, theoretically novel direct thrombin inhibitors[69] might be more effective than currently used heparin as suppressors of rtPA-induced coagulation.

Contrary to these considerations are observations that the concomitant use of heparin may increase the thrombolytic potential otherwise confined to the thrombus.[70,71] In particular, in a canine femoral artery thrombosis model, rproUK plus heparin produced a significant increase in thrombus lysis compared with rproUK, vehicle plus heparin, and vehicle alone,[71] and minimized further thrombus accretion. Other experimental data suggest that heparin doses sufficient to increase the aPTT time to 1.5 times control values markedly increase the recanalization efficacy of rproUK.[72] The combination of rproUK and heparin would, therefore, be expected to enhance thrombus lysis by direct intra-arterial infusion.

Combined thrombolysis and neuroprotection

One of the most disappointing results of stroke clinical research has been the failure of clinical trials with neuroprotective agents, which had been demonstrated to be effective by experimental studies.[73] Among the explanations for this, the crucial element is that the most a neuroprotectant can do is 'freeze' the ischemic penumbra while waiting for reperfusion. Spontaneous reperfusion does happen, but often too late to save the ischemic tissue. Harmful events are most likely to occur in brain tissue with the lowest residual blood flows, but, as time goes on, injury also occurs in tissue with higher residual blood flow within the ischemic penumbra.[74] This means that in order to obtain maximal benefit for a given neuroprotectant, immediate brain reperfusion would be ideal. This is supported by the observation that many neuroprotective agents have their best effects in experimental models of focal temporary ischemia.

For thrombolysis, the low number of treatable patients is largely due to the very narrow available time window of 3 h, together with the fear of hemorrhagic transformation. Many neuroprotective agents would be ideal candidates to improve the efficacy of thrombolysis and minimize side-effects. Again, this is well supported by evidence from animal stroke models (Table 19.3). Eliprodil, which blocks both the modulatory polyamine site of the N-methyl-D-aspartate (NMDA) receptor and neuronal voltage-sensitive calcium channels, combined with rtPA markedly reduced the volume of brain damage and the neurological deficit better than either therapy alone.[75] Dizocilpine, another excitatory amino-acid antagonist, combined with rtPA yielded additional benefit in treatment of rat thromboembolic stroke, with improvement of clinical score and infarct size.[76]

Topiramate enhances the inhibitory effects of γ-amino butyric acid (GABA), which antagonizes the excitotoxic effects of glutamate released during ischemia, and added to low-dose urokinase improved neurological recovery and reduced infarct size more than any single drug.[77,78]

Citicoline (cytidine-5′-diphosphocholine) provides both choline and cytidine, which serve as substrates for the synthesis of phosphatidylcholine, a primary neuronal membrane component thought to promote membrane synthesis and repair, which is essential for recovery from stroke. Moreover in models of transient global ischemia, citicoline reduced the production of neurotoxic free fatty acids. Its combination with IV rtPA[79] or IA urokinase[80] was effective in further reducing infarct size.

An additive effect was also shown by combining rtPA with monoclonal antibodies directed against leukocyte adhesion molecules,[81,82] whose upregulation during ischemia plays an important role in the inflammation mediated neuronal damage and no-reflow phenomenon.

In a rat model of stroke, the combination of rtPA with the proteasome inhibitor PS-519, which blocks activation of nuclear factor κB (NFκB), a major mediator of inflammation, even at 6 h significantly reduced infarct volume, improved neurological recovery, and did not increase the incidence of hemorrhagic transformation, compared with the control group or the group treated with PS-519 alone.[83] Further, the anti-inflammatory properties of unfractionated heparin[84] would make it an interesting drug

Table 19.3 Experimental studies combining thrombolysis and neuroprotection

Authors	Neuroprotectant drug combined with thrombolysis	Outcome measures
	NMDA receptor antagonist/neuronal voltage-sensitive calcium channel blocker	
Lekieffre et al[75]	Eliprodil + rtPA	• Significant reduction of neurological deficit • Significant reduction of infarct volume
	Excitatory amino-acid antagonist	
Sereghy et al[76]	Dizocilpine	• Significant reduction of infarct volume • Significant improvement of clinical score
	GABA agonist	
Yang et al[77]	Topiramate (enhances inhibitor effects of GABA, which antagonizes the excitotoxic effects of glutamate released during ischemia) + low-dose urokinase	• Significant reduction of infarct volume • Reduction of risk of cerebral hemorrhage
Yang et al[78]	Topiramate + low-dose urokinase	• Significant reduction of infarct volume • Reduction of risk of cerebral hemorrhage
	Citicoline	
Andersen et al[79]	Cytidine-5′-diphosphocholine (which provides both choline and cytidine, to serve as substrates for the synthesis of phosphatidylcholine to promote membrane synthesis and repair) + rtPA	• Significant reduction of infarct size
	Anti-ICAM-1 (intercellular adhesion molecule 1) antibody	
Zhang et al[82]	Anti-ICAM-1 antibody + rtPA	• Significant reduction of neurological deficit • Significant reduction of infarct volume
Bowes et al[81]	Anti-ICAM-1 antibody + rtPA Proteasome inhibitor (PS-519)	• Significant improvement of neurological outcome
Zangh et al[83]	PS-519 (which blocks activation of NFκB, a major mediator of inflammation) + rtPA	• Significant reduction of infarct volume • Significant improvement of neurological recovery • Did not increase the incidence of hemorrhagic transformation
	Compounds interfering with oxygen free radicals	
Sanchez et al[88]	U-74389-G (a free-radical scavenger) + rtPA	• No significant reduction of mortality • No significant reduction of cerebral lesion
Orozco et al[89]	U74006F (a 21-aminosteroid) + rtPA	• No significant reduction of infarct volume
	Matrix me talloproteinase (MMP) inhibitors	
Sumii and Lo[94] Lapchak and Araujo[95]	BB-94 (which inhibits degradation of components of the extracellular matrix mediated by MMPs)	• Significant reduction of rtPA-associated cerebral hemorrhage

to be combined with thrombolysis, irrespective of its antithrombotic activity.

Because of the key role played by oxygen free radicals,[85–87] compounds that interfere with these radicals would also be ideal for combination with thrombolysis. Unfortunately, the experimental studies where this approach was used were disappointing since combinations of rtPA both with the free-radical scavenger U-74389-G[88] and with the 21-aminosteroid U74006F[89] were ineffective in reducing infarct volume more than the single drugs alone.

While experimental interventions using free-radical scavengers effectively reduce the severity of hemorrhagic transformation after thrombolytic reperfusion, another emerging candidate mechanism involves a class of zinc-dependent matrix metalloproteinases (MMPs). It has been shown that MMPs are upregulated in the central nervous system after acute ischemia, hemorrhage, and trauma. As a family of extracellular proteinases, MMPs can degrade almost all components of the extracellular matrix. In the context of hemorrhagic transformation, uncontrolled MMP activation after rtPA reperfusion can degrade critical proteins, including collagen and laminin in the basal lamina. Degradation of these critical components may disrupt vascular structural integrity and lead to leakage and rupture. Interestingly, it has been shown that free-radical injury is mechanistically linked to MMP upregulation.[90,91] Hence, the involvement of MMPs in the pathophysiology of hemorrhage fits well in the context of oxidative damage and reperfusion injury. Data also suggest that rtPA is biochemically linked to the MMP axis of extracellular proteolysis, with plasmin acting as an upstream activator of the MMP cascade.[92,93] This provides another potential mechanism for the role of MMP-mediated hemorrhage after rtPA thrombolysis. It will be critical in future studies to carefully examine the mechanisms and effects of rtPA on all potential sources of MMP activity, including inflammatory cells that may infiltrate through the disrupted blood–brain barrier. The experimental efficacy of the MMP inhibitor BB-94[94,95] and of a spin-trapping agent[96] in reducing rtPA-associated cerebral hemorrhage encourages further research in this area.

Despite the reported experimental data in favor of the combination of neuroprotective agents and thrombolysis, this approach has been tested in only two clinical studies (Table 19.4). In a prospective randomized double-blinded multicenter placebo-controlled trial Grotta et al[97] randomized 44 patients to placebo plus rtPA (0.9 mg/kg, maximum 90 mg), and 45 to rtPA plus lubeluzole 7.5 mg IV then 10 mg/day IV for 5 days. The inclusion and exclusion criteria were those of the NINDS study. The median NIHSS Score at admission was 13 in the combined group and 14 in the rtPA alone group. The mean time to IV rtPA treatment was 2.5 h and that to IV lubeluzole or placebo was 3.2 h. No significant differences were found between the two treatment groups in the rate of ICH (5% in the rtPA-plus-lubeluzole group vs 16% in the rtPA-alone group), serious adverse events (51% vs 50%), and deaths (24% vs 29%), which indicates that the combination was safe. With regard to efficacy, at 3 months, 41% of patients receiving lubeluzole plus rtPA and 33% of those given rtPA plus placebo had an mRS of 0–2, and 44% of the former and 48% of the latter had a Barthel Index greater than 70. Although there were no safety concerns, this study was prematurely terminated by the sponsor before the planned enrolment of 200 patients, when a concurrent phase III trial of lubeluzole versus placebo given up to 6 h after stroke was negative.[98] Therefore, the sample of studied patients is too small to allow interpretation of the safety and efficacy data.

Lyden et al[99] performed a somewhat larger multicenter prospective randomized double-blinded placebo-controlled trial to explore the feasibility and safety of treatment with clomethiazole given within 12 h of symptom onset to patients who had received rtPA within 3 h. There were 101 patients randomized to rtPA (0.9 mg/kg, maximum 90 mg) plus clomethiazole (68 mg/kg IV) and 99 to rtPA plus placebo. The inclusion and exclusion criteria were the same as those used in the NINDS study. The median NIHSS Score at admission was 14 in the rtPA-plus-clomethiazole group and 13 in the rtPA-alone group. The mean time to treatment with clomethiazole was 5.4 h. Hemorrhagic transformation was observed in 9.4% of rtPA-plus-clomethiazole patients and in 14.3% of rtPA-alone patients, while the fatality rate was 15% in the former and 10% in the latter. Better outcome (3-month Barthel Index >70) was not significantly more frequent in either of the two groups.

From the data reviewed, it seems that combination therapy with thrombolysis and neuroprotection has yet to be adequately tested in human stroke. Larger

Table 19.4   Clinical studies combining thrombolysis and neuroprotection

Authors	No. of patients	NIHSS Score on admission	Treatment dose	Time to treatment	ICH	HI	Serious adverse events	Deaths	RS 0–2 at 3 months	BI > 70 at 3 months
Grotta[97] (prospective randomized double-blinded multicenter placebo-controlled trial)	89: 45 IV rtPA/lubeluzole 44 IV rtPA/placebo	13 (median) 14 (median)	0.9 mg/kg IV rtPA + lubeluzole 7.5 mg IV within 3 h then 10 mg/day IV for 5 days	2.5 h (mean)	5% 16%		51% 50%	24% 29%	41% 33%	44% 48%
Lyden et al[99] (randomized double-blinded trial)	190: 97: IV rtPA/clomethiazole 93: IV rtPA/placebo	14 (median) 13 (median)	0.9 mg/kg IV rtPA within 3 h then 68 mg/kg IV clomethiazole within 12 h	5.4 h (mean)		9.4% 14.3%	47% 49%	15% 10%		66% 67%

NIHSS, National Institutes of Health Stroke Scale; ICH, intracerebral hemorrhage; HI, hemorrhagic infarction; RS, Rankin Score; BI, Barthel Index; IV, intravenous; rtPA, recombinant tissue-type plasminogen activator.

trials are needed that take into due consideration dose, timing of administration, and possible pharmacological interactions of a given neuroprotectant with rtPA.

Conclusions

We are only at the beginning of advancing the utility of intravenously administered thrombolytic therapy using various combination strategies. Of the four approaches discussed here (with IA rtPA, antithrombotic agents, anticoagulants, or neuroprotection), the combination of IV with IA rtPA seems most likely to be the first to come to fruition. This is because of the logic of IA recanalization of arteries if IV approaches have failed, as well as the demonstrated success using surrogate outcome measures. Hopefully, a number of strategies will quickly prove effective and thus expand our repertoire of acute stroke therapies.

References

1. Wardlaw J, del Zoppo G, Yamaguchi T. Thrombolysis for acute ischaemic stroke. In: The Cochrane Library. Oxford: Update Software, 1999.
2. Katzan IL, Sila CA, Furlan AJ. Community use of intravenous tissue plasminogen activator for acute stroke: results of the brain matters stroke management survey. Stroke 2001;32:861–5.
3. Marler JR, Tilley BC, Lu M, et al. Early stroke treatment associated with better outcome: the NINDS rt-PA stroke study. Neurology 2000;55:1649–55.
4. Wolpert SM, Bruckmann H, Greenlee R, et al. Neuroradiologic evaluation of patients with acute stroke treated with recombinant tissue plasminogen activator. The rt-PA Acute Stroke Study Group. AJNR Am J Neuroradiol 1993;14:3–13.
5. Zeumer H, Freitag HJ, Zanella F, et al. Local intra-arterial fibrinolytic therapy in patients with stroke: urokinase versus recombinant tissue plasminogen activator (r-TPA). Neuroradiology 1993;35:159–62.
6. Freitag HJ, Becker VU, Thie A, et al. Lys-plasminogen as an adjunct to local intra-arterial fibrinolysis for carotid territory stroke: laboratory and clinical findings. Neuroradiology 1996;38:181–5.
7. Lewandowski CA, Frankel M, Tomsick TA, et al. Combined intravenous and intra-arterial r-TPA versus intra-arterial therapy of acute ischemic stroke: Emergency Management of Stroke (EMS) bridging trial. Stroke 1999;30:2598–605.
8. The National Institute of Neurological Disorders and Stroke rt-PA Stroke Study Group. Tissue plasminogen activator for acute ischemic stroke. N Engl J Med 1995;333:1581–7.
9. Hacke W, Kaste M, Fieschi C, et al. Intravenous thrombolysis with recombinant tissue plasminogen activator for acute hemispheric stroke. The European Cooperative Acute Stroke Study (ECASS). JAMA 1995;274:1017–25.
10. Hacke W, Kaste M, Fieschi C, et al. Randomised double-blind placebo-controlled trial of thrombolytic therapy with intravenous alteplase in acute ischaemic stroke (ECASS II). Second European–Australasian Acute Stroke Study Investigators. Lancet 1998;352:1245–51.
11. Ernst R, Pancioli A, Tomsick T, et al. Combined intravenous and intra-arterial recombinant tissue plasminogen activator in acute ischemic stroke. Stroke 2000;31:2552–7.
12. Furlan A, Higashida R, Wechsler L, et al. Intra-arterial prourokinase for acute ischemic stroke. The PROACT II study: a randomized controlled trial. Prolyse in Acute Cerebral Thromboembolism. JAMA 1999;282: 2003–11.
13. Zaidat OO, Suarez JI, Santillan C, et al. Response to intra-arterial and combined intravenous and intra-arterial thrombolytic therapy in patients with distal internal carotid artery occlusion. Stroke 2002; 33:1821–7.
14. Tong DD. Intra-arterial thrombolytic therapy for acute stroke: the debate continues. Stroke 2002;33: 1821–7.
15. Suarez JI, Zaidat OO, Sunshine JL, et al. Endovascular administration after intravenous infusion of thrombolytic agents for the treatment of patients with acute ischemic strokes. Neurosurgery 2002;50:251–9; discussion 259–60.
16. Hill MD, Barber PA, Demchuk AM, et al. Acute intravenous–intra-arterial revascularization therapy for severe ischemic stroke. Stroke 2002;33:279–82.

17. Keris V, Rudnicka S, Vorona V, et al. Combined intraarterial/intravenous thrombolysis for acute ischemic stroke. AJNR Am J Neuroradiol 2001;22: 352–8.

18. Qureshi AI. New grading system for angiographic evaluation of arterial occlusions and recanalization response to intra-arterial thrombolysis in acute ischemic stroke. Neurosurgery 2002;50:1405–14; discussion 1414–15.

19. Christou I, Burgin WS, Alexandrov AV, Grotta JC. Arterial status after intravenous TPA therapy for ischaemic stroke. A need for further interventions. Int Angiol 2001;20:208–13.

20. Demchuk AM, Burgin WS, Christou I, et al. Thrombolysis in brain ischemia (TIBI) transcranial Doppler flow grades predict clinical severity, early recovery, and mortality in patients treated with intravenous tissue plasminogen activator. Stroke 2001;32: 89–93.

21. Fieschi C, Argentino C, Lenzi GL, et al. Clinical and instrumental evaluation of patiens with ischemic stroke within the first six hours. J Neurol Sci 1989; 91:311–21.

22. del Zoppo GJ, Higashida RT, Furlan AJ, et al. PROACT: a phase II randomized trial of recombinant pro-urokinase by direct arterial delivery in acute middle cerebral artery stroke. PROACT Investigators. Prolyse in Acute Cerebral Thromboembolism. Stroke 1998,29.4–11.

23. Italy (MAST-I) Group. Randomised controlled trial of streptokinase, aspirin, and combination of both in treatment of acute ischaemic stroke. Multicentre Acute Stroke Trial. Lancet 1995;346:1509–14.

24. Ciccone A, Motto C, Aritzu E, et al. Negative interaction of aspirin and streptokinase in acute ischemic stroke: further analysis of the Multicenter Acute Stroke Trial – Italy. Cerebrovasc Dis 2000;10:61–4.

25. Coller BS. Platelets and thrombolytic therapy. N Engl J Med 1990;322:33–42.

26. Patrono C. Aspirin as an antiplatelet drug. N Engl J Med 1994;330:1287–94.

27. Motto C, Ciccone A, Aritzu E, et al. Hemorrhage after an acute ischemic stroke. MAST-I Collaborative Group. Stroke 1999;30:761–4.

28. Cornu C, Boutitie F, Candelise L, et al. Streptokinase in acute ischemic stroke: an individual patient data meta-analysis: the Thrombolysis in Acute Stroke Pooling Project. Stroke 2000;31:1555–60.

29. Donnan GA, Davis SM, Chambers BR, et al. Streptokinase for acute ischemic stroke with relationship to time of administration: Australian Streptokinase (ASK) Trial Study Group. JAMA 1996; 276:961–6.

30. Europe Study Group. Thrombolytic therapy with streptokinase in acute ischemic stroke. The Multicenter Acute Stroke Trial. N Engl J Med 1996;335:145–50.

31. Morris AD, Ritchie C, Grosset DG, et al. A pilot study of streptokinase for acute cerebral infarction. Q J Med 1995;88:727–31.

32. Thomas GR, Thibodeaux H, Errett CJ, et al. Intravenous aspirin causes a paradoxical attenuation of cerebrovascular thrombolysis. Stroke 1995;26:1039–46.

33. Abel-Halim M, von Holst H, Meyerson B, et al. Prostaglandin profiles in tissue and blood vessels from human brain. J Neurochem 1980;34:1331–3.

34. Leffler C, Armstead W, Shibata M. Role of eicosanoids in cerebral hemodynamics. In: Philips J (ed). The Regulation of Cerebral Blood Flow. Boca Raton, FL: CRC Press, 1993: 297–313.

35. Bednar MM, Gross CE. Aspirin reduces experimental cerebral blood flow in vivo. Neurol Res 1999;21: 488–90.

36. Bednar MM, Gross CE, Howard DB, et al. Nitric oxide reverses aspirin antagonism of t-PA thrombolysis in a rabbit model of thromboembolic stroke. Exp Neurol 1997;146:513–17.

37. Bednar MM, Gross CE, Howard DB, et al. The effect of vasodilators on aspirin-induced antagonism of t-PA thrombolysis. Neurol Res 2001;23:745–50.

38. Crutchley DJ, Conanan LB, Maynard JR. Stimulation of fibrinolytic activity in human skin fibroblasts by prostaglandins E1, E2 and I2. J Pharmacol Exp Ther 1982;222:544–9.

39. Ellis E. Editorial comment. Stroke 1995;26:1046.

40. Bednar MM, Quilley J, Russell SR, et al. The effect of oral antiplatelet agents on tissue plasminogen activator-mediated thrombolysis in a rabbit model of thromboembolic stroke. Neurosurgery 1996;39:352–9.

41. Bednar MM, Raymond-Russell SJ, Booth CL, Gross CE. Combination tissue plasminogen activator and ticlopidine therapy in a rabbit model of acute thromboembolic stroke. Neurol Res 1996;18:45–8.

42. Bevers EM, Comfurius P, van Rijn JL, et al. Generation of prothrombin-converting activity and the exposure of phosphatidylserine at the outer surface of platelets. Eur J Biochem 1982;122:429–36.

43. Osterud B, Rapaport SI, Lavine KK. Factor V activity of platelets: evidence for an activated factor V molecule and for a platelet activator. Blood 1977;49:819–34.

44. Reed GL, Matsueda GR, Haber E. Platelet factor XIII increases the fibrinolytic resistance of platelet-rich clots by accelerating the crosslinking of α_2-antiplasmin to fibrin. Thromb Haemost 1992;68:315–20.

45. Coller BS. GPIIb/IIIa antagonists: pathophysiologic and therapeutic insights from studies of c7E3 Fab. Thromb Haemost 1997;78:730–5.

46. Muhlestein JB, Karagounis LA, Treehan S, Anderson JL. 'Rescue' utilization of abciximab for the dissolution of coronary thrombus developing as a complication of coronary angioplasty. J Am Coll Cardiol 1997; 30:1729–34.

47. Neumann FJ, Blasini R, Schmitt C, et al. Effect of glycoprotein IIb/IIIa receptor blockade on recovery of coronary flow and left ventricular function after the placement of coronary-artery stents in acute myocardial infarction. Circulation 1998;98:2695–701.

48. Kaku S, Umemura K, Mizuno A, et al. Evaluation of a GPIIb/IIIa antagonist YM337 in a primate model of middle cerebral artery thrombosis. Eur J Pharmacol 1998;345:185–92.

49. Ohman EM, Kleiman NS, Gacioch G, et al. Combined accelerated tissue-plasminogen activator and platelet glycoprotein IIb/IIIa integrin receptor blockade with Integrilin in acute myocardial infarction. Results of a randomized, placebo-controlled, dose-ranging trial. IMPACT-AMI Investigators. Circulation 1997; 95:846–54.

50. van den Merkhof LF, Zijlstra F, Olsson H, et al. Abciximab in the treatment of acute myocardial infarction eligible for primary percutaneous transluminal coronary angioplasty. Results of the Glycoprotein Receptor Antagonist Patency Evaluation (GRAPE) pilot study. J Am Coll Cardiol 1999;33:1528–32.

51. Antman EM, Gibson CM, de Lemos JA, et al. Combination reperfusion therapy with abciximab and reduced dose reteplase: results from TIMI 14. The Thrombolysis in Myocardial Infarction (TIMI) 14 Investigators. Eur Heart J 2000;21:1944–53.

52. Wallace RC, Furlan AJ, Moliterno DJ, et al. Basilar artery rethrombosis: successful treatment with platelet glycoprotein IIB/IIIA receptor inhibitor. AJNR Am J Neuroradiol 1997;18:1257–60.

53. Eckert B, Koch C, Thomalla G, et al. Acute basilar artery occlusion treated with combined intravenous Abciximab and intra-arterial tissue plasminogen activator: report of 3 cases. Stroke 2002;33:1424–7.

54. Kwon OK, Lee KJ, Han MH, et al. Intraarterially administered abciximab as an adjuvant thrombolytic therapy: report of three cases. AJNR Am J Neuroradiol 2002;23:447–51.

55. Mahaffey KW, Granger CB, Collins R, et al. Overview of randomized trials of intravenous heparin in patients with acute myocardial infarction treated with thrombolytic therapy. Am J Cardiol 1996;77:551–6.

56. von Kummer R, Hacke W. Safety and efficacy of intravenous tissue plasminogen activator and heparin in acute middle cerebral artery stroke. Stroke 1992;23: 646–52.

57. Trouillas P, Nighoghossian N, Getenet J, et al. Open trial of intravenous tissue plasminogen activator in acute carotid territory stroke: correlations of outcome with clinical and radiological data. Stroke 1996;27: 882–90.

58. Trouillas P, Nighoghossian N, Derex L, et al. Thrombolysis with intravenous rtPA in a series of 100 cases of acute carotid territory stroke: determination of etiological, topographic, and radiological outcome factors. Stroke 1998;29:2529–40.

59. Grond M, Stenzel C, Schmulling S, et al. Early intravenous thrombolysis for acute ischemic stroke in a community-based approach. Stroke 1998;29:1544–9.

60. Rudolf J, Schmuelling S, Strotmann-Tack T, et al. ASA-pretreatment, concomitant heparin therapy and the risk of early intracranial hemorrhage following intravenous thrombolysis for acute ischemic stroke. Cerebrovasc Dis 2002:54(abst).

61. Kase CS, Furlan AJ, Wechsler LR, et al. Cerebral hemorrhage after intra-arterial thrombolysis for ischemic stroke: the PROACT II trial. Neurology 2001;57: 1603–10.

62. Fassbender K, Dempfle CE, Mielke O, et al. Changes in coagulation and fibrinolysis markers in acute ischemic stroke treated with recombinant tissue plasminogen activator. Stroke 1999;30:2101–4.

63. Aronson DL, Chang P, Kessler CM. Platelet-dependent thrombin generation after in vitro fibrinolytic treatment. Circulation 1992;85:1706–12.

64. Rapold HJ, de Bono D, Arnold AE, et al. Plasma fibrinopeptide A levels in patients with acute myocardial infarction treated with alteplase. Correlation with concomitant heparin, coronary artery patency, and recurrent ischemia. The European Cooperative Study Group. Circulation 1992;85:928–34.

65. Scharfstein JS, Abendschein DR, Eisenberg PR, et al. Usefulness of fibrinogenolytic and procoagulant markers during thrombolytic therapy in predicting clinical outcomes in acute myocardial infarction. TIMI-5 Investigators. Thrombolysis in Myocardial Infarction. Am J Cardiol 1996;78:503–10.

66. Stangl K, Laule M, Tenckhoff B, et al. Fibrinogen breakdown, long-lasting systemic fibrinolysis, and procoagulant activation during alteplase double-bolus regimen in acute myocardial infarction. Am J Cardiol 1998;81:841–7.

67. Galvani M, Abendschein DR, Ferrini D, et al. Failure of fixed dose intravenous heparin to suppress increases in thrombin activity after coronary thrombolysis with streptokinase. J Am Coll Cardiol 1994;24:1445–52.

68. Weitz J, Leslie B, Hudoba M. Thrombin binds to soluble fibrin degradation products where it is protected

from inhibition by heparin–antithrombin but susceptible by antithrombin-independent inhibitors. Circulation 1998;97:544–52.

69. Kaplan KL, Francis CW. Direct thrombin inhibitors. Semin Hematol 2002;39:187–96.

70. Pannell R, Gurewich V. Activation of plasminogen by single-chain urokinase or by two-chain urokinase – a demonstration that single-chain urokinase has a low catalytic activity (pro-urokinase). Blood 1987;69:22–6.

71. Burke SE, Lubbers NL, Nelson RA, Henkin J. Recombinant pro-urokinase requires heparin for optimal clot lysis and restoration of blood flow in a canine femoral artery thrombosis model. Thromb Haemost 1993;69:375–80.

72. IND 3472 Serial No. 000.1989. Evaluation of recombinant pro-urokinase (ABBOTT-74187) in the canine femoral artery clot lysis model. Abbott Laboratories Scientific Report PPRd/89/541, 1989: December 27.

73. Sacchetti ML, Toni D, Fiorelli M, Argentino C, Fieschi C. The concept of combination therapy in acute ischemic stroke. Neurology 1997;49(Suppl 4):S70–4.

74. Hossmann KA. Viability thresholds and the penumbra of focal ischemia. Ann Neurol 1994;36:557–65.

75. Lekieffre D, Benavides J, Scatton B, Nowicki JP. Neuroprotection afforded by a combination of eliprodil and a thrombolytic agent, rt-PA, in a rat thromboembolic stroke model. Brain Res 1997;776:88–95.

76. Sereghy T, Overgaard K, Boysen G. Neuroprotection by excitatory amino acid antagonist augments the benefit of thrombolysis in embolic stroke in rats. Stroke 1993;24:1702–8.

77. Yang Y, Li Q, Miyashita H, et al. Usefulness of postischemic thrombolysis with or without neuroprotection in a focal embolic model of cerebral ischemia. J Neurosurg 2000;92:841–7.

78. Yang Y, Li Q, Shuaib A. Enhanced neuroprotection and reduced hemorrhagic incidence in focal cerebral ischemia of rat by low dose combination therapy of urokinase and topiramate. Neuropharmacology 2000;39:881–8.

79. Andersen M, Overgaard K, Meden P, et al. Effects of citicoline combined with thrombolytic therapy in a rat embolic stroke model. Stroke 1999;30:1464–71.

80. Shuaib A, Yang Y, Li Q. Evaluating the efficacy of citicoline in embolic ischemic stroke in rats: neuroprotective effects when used alone or in combination with urokinase. Exp Neurol 2000;161:733–9.

81. Bowes MP, Rothlein R, Fagan SC, Zivin JA. Monoclonal antibodies preventing leukocyte activation reduce experimental neurologic injury and enhance efficacy of thrombolytic therapy. Neurology 1995;45:815–19.

82. Zhang RL, Zhang ZG, Chopp M, Zivin JA. Thrombolysis with tissue plasminogen activator alters adhesion molecule expression in the ischemic rat brain. Stroke 1999;30:624–9.

83. Zhang L, Zhang ZG, Zhang RL, et al. Postischemic (6-hour) treatment with recombinant human tissue plasminogen activator and proteasome inhibitor PS-519 reduces infarction in a rat model of embolic focal cerebral ischemia. Stroke 2001;32:2926–31.

84. Chamorro A. Immediate anticoagulation in acute focal brain ischemia revisited: gathering the evidence. Stroke 2001;32:577–8.

85. Siesjo BK. Pathophysiology and treatment of focal cerebral ischemia. Part II: Mechanisms of damage and treatment. J Neurosurg 1992;77:337–54.

86. Globus MY, Busto R, Lin B, et al. Detection of free radical activity during transient global ischemia and recirculation: effects of intraischemic brain temperature modulation. J Neurochem 1995;65:1250–6.

87. Busch E, Kruger K, Allegrini PR, et al. Reperfusion after thrombolytic therapy of embolic stroke in the rat: magnetic resonance and biochemical imaging. J Cereb Blood Flow Metab 1998;18:407–18.

88. Sanchez C, Alonso de Lecinana M, Diez-Tejedor E, et al. [Treatment of embolic cerebral infarct via thrombolysis and cytoprotection with U-74389-G in rats]. Rev Neurol 1998;27:653–8.

89. Orozco J, Mendel RC, Hahn MR, et al. Influence of a 'brain protector' drug 21-amino steroid on the effects of experimental embolic stroke treated by thrombolysis. Neurol Res 1995;17:423–5.

90. Morita-Fujimura Y, Fujimura M, Gasche Y, et al. Overexpression of copper and zinc superoxide dismutase in transgenic mice prevents the induction and activation of matrix metalloproteinases after cold injury-induced brain trauma. J Cereb Blood Flow Metab 2000;20:130–8.

91. Gasche Y, Copin JC, Sugawara T, et al. Matrix metalloproteinase inhibition prevents oxidative stress–associated blood–brain barrier disruption after transient focal cerebral ischemia. J Cereb Blood Flow Metab 2001;21:1393–400.

92. Cuzner ML, Opdenakker G. Plasminogen activators and matrix metalloproteases, mediators of extracellular proteolysis in inflammatory demyelination of the central nervous system. J Neuroimmunol 1999;94:1–14.

93. Hartung HP, Kieseier BC. The role of matrix metalloproteinases in autoimmune damage to the central and peripheral nervous system. J Neuroimmunol 2000; 107:140–7.

94. Sumii T, Lo EH. Involvement of matrix metalloproteinase in thrombolysis-associated hemorrhagic

transformation after embolic focal ischemia in rats. Stroke 2002;33:831–6.

95. Lapchak PA, Araujo DM. Reducing bleeding complications after thrombolytic therapy for stroke: clinical potential of metalloproteinase inhibitors and spin trap agents. CNS Drugs 2001;15:819–29.

96. Lapchak PA, Araujo DM, Song D, et al. Effects of the spin trap agent disodium-[(*tert*-butylimino)methyl] benzene-1,3-disulfonate *N*-oxide (generic NXY-059) on intracerebral hemorrhage in a rabbit large clot embolic stroke model: combination studies with tissue plasminogen activator. Stroke 2002;33:1665–70.

97. Grotta J. Combination Therapy Stroke Trial: recombinant tissue-type plasminogen activator with/without lubeluzole. Cerebrovasc Dis 2001;12:258–63.

98. Diener HC, Cortens M, Ford G, et al. Lubeluzole in acute ischemic stroke treatment: A double-blind study with an 8-hour inclusion window comparing a 10-mg daily dose of lubeluzole with placebo. Stroke 2000;31:2543–51.

99. Lyden P, Jacoby M, Schim J, et al. The Clomethiazole Acute Stroke Study in tissue-type plasminogen activator-treated stroke (CLASS-T): final results. Neurology 2001;57:1199–205.

20

Cerebral venous thrombosis

José M Ferro and Patrícia Canhão

Introduction

Thrombosis of the dural sinus and encephalic veins (cerebral venous thrombosis: CVT) was until recently considered a rare, often fatal, disease. With the introduction of magnetic resonance imaging (MRI) into clinical practice, CVT became recognized with increasing frequency. The incidence of CVT is probably underestimated, because it has a rather variable clinical presentation and it is necessary to perform magnetic resonance angiography (MRA) to confirm the diagnosis.[1–4] CVT is more common in neonates and in children than in adults.[5,6] Adult patients with CVT are predominantly females and are usually younger than those with other types of stroke.[2,7]

The clinical symptoms and signs of CVT depend on the site and number of occluded sinuses and veins, on the presence of parenchymal lesions,[1,2,7] on the age of the patient,[5,6,8] and on the interval from onset to presentation.[9] Headache is the most frequent symptom of CVT.[10–14] Patients with a chronic course or delayed clinical presentation may show papilloedema on fundoscopy.[9] In severe acute cases, disturbances of consciousness and mental problems (e.g. delirium, apathy, or a frontal lobe syndrome) are often present. Motor deficits and aphasia are the most frequent focal deficits. Focal or generalized seizures, including status epilepticus, are more frequent than in other stroke types.[15] Symptoms and signs of CVT can be grouped in three major syndromes: isolated intracranial hypertension syndrome (headache with or without vomiting, papilloedema, and visual problems),[16] focal syndrome (focal deficits, seizures, or both) and encephalopathy (multifocal signs, mental status changes, and stupor/coma).[2,17]

MRI, including MR venography, is necessary to confirm the diagnosis,[2,18,19] by demonstrating the thrombus and the occluded sinus or vein (Figure 20.1). Alternative techniques to demonstrate the filling defect of the thrombosed sinus are digital intra-arterial venography and computed tomography (CT) venography.[20,21] Confirmation of the diagnosis of cortical vein thrombosis is particularly difficult.[22–24] CT and MRI can also show edema, venous infarcts, and intracerebral haemorrhages.

Many medical conditions and risk factors are associated with CVT.[2,7,25] The most common are oral contraceptive use,[26,27] puerperium,[28,29] cancer, or other acquired prothrombotic conditions. In addition, many patients also have an inherited prothrombotic condition.[30]

Several recent prospective series, in particular the large ISCVT (International Study on Cerebral Vein and Dural Sinus Thrombosis) cohort[7] confidently established the vital and functional prognosis of patients with acute CVT. The overall death or dependency rate is 15%. Long-term predictors of poor prognosis are central nervous system infection, malignancy, deep cerebral venous system thrombosis, hemorrhage on CT/MRI, Glasgow Coma Scale (GCS) Score less than 9 on admission, mental status disorder, age more than 37 years and male gender.[7,31–37] Despite the overall favorable prognosis, 4% of CVT patients die in the acute phase.[7,38] The main cause of death is transtentorial herniation secondary to large hemorrhagic lesions.[38] Other causes of death are herniation due to multiple lesions or to diffuse brain edema, status epilepticus, medical complications, and pulmonary embolism.[39]

Recanalization occurs in 40–90% of patients, depending on the occluded sinus (less often in the lateral sinus), mostly within the first 4 months.[40]

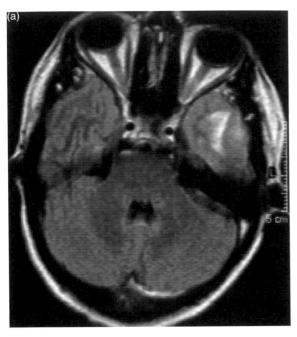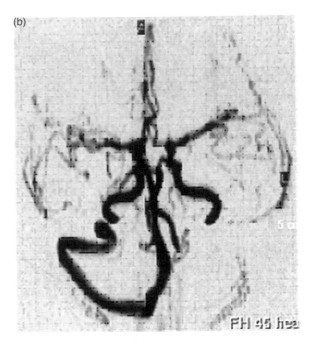

Figure 20.1
Thrombosis of the left lateral sinus. (a) T1-weighted MRI showing a hemorrhagic lesion in the temporal lobe and hyperintense signals in the lateral sinus. (b) MR-angiography: there is no flow in the left lateral sinus.

Recanalization of the occluded sinus is not related to outcome.

CVT patients who survive the acute phase may later die due to the underlying disease. Recurrent CVT is very rare. Long-term complications include deep venous thrombosis (DVT) of the limbs or pelvis, seizures, and headaches. Severe visual loss is very rare nowadays.[7]

Treatment of CVT includes (1) etiological treatment to manage the associated condition and risk factors, (2) symptomatic treatment, including treatment of intracranial hypertension, seizures, headache, and visual failure, and (3) antithrombotic treatment.[41]

Aims and modalities of antithrombotic treatment in CVT

The purposes of antithrombotic treatment, be this with antiplatelet drugs, anticoagulants (intravenous) heparin or low-molecular-weight heparins (LMWH)

or with thrombolytics,[41–43] are fourfold: (1) to recanalize the occluded sinus/vein, (2) to prevent propagation of the thrombus, namely to the bridging cerebral veins, (3) to prevent pulmonary embolism,[39] and (4) to treat the underlying prothrombotic state, in order to prevent venous thrombosis in other parts of the body and the recurrence of CVT.

Evidence for the efficacy of heparins in acute CVT

Only two randomized controlled trials of anticoagulation in acute CVT have been performed[44,45] (Tables 20.1 and 20.2). Both have some methodological problems, namely their modest sample size. The German trial[44] (intravenous heparin vs placebo) was stopped prematurely because of excess mortality in the placebo arm. This trial showed a significant better outcome in the heparin arm. However, its outcome measure was a nonvalidated composite CVT severity scale. In the Dutch trial[45] (subcutaneous nadroparin vs placebo), patients who would need lumbar punctures for the

Table 20.1   Randomized controlled trial of heparin anticoagulation in acute CVT[44]

	Outcome at 3 months
Heparin group	
Total recovery	8 (80%)
Residual motor deficit	2 (20%)
Placebo group	
Total recovery	1 (10%)
Minor residual deficit	6 (60%)
Deaths	3 (30%)

relief of intracranial pressure were excluded. Despite randomization, there were more cases with isolated intracranial hypertension in the control group and more patients with infarcts in the nadroparin group. A meta-analysis of the two trials shows a 6% relative risk reduction of death or dependency on anticoagulants compared with placebo.[46] Two other trials,[47,48] including 57 and 40 patients and performed in India, were not included in the meta-analysis, because the diagnosis of CVT was confirmed by CT only and information was available only in abstract form. Both favored heparin: 15% versus 40% mortality in the Maiti and Chakrabarti trial[47] and recovery in all heparin-treated patients contrasting with two deaths and one patient with a residual hemiparesis in the control group in the Nagajara et al trial.[48]

Is heparin safe in CVT?

In the two trials[44,45] mentioned above, no new intracranial hemorrhages were detected in patients randomized to heparin and only one case of major extracranial bleeding was reported. In other series, the risks of intracranial hemorrhage (<5%) and systemic hemorrhage (<2%) were also low. More importantly, such hemorrhages did not influence outcome.[1,17,33,49]

Anticoagulants are also safe to use in patients with intracranial hemorrhages, either intracerebral or subarachnoid. This is in accordance with the fact that such intracranial hemorrhages are secondary to venous outflow blockage.

Anticoagulant therapy is also safe in children.[50]

Anticoagulation of acute CVT in current practice

Nowadays, there is wide consensus on the use of heparin or LMWH in acute CVT. For instance, in the ISCVT trial, more than 80% of the patients were anticoagulated.[7] Despite the available evidence, physicians are still somewhat reluctant to prescribe heparin to older patients and to patients with intracranial hemorrhages, and also, in some countries, to puerperal CVT.[51,52]

Antiplatelet drugs in CVT

Although antiplatelet drugs are used as alternatives to anticoagulants when these are contraindicated, there is no evidence, even from uncontrolled series, regarding their efficacy and safety in CVT.

Table 20.2   Randomized controlled trial of nadroparin anticoagulation for acute CVT[45]

Outcome	Nadroparin	Placebo	Risk difference
At 3 weeks			
Deaths	2	4	
BI <15	4	3	
Death or BI <15	6 (20%)	7 (24%)	4% (−25 to 17)
At 12 weeks			
Deaths	2	4	
Dependent (RS 3–5)	2	2	
Death or dependent (RS 3–5)	4 (13%)	6 (21%)	7% (−26 to 12)

BI, Barthel Index; RS, Rankin Score.

Is there a place for thrombolysis in CVT?

Although the majority of patients with CVT have a good outcome, approximately 4% die during the acute phase.[7] Several patients worsen despite anticoagulant therapy. It therefore seems justified to attempt a more aggressive treatment to improve the prognosis of CVT patients.

How can thrombolytic agents reach the thrombus?

Direct thrombolysis aims to dissolve the thrombus by delivering a thrombolytic agent within the occluded sinus. To introduce the agent into the sinus, a catheter has to be located in the thrombus, usually via a femoral or jugular approach, and gradually advanced to a more distal location while the thrombus is dissolved. Often, the catheter is left in the sinus, and infusion of the thrombolytic agent ensues for a variable period of time, with repeated radiological assessments to evaluate the rate of recanalization.

There are a small number of published cases of CVT treated with intravenous delivery of thrombolytic drugs. This route is less attractive, since the concentration of thrombolytic agent in the thrombus is considerably less than when it is administered directly within the thrombus.

In some cases, mechanical endovascular disruption of the thrombus has also been reported as useful in enhancing the recanalization of thrombosed dural sinuses. Mechanical methods may include the use of guiding catheters, thrombosuction with a rheolytic catheter, or thrombus removal with a balloon catheter.[53,54]

Which thrombolytic drugs are used in CVT treatment?

The first thrombolytic drug to be used in CVT was urokinase. More recently, recombinant tissue-type plasminogen activator (rtPA) has been used. There has been a wide variety of management according to the type and dosage of thrombolytic drug. Total doses of local urokinase reported in the literature range between 12 000 IU (in newborns) and 13 790 000 IU, with a mean dose of 2 292 448 ± 2 269 174 IU. Total doses of local rtPA range between 8 and 300 mg, with a mean dose of 78.4 ± 64.7 mg. The mean duration of treatment was 41 ± 49 h, with a range between less than a hour and 244 h.[55]

What is the evidence of efficacy of local thrombolysis in CVT?

There is currently no evidence from randomized controlled trials concerning the efficacy of systemic or local thrombolysis in CVT patients. Many case reports or case series have been published suggesting that thrombolytics might be useful and safe.[56–59] In a systematic review of patients treated with local thrombolysis,[55] only 5% patients died during the acute phase of CVT and 8% were dependent at discharge. The results of this review suggest a possible benefit for severe CVT cases, indicating that thrombolytics may reduce case fatality in critically ill patients.

What is the evidence of safety of local thrombolysis in CVT?

Due to a lack of randomized controlled trials, the hemorrhagic complications of local thrombolysis and the benefit/risk ratio of this treatment are not established.

In the above-mentioned systematic review,[55] thrombolytic treatment was considered safe, with few serious hemorrhagic complications. Intracranial hemorrhages were reported in 16% of cases, but only in 5% were they associated with clinical deterioration. In 19% of patients, extracranial hemorrhages were reported, but they were severe in only 2%.

Is local thrombolysis safe in CVT patients with intracranial hemorrhage?

The systematic review[55] identified 39 patients with brain hemorrhage treated with local thrombolysis.

Case fatality was no higher in cases with CT/MRI hemorrhage (7%). Hemorrhagic complications were not significantly higher in cases with previous hemorrhage on CT/MRI.

Do the literature results of thrombolytic therapy in CVT match those of the clinical practice?

There is a potential publication bias in the literature, with possible underestimation of poor outcomes and complications. Treatment and evaluation were non-blinded, leading to bias in evaluating outcomes. In the ISCVT trial, 13 patients were treated with local thrombolysis. Five (38.5%) were dead or dependent 6 months after CVT. These results are worse than the results in the published literature, but may reflect the prevailing results in clinical practice.

Should thrombolytics be used routinely?

There is no evidence to support the routine use of thrombolysis. Until better evidence is available, endovascular thrombolysis may be performed in selective centers with expertise in interventional radiology, in patients with a poor prognosis, such as those who worsen despite best medical treatment and anticoagulation, provided that other causes of worsening are excluded and treated.

Duration of antithrombotic treatment after CVT

The aim of continuing anticoagulation after the acute phase is to prevent recurrent CVT (a very rare event) and other venous thrombosis, including pulmonary embolism. Following the evidence and recommendations for systemic DVT, anticoagulation

with warfarin for 6–12 months is used in survivors of acute CVT, aiming at an International Normalized Ratio (INR) of 2–3.[60] Prolonged, continuous, anticoagulation is reserved for patients with inherited or acquired prothrombotic conditions. Patients with antiphospholipid syndrome must be on a higher INR range.

The risk of complications, including recurrent CVT or other venous thrombosis during future pregnancies, is low.[7,17,61–63] Unless a prothrombotic condition or a previous thromboembolism has been identified, antithrombotic prophylaxis during pregnancy is probably unnecessary. Women should be advised not to become pregnant while on warfarin, because of its teratogenic effects.[64]

Do we need new randomized controlled trials in CVT?

Published experience with local thrombolysis is promising, but is only based on case reports or case series. A randomized control trial is justified and needed to compare the efficacy and safety of endovascular thrombolysis versus heparins.

The duration of anticoagulation after acute CVT is also uncertain. There is growing evidence from DVT trials that more prolonged anticoagulation may prevent late recurrent venous thrombosis.[65–68] In the case of CVT, this risk has to be balanced against the hazard of intracranial hemorrhage. A randomized controlled trial comparing short (3 months) and long (1 year) oral anticoagulation after acute CVT is warranted.

Conclusions

Although CVT is a rare type of stroke, it may be fatal in about 5% of patients, who in general are young and active. Intravenous heparin or LMWH is the recommended antithrombotic treatment for all patients, including those with intracranial hemorrhages (level II evidence). Local thrombolysis is an alternative treatment in comatose patients and in those who deteriorate despite anticoagulation (level IV evidence).

References

1. Bousser MG, Chiras J, Bories J, et al. Cerebral venous thrombosis – a review of 38 cases. Stroke 1985;16: 199–213.
2. Bousser MG, Russell RR. Cerebral venous thrombosis. In: Warlow CP, Van Gijn J (eds). Major Problems in Neurology, Vol 33. London: Saunders, 1997:27–9 and 104–26.
3. Einhäupl KM, Villringer A, Haberl RL, et al. Clinical spectrum of sinus venous thrombosis. In: Einhäupl KM, Kempski O, Baethmann A (eds). Cerebral Sinus Thrombosis: Experimental and Clinical Aspects. New York: Plenum Press, 1990:149–55.
4. Kalbag RM, Woolf AL. Cerebral Venous Thrombosis, Vol 1. Oxford: Oxford University Press: 1967.
5. deVeber G, Andrew M, Adams C, et al, and the Canadian Pediatric Ischemic Stroke Study Group. Cerebral sinovenous thrombosis in children. N Engl J Med 2000;345:417–23.
6. Lancon JA, Killough KR, Tibbs RE, et al. Spontaneous dural sinus thrombosis in children. Pediatr Neurosurg 1999;30:23–9.
7. Ferro JM, Canhão P, Stam J, et al, and the ISCVT Investigators. Prognosis of cerebral vein and dural sinus thrombosis: results of the International Study on Cerebral Vein and Dural Sinus Thrombosis (ISCVT). Stroke 2004;35:664–70.
8. Ferro JM, Canhão P, Bousser MG, et al. Cerebral vein and dural sinus thrombosis in elderly patients. Stroke 2005;36:1927–32.
9. Ferro JM, Lopes MG, Rosas MJ, et al, and the VENO-PORT Investigators. Delay in hospital admission of patients with cerebral vein and dural sinus thrombosis. Cerebrovasc Dis 2005;19:152–6.
10. Ameri A, Bousser MG. Headache in cerebral venous thrombosis: a study of 110 cases. Cephalalgia 1993;13(Suppl 13):110.
11. De Bruijn SF, Stam J, Kappelle LJ. Thunderclap headache as first symptom of cerebral venous sinus thrombosis. CVST Study Group. Lancet 1996;348:1623–5.
12. Lopes MG, Ferro J, Pontes C, et al. for the Venoport Investigators. Headache and cerebral venous thrombosis. Cephalalgia 2000;20:292.
13. Martins IP, Sá J, Pereira RC, et al. Cerebral venous. thrombosis – may mimic migraine with aura. Headache Q 2001;12:121–4.
14. Newman DS, Levine SR, Curtis VL, et al. Migraine-like visual phenomena associated with cerebral venous thrombosis. Headache 1989;29:82–5.
15. Ferro JM, Correia M, Rosas MJ, et al, and the Cerebral Venous Thrombosis Portuguese Collaborative Study Group (VENOPORT). Seizures in cerebral vein and dural sinus thrombosis. Cerebrovasc Dis 2003;15: 78–83.
16. Biousse V, Ameri A, Bousser MG. Isolated intracranial hypertension as the only sign of cerebral venous thrombosis. Neurology 1999;53:1537–42.
17. Ferro JM, Correia M, Pontes C, et al, for the Cerebral Venous Thrombosis Portuguese Collaboration Study Group (VENOPORT). Cerebral venous thrombosis in Portugal 1980–98. Cerebrovasc Dis 2001;11:177–82.
18. Chu K, Kang DW, Yoon BW, et al. Diffusion-weighted MR in cerebral venous thrombosis. Arch Neurol 2001;58:1569–76.
19. Selim M, Fink J, Linfante I, et al. Diagnosis of cerebral venous thrombosis with echo-planar T2*-weighted magnetic resonance imaging. Arch Neurol 2002 59:1021–6.
20. Ozsvath RR, Casey SO, Lustrin ES, et al. Cerebral venography: comparison of CT and MR projection venography. AJR Am J Roentgenol 1997;169:1699–707.
21. Wetzel SG, Kirsch E, Stock KW. Cerebral veins: comparative study of CT venography with intra-arterial digital subtraction angiography. AJNR Am J Neuroradiol 1999;20:249–55.
22. Ahn TB, Roh JK. A case of cortical vein thrombosis with the cord sign. Arch Neurol 2003;60:1314–16.
23. Cakmak S, Hermier M, Montavont A, et al. T2*-weighted MRI in cortical venous thrombosis. Neurology 2004;63:1698.
24. Jacobs K, Moulin T, Bogousslavsky J, et al. The stroke syndrome of cortical vein thrombosis. Neurology 1996;47:376–82.
25. Bousser MG. Cerebral venous thrombosis: diagnosis and management. J Neurol 2000;247:252–8.
26. de Bruijn SF, Stam J, Koopman MM, et al. Case–control study of risk of cerebral sinus thrombosis in oral contraceptive users who are carriers of hereditary prothrombotic conditions. The Cerebral Venous Sinus Thrombosis Study Group. BMJ 1998;316:589–92.
27. Martinelli I, Sacchi E, Landi G. High-risk of cerebral-vein thrombosis in carriers of a prothrombin-gene mutation and in users of oral contraceptives. N Engl J Med 1998;338:1793–7.
28. Cantu C, Barinagarrementeria F. Cerebral venous thrombosis associated with pregnancy and puerperium; review of 67 cases. Stroke 1993;24:1880–4.

29. Lanska DJ, Kryscio RJ. Risk factors for peripartum and postpartum stroke and intracranial venous thrombosis. Stroke 2000;31:1274–82.

30. Biousse V, Conard J, Brouzes C. Frequency of 20210 G→A mutation in the 3′-untranslated region of the prothrombin gene in 35 cases of cerebral venous thrombosis. Stroke 1998;29:1398–400.

31. Cakmak S, Derex L, Berruyer M, et al. Cerebral venous thrombosis: clinical outcome and systematic screening of prothrombotic factors. Neurology 2003;60: 1175–8.

32. Breteau G, Mounier-Vehier F, Godefroy O, et al. Cerebral venous thrombosis: 3-year clinical outcome in 55 consecutive patients. J Neurol 2003;250:29–35.

33. Brucker AB, Vollert-Rogenhofer H, Wagner M, et al. Heparin treatment in acute cerebral sinus venous thrombosis: a retrospective clinical and MR analysis of 42 cases. Cerebrovasc Dis 1998;8:331–7.

34. de Bruijn SFTM, de Haan RJ, Stam J, for the Cerebral Venous Sinus Thrombosis Study Group. Clinical features and prognostic factors of cerebral venous sinus thrombosis in a prospective series of 59 patients. J Neurol Neurosurg Psychiatry 2001;70:105–8.

35. Ferro JM, Lopes MG, Rosas MJ, et al, for the Cerebral Venous Thrombosis Portuguese Collaborative Study Group (VENOPORT). Long-term prognosis of cerebral vein and dural sinus thrombosis: results of the VENOPORT study. Cerebrovasc Dis 2002;13:272–8.

36. Preter M, Tzourio CH, Ameri A, et al. Long term prognosis in cerebral venous thrombosis: a follow-up of 77 patients. Stroke 1996;27:243–6.

37. Rondepierre P, Hamon M, Leys D, et al. Thromboses veineuses cérébrales: étude de l'évolution. Rev Neurol (Paris) 1995;151:100 4.

38. Canhão P, Ferro JM, Lindgren AG, et al. ISCVT Investigators. Causes and predictors of death in cerebral venous thrombosis. Stroke 2005;36:1720–5.

39. Diaz JM, Schiffman JS, Urban ES, et al. Superior sagittal sinus thrombosis and pulmonary embolism: a syndrome rediscovered. Acta Neurol Scand 1992;86: 390–6.

40. Baumgartner RW, Studer A, Arnold M, et al. Recanalisation of cerebral venous thrombosis. J Neurol Neurosurg Psychiatry 2003;74:459–61.

41. Einhäupl K, Bousser MG, de Bruijn SFTM, et al. EFNS guideline on the treatment of cerebral venous and sinus thrombosis. Eur J Neurol (accepted for publication).

42. Benamer HT, Bone I. Cerebral venous thrombosis: anticoagulants or thrombolyic therapy? J Neurol Neurosurg Psychiatry 2000;69:427–30.

43. Bousser MG. Cerebral venous thrombosis. Nothing, heparin, or local thrombolysis? Stroke 1999;30:481–3.

44. Einhäupl KM, Villringer A, Meister W, et al. Heparin treatment in sinus venous thrombosis. Lancet 1991;338:597–600.

45. de Bruijin SF, Stam J. Randomized, placebo-controlled trial of anticoagulant treatment with low-molecular-weight heparin for cerebral sinus thrombosis. Stroke 1999;30:484–8.

46. Stam J, De Bruijn SF, DeVeber G. Anticoagulation for cerebral sinus thrombosis. Cochrane Database Syst Rev 2002;4:CD002005.

47. Maiti B, Chakrabarti I. Study on cerebral venous thrombosis with special reference to efficacy of heparin. J Neurol Sci 1997;150(Suppl):s147.

48. Nagaraja D, Rao BSS, Taly AB. Randomized controlled trial of heparin in puerperal cerebral venous/sinus thrombosis. Nimhans J 1995;13:111–15.

49. Wingerchuk DM, Wijdicks EF, Fulgham JR. Cerebral venous thrombosis complicated by hemorrhagic infarction: factors affecting the initiation and safety of anticoagulation. Cerebrovasc Dis 1998;8: 25 30.

50. deVeber G, Chan A, Monagle P, et al. Anticoagulation therapy in pediatric patients with sinovenous thrombosis: a cohort study. Arch Neurol 1998;55: 1533–7.

51. Ferro JM, Lopes GC, Rosas MJ, et al. Do randomised clinical trials influence practice? The example of cerebral vein and dural sinus thrombosis. J Neurol 2002; 249:1595–6.

52. Ferro JM, Bousser MG, Barinagarrementeria F, et al, and the ISCVT Collaborators. Variation in management of acute cerebral vein and dural sinus thrombosis. Cerebrovasc Dis 2002;13(Suppl 3):60.

53. Bagley LJ, Hurst RW, Galetta S, et al. Use of a microsnare to aid direct thrombolytic therapy of dural sinus thrombosis. AJR Am J Roentgenol 1998; 170:784–6.

54. Scarrow AM, Williams RL, Jungreis CA, et al. Removal of a thrombus from the sigmoid and transverse sinuses with a rheolytic thrombectomy catheter. AJNR Am J Neuroradiol 1999;20:1467–9.

55. Canhão P, Falcão F, Ferro JM. Thrombolytics for cerebral sinus thrombosis: a systematic review. Cerebrovasc Dis 2003;15:159–66.

56. Horowitz M, Purdy P, Unwin H, et al. Treatment of dural sinus thrombosis using elective catheterization and urokinase. Ann Neurol 1995;38:58–67.

57. Frey JL, Muro GJ, Mcdougall CG, et al. Cerebral venous thrombosis. Combined intrathrombus rtPA and intravenous heparin. Stroke 1999;30:489–94.

58. Kim SY, Suh JH. Direct endovascular thrombolytic therapy for dural sinus thrombosis: infusion of alteplase. AJNR Am J Neuroradiol 1997;18:639–645.

59. Wasay M, Bakshi R, Kojan S, et al. Nonrandomized comparison of local urokinase thrombolysis versus systemic heparin anticoagulation for superior sagittal sinus thrombosis. Stroke 2001;32:2310–7.

60. Büller HR, Agnelli G, Hull RD, et al. Antithrombotic therapy for venous thromboembolic disease: the Seventh ACCP Conference on antithrombotic and thrombolytic therapy. Chest 2004;12:401S–28S.

61. Lamy C, Hamon JB, Coste J, et al. Ischemic stroke in young women: risk of recurrence during subsequent pregnancies. French Study Group on Stroke in Pregnancy. Neurology 2000;55:269–74.

62. Mehraein S, Ortwein H, Busch M, et al. Risk of recurrence of cerebral venous and sinus thrombosis during subsequent pregnancy and puerperium. J Neurol Neurosurg Psychiatry 2003;74:814–16.

63. Srinivasan K. Cerebral venous and arterial thrombosis in pregnancy and puerperium. A study of 135 patients. Angiology 1983;34:731–46.

64. Jilma B, Kamath S, Lip GY. Antithrombotic therapy in special circumstances. I – pregnancy and cancer. BMJ 2003;326:37–40.

65. Agnelli G, Prandoni P, Santamaria MG, et al. Three months versus one year of oral anticoagulant therapy for idiopathic deep venous thrombosis. Warfarin Optimal Duration Italian Trial Investigators. N Engl J Med 2001;345:165–9.

66. Hutten BA, Prins MH. Duration of treatment with vitamin K antagonists in symptomatic venous thromboembolism. Cochrane Database Syst Rev (2000)3: CD001367.

67. Ridker PM, Goldhaber SZ, Danielson E, et al. PREVENT Investigators. Long-term, low-intensity warfarin therapy for the prevention of recurrent venous thromboembolism. N Engl J Med (2003)348:1425–34.

68. Schafer AI. Warfarin for venous thromboembolism – walking the dosing tightrope. N Engl J Med 2003; 348:1478–80.

Index

Page numbers in *italics* refer to tables and figures.